EXTENDED STABILITY FOR PARENTERAL DRUGS

EXTENDED STABILITY FOR PARENTERAL DRUGS

7th Edition

Michelle C. Simpson, PharmD, BCSCP
Clinical Program Manager
National Home Infusion Association
Alexandria, Virginia

Eric G. Schaefer, PharmD, MHSA
Director of Pharmacy Operations
Chartwell Pennsylvania, LP
Pittsburgh, Pennsylvania

ashp®

Any correspondence regarding this publication should be sent to the publisher, American Society of Health-System Pharmacists, 4500 East-West Highway, Suite 900, Bethesda, MD 20814, attention: Special Publishing.

Vice President, Publishing Office: Daniel J. Cobaugh, PharmD, DABAT, FAACT

Editorial Director, Special Publishing: Ryan E. Owens, PharmD, BCPS

Editorial Coordinator, Special Publishing: Elaine Jimenez

Director, Production and Platform Services, Publishing Operations: Johnna M. Hershey, BA

Cover Design: DeVall Advertising

Cover Art: Sergign - stock.adobe.com

Page Design: David Wade

Library of Congress Cataloging-in-Publication Data

Names: Simpson, Michelle C., editor. | Schaefer, Eric George, editor. | American Society of Health-System Pharmacists, issuing body.
Title: Extended stability for parenteral drugs / [edited by] Michelle C. Simpson, Eric G. Schaefer.
Description: Seventh edition. | Bethesda, MD : ASHP, [2023] | Includes bibliographical references and index. | Summary: "In the twenty-year span since publishing the first edition of Extended Stability for Parenteral Drugs, compounding of sterile preparations has been studied, reported, and regulated with increasing emphasis on sterility and patient safety risks. The need for compiling extended stability of parenteral drugs continues today, as pharmacists search for innovative solutions to improve patient access, manage medication shortages, and utilize compounded medications in a cost-effective way. As new drugs are approved, infusion pharmacists start seeking extended stability, and it takes considerable resources to organize and maintain an internal library of drug information for the medications compounded in a particular pharmacy. The requirement for reliable and relevant drug stability information remains a direct contributor to any pharmacy operation that compounds sterile preparations. The editors of the 7th edition worked diligently to expand the list of medications to include those beyond home infusion to be inclusive of all clinical settings where parenteral drugs are stored or compounded. The extended stability information provided is intended to be used as part of a risk-based approach to decrease risks posed to patients of physical or chemical degradation, and microbial contamination of parenteral medications"—Provided by publisher.
Identifiers: LCCN 2021060309 (print) | LCCN 2021060310 (ebook) | ISBN 9781585286713 (paperback) | ISBN 9781585286720 (adobe pdf) | ISBN 9781585286737 (epub)
Subjects: MESH: Drug Stability | Drug Storage | Home Infusion Therapy | Parenteral Nutrition | Time Factors | Handbook
Classification: LCC RS424 (print) | LCC RS424 (ebook) | NLM QV 735 | DDC 615.8/55—dc23/eng/20220112
LC record available at https://lccn.loc.gov/2021060309
LC ebook record available at https://lccn.loc.gov/2021060310

ISBN: 978-1-58528-671-3 (paperback)
ISBN: 978-1-58528-672-0 (Adobe pdf)
ISBN: 978-1-58528-673-7 (ePub)

DOI: 10.37573/9781585286720

10 9 8 7 6 5 4 3 2 1

DEDICATION

To the American Society of Health-System Pharmacists for seeing the potential in us, and believing we could bring a fresh perspective while maintaining the tradition of excellence of previous editions.

TABLE OF CONTENTS

DOI 10.37573/9781585286720.FM

PART II

PART III: APPENDICES

PREFACE

In the twenty-year span since publishing the first edition of *Extended Stability for Parenteral Drugs*, compounding of sterile preparations has been studied, reported, and regulated with increasing emphasis on sterility and patient safety. The first edition focused on maximum length of time to store compounded preparations. Future editions were transformed by United States Pharmacopeia *General Chapter <797> Pharmaceutical Compounding – Sterile Preparations* (USP <797>). The focus pivoted from maximizing the time until the compounded drug concentration fell below 90%, to include risk for microbial contamination during compounding related to the quality components of the environment where the medication was compounded. Home infusion providers advocated for revisions to the initial version of USP <797> to allow for continuation of care established over decades of experience with extended stability of parenteral drugs safely administered in the residential setting. After USP <797> became official in 2004, the USP collected thousands of comments. Many comments were submitted in response to the introduction and sudden limitation of beyond-use dates for each compounded preparation. Extended stability was called into question, and the USP was tasked with defining how long was too long to store compounded drugs. The home infusion industry consistently reported a low incidence of patient events related to their infusion therapy, which helped influence the revision to USP <797> in 2008 increasing the allowable beyond-use date to 9 days.

The need for compiling extended stability of parenteral drugs continues today, 20 years later, as pharmacists search for innovative solutions to improve patient access, manage medication shortages, and utilize compounded medications in a cost-effective way. As new drugs are approved, infusion pharmacists start seeking extended stability, and it takes considerable resources to organize and maintain an internal library of drug information for the medications compounded in a particular pharmacy. The requirement for reliable and relevant drug stability information remains a direct contributor to any pharmacy operation that compounds sterile preparations. Having a publication dedicated to extended stability for parenteral drugs supports the standardization and labeling of beyond-use dates for pharmacists who use the reference.

When starting the revision process for this 7th edition of *Extended Stability for Parenteral Drugs*, co-editors performed an assessment determining what information infusion pharmacists need to expedite decisions during the compounding and dispensing process. Through surveys, we collected ideas for developing the content to serve as an organized reference where a pharmacist can quickly and easily find information. Along with the reader survey, we performed a comprehensive review of available injectable drugs, paying particular attention to any that had stability longer than 24 hours, and especially those with stability of 9 days or more. Once we had the full list of injectable medications sorted by stability data, we had to decide which ones would be added to this edition. Basing the decision on past editions, our current team of editors and writers, and our vision for the future, we decided upon the list of medication monographs included in this 7th edition.

From initial conversations and meetings to the final submission for publication, our team maintained an ambitious schedule and assignment load. Bringing together pharmacist writers from a variety of practice settings added to the diversity of the content. We expanded beyond home infusion to be inclusive of all clinical settings where parenteral drugs are stored or compounded. The extended stability information provided is intended to be used as part of a risk-based approach to decrease risks posed to patients of physical or chemical degradation, and microbial contamination of parenteral medications.

Michelle C. Simpson, PharmD, BCSCP
June 2022, Atlanta, Georgia

DOI 10.37573/9781585286720.FM

ACKNOWLEDGMENTS

We want to thank Daniel J. Cobaugh, who brought together two editors with contrasting backgrounds and encouraged our excitement and vision. We appreciate Lori Justice and Elaine Jimenez, who have expedited our requests and supported us throughout the process. Preparing this edition has been a team effort that would not be possible without our writers, contributors, and professionals, who continue to collaborate and advise us. We are grateful to Caryn Dellamorte Bing and the contributors of previous editions, who kept the reference relevant and brought us to a 7th edition.

DOI 10.37573/9781585286720.FM

WHAT'S NEW IN THIS EDITION

The 196 monographs in this 7th edition include updates to all previous monographs, and 37 new drug monographs: alprostadil, alteplase, aminocaproic acid, ascorbic acid, azathioprine sodium, calcium chloride, cetuximab, cisatracurium besylate, dexMEDEtomidine, diazePAM, diltiazem hydrochloride, droperidol, ePHEDrine, EPINEPHrine, eravacycline dihydrochloride, ferric gluconate, insulin (regular), isoproterenol, lacosamide, levETIRAcetam, LEVOleucovorin, levothyroxine sodium, lidocaine, lipid emulsion, magnesium sulfate, meropenem-vaborbactam, mycophenolate mofetil, NORepinephrine, omadacycline, palonsetron hydrochloride, phenylephrine hydrochloride, plazomicin, rifAMPin, sodium bicarbonate, succinylcholine chloride, tacrolimus, and tranexamic acid. Monograph updates incorporated formulation differences, biosimilars, and specific brands where applicable. The section, Applying Stability Data in Sterile Compounding, provides information using comparison tables and charts for the following: Conditions Affecting Drug Stability, Extrapolating Stability Data, Comparison of Plastics for Compounding and Storage of Parenteral Drugs, Quality Assurance of Sterile Compounding, Temperature Excursion Stability Data for Refrigerated Intact Vials Stored at Room Temperature, Storage of Commercial IV Solution Containers After Removal From Protective Overwrap, Overfill Volumes of Commercial IV Solution Containers, Beyond-Use Date for Point-of-Care Activated Devices After Assembly, and Vascular Access Device Lumen Volume. Similarly, the section on Applying Stability Data in Compounding Parenteral Nutrition uses comparison charts and tables for the following: Conditions Affecting Parenteral Nutrition Stability and Extrapolation Considerations for Compounding Parenteral Nutrition. We decided to retain stability data on some devices that were previously widely used and are no longer marketed in the United States, but are still available internationally and in Puerto Rico; monograph footnotes clarify this status. As with prior editions, the publisher, editors, and writers welcome your feedback and suggestions.

DOI 10.37573/9781585286720.FM

ABOUT THE EDITORS

Michelle C. Simpson, PharmD, BCSCP, is a board certified Sterile Compounding Pharmacist with an established career in home infusion. She is the Clinical Program Manager for the National Home Infusion Association (NHIA), where she is responsible for continuing education accreditation, research through the National Home Infusion Foundation (NHIF), clinical education development, and implementation of resident and fellow programs. Previously, Simpson spent most of her time working as a clinical pharmacist at a corporate level for national home infusion providers. Her responsibilities in corporate home infusion included directing a drug information service for a large network of pharmacies, focusing on quality improvement by implementing a training program for handling drug information inquiries, which included a team of pharmacy residents. She assisted heavily in the pharmacy residency program as preceptor and advisor, consistently producing posters, presentations, and manuscripts associated with residency projects. She founded and was Chair of the Residency Advisory Committee for 2 years and founded and led the committee responsible for corporate clinical documents (monographs, policies, procedures) for 4 years. Simpson is active in association conferences and has both presented and hosted a round table discussion at NHIA annual meetings on the topics of parenteral nutrition and pharmacy-generated waste. She is a member of NHIA, American Medical Writers Association, and ASHP; Simpson assists as a peer-review pharmacist for article submissions for *American Journal of Health-System Pharmacy*. She received a PharmD degree from Mercer University, School of Pharmacy, in Atlanta, Georgia. She is board certified in compounded sterile preparations with the Board of Pharmacy Specialties.

Eric G. Schaefer, PharmD, MHSA, is the Director of Pharmacy Operations at Chartwell Pennsylvania, LP in Pittsburgh, Pennsylvania. Previously, Schaefer was a Manager of Pharmacy Operations at Allegheny General Hospital, the flagship hospital of the Allegheny Health Network in Pittsburgh, Pennsylvania, and prior to that, he was a Manager of Pharmacy Operations at the Presbyterian campus of UPMC Presbyterian-Shadyside, which is the flagship hospital for the University of Pittsburgh Medical Center Health Services Division. During his time at UPMC Presbyterian, Schaefer oversaw operations of the inpatient pharmacy department, with specific oversight of operations related to sterile compounding, non-sterile compounding, perioperative and operative pharmacy services, inventory management services, after-hours services, and central medication distribution services. He served as a program coordinator of the UPMC Presbyterian HSPAL Residency Program and the Pharmacy Administration Fellowship Program. He was co-author of a journal article in *Surgery* and a co-author of a white paper for Kit Check, Incorporated. Schaefer is a member of ACCP, ASHP, Pittsburgh Young Professionals, and PSHP. He was President-Elect of the western chapter of PSHP in January 2021. Schaefer received his Doctor of Pharmacy degree from the Lake Erie College of Osteopathic Medicine School of Pharmacy, in Erie, Pennsylvania. After graduation, he completed an ASHP-accredited Post Graduate Year One Pharmacy Practice Residency at Millcreek Community Hospital in affiliation with the Lake Erie College of Osteopathic Medicine School of Pharmacy. Schaefer received his Masters in Health Services Administration degree from the Lake Erie College of Osteopathic Medicine School of Health Services Administration, in Erie, Pennsylvania. He served as an Aircraft Fuel Systems Journeyman in the Pennsylvania Air National Guard for 9 years, during which time he deployed overseas to maintain the fuel systems of KC-135 Stratotankers utilized for aerial refueling missions. Schaefer had achieved the rank of Staff Sargent by the time he separated with an honorable discharge.

DOI 10.37573/9781585286720.FM

WRITERS' AFFILIATIONS

CO-EDITORS

Michelle C. Simpson, PharmD, BCSCP

Clinical Program Manager: National Home Infusion Association, Alexandria, Virginia

Eric G. Schaefer, PharmD, MHSA

Director of Pharmacy Operations: Chartwell Pennsylvania, LP, Pittsburgh, Pennsylvania

WRITERS

Gene Bernieri, PharmD, CNSC

Staff Pharmacist: Kaiser Permanente, San Diego, California

Marissa A. Davis, PharmD, BCSCP

Lead Pharmacist – Sterile Products: UPMC Presbyterian-Shadyside – Presbyterian Campus, Pittsburgh, Pennsylvania

Ernest H. Faucher III, PharmD

Area Clinical Director: Option Care Health, Round Rock, Texas

Brenda L. Gray, PharmD, BCNSP, CNSC, VA-BC, CVAA(c), PRS, BCSCP

Owner and Senior Pharmacy and Accreditation Consultant: Clinical Pharmacy Partners, Tampa, Florida

J. Michael Hayes, PharmD

Pharmacotherapy Specialist, Investigational Drug Service: Tampa General Hospital, Tampa, Florida

Annemarie Hocking, PharmD

Clinical Pharmacist & Lead Preceptor PGY1 Residency: Option Care Health, Wood Dale, Illinois

Alexandre Ivanov, PharmD, MS, RD, BCNSP

Pharmacy Specialist: Emory St. Joseph's Hospital, Atlanta, Georgia

Margaret Kronz, PharmD

Health-System Pharmacy Administration & Leadership Resident: Allegheny Health Network - Allegheny General Hospital, Pittsburgh, Pennsylvania

Drew Lambert, PharmD, BCPS

Associate Professor of Pharmacy Practice: Husson University School of Pharmacy, Bangor, Maine

Rachel V. Marini, PharmD, BCIDP

Lead Pharmacist – Antimicrobial Stewardship: UPMC Presbyterian-Shadyside – Presbyterian Campus, Pittsburgh, Pennsylvania

Kevn M. McNamara, PharmD, CSP, PRS, BCSCP

Director of Accreditation: Comprehensive Pharmacy Services, Fort Myers, Florida

Julie Wurdeman, PharmD

Manager of Home Health Pharmacy: Children's Hospital and Medical Center, Omaha, Nebraska

Paula Zelle, PharmD, FASHP, FNHIA

President: Infusion Consultant Services, Inc., Canton, Ohio
Consultant: Accreditation Resources, Canton, Ohio

DOI 10.37573/9781585286720.FM

CLINICAL PROOFREADERS

Bethany Baker, PharmD, MHA
Director of Pharmacy Clinical Services
Children's Mercy Kansas City
Kansas City, Missouri

Johanna Bezjak, PharmD, BCNSP
PGY1 Residency Program Director
Clinical Pharmacy Manager
CarePathRx
Pittsburgh, Pennsylvania

Michael Bunn, PharmD
Pittsburgh, Pennsylvania

Julia Conforti, PharmD
Atlanta, Georgia

Julia Cowell, MHS, PharmD
Pharmacy Supervisor
Clinical Pharmacist – Intake
Option Care Health
Florham Park, New Jersey

Elena Echenique, RPh
Independent Consultant
Shepherdstown, West Virginia

Maria Giannakos, PharmD, MBA, BCPS, BCSCP
Clinical Pharmacy Services Manager
PGY1 Pharmacy Residency Program Director
Option Care Health
Cleveland, Ohio

Mort Goldman, PharmD
Independent Consultant
Cleveland, Ohio

Adam Hussain, PharmD, MS, RPh
Senior Manager
Advertising and Promotion
Sobi – North America
Waltham, Massachusetts

Janet Misko, RPh
Senior Software Quality Assurance Analyst
McKesson Pharmacy Systems
Pittsburgh, Pennsylvania

Alexandros Pitsakis, PharmD, MBA, BS
Pharmacy Supervisor
Option Care Health
Schwenksville, Pennsylvania

Lisa Linn Siefert, RPh, FASHP, ASQ-CMQ/OE
Vice President of Pharmacy Services
Palmetto Infusion Services
Duluth, Georgia

Nicholas A. Skezas, PharmD, BCPS
Supervisor of Pharmacy Operations Chartwell
Pennsylvania, LP
Pittsburgh, Pennsylvania

Andrew Sobek, PharmD
Pharmacy Supervisor
CarepathRX
Pittsburgh, Pennsylvania

DOI 10.37573/9781585286720.FM

EXTENDED STABILITY FOR PARENTERAL DRUGS USERS GUIDE

Extended Stability for Parenteral Drugs is comprised of parenteral medication monographs with published stability or manufacturer stability data. Information from 808 references and communication documents is presented in a standardized structure and format to facilitate clinical decision making for the purpose of patient safety. Stability monographs are alphabetical by generic drug name. Each monograph includes drug stability data measured over time for various container systems, solutions, concentrations, and temperature conditions. Stability data indicate at least 90% of the drug is measurable in the container specified under the conditions listed, with the exception of factor products, which are required to retain at least 80% activity. Where applicable, brand, product, and manufacturer names are provided for the purpose of clinical considerations, and are not intended to be an endorsement of any product or manufacturer.

						Temperature			Post-Thaw			
Container	*Drug Manufacturer*	*Concentration*	*Diluents*	*Osmolality*	*pH*	*Room*	*Refrig*	*Frozen*	*Room*	*Refrig*	*Body Temp*	*Refer.*
1	*2*	*3*	*4*	*5*	*6*	*7*	*8*	*9*	*10*	*11*	*12*	*13*

1. Container: container material used for storage of the compounded drug
2. Drug manufacturer: manufacturer of the primary drug
3. Concentration: shown in terms of concentration per milliliter
4. Diluents: infusion solution used in the stability test
5. Osmolality: shown in mOsm/kg
6. pH: pH of the studied solution
7. Room temperature: 15°C to 30°C
8. Refrigerated temperature: 2°C to 8°C
9. Frozen temperature: –25°C to –10°C
10. Post-thaw room temperature: time stored at room temperature after thawing
11. Post-thaw refrigerated temperature: time stored at refrigerated temperature after thawing
12. Body temperature: 37°C
13. Reference: reference to the original source of the information

*When n/a is used in any field, no information is available.

Flush Compatibility: The Flush Compatibility section reflects compatibility with common solutions used to flush vascular access devices. Compatible solutions for flushing drugs incompatible with sodium chloride 0.9% are provided.

Special Considerations: The Special Considerations section includes information on drug storage and preparation as it relates to stability.

Notes: The Notes section highlights important information. Lowercase superscript letters are used within the monographs.

DOI 10.37573/9781585286720.FM

USE OF ADDITIONAL RESOURCES

The information contained in these monographs is a compilation of extended stability data from multiple sources. This information is not a substitute for the official product literature. Practitioners should consult the primary literature and the product manufacturer to determine the applicability of stability data to a particular patient and practice scenario. Practitioners should maintain current drug reference resources as well as the most current edition of a comprehensive reference on drug stability and compatibility. Every pharmacy that compounds or provides sterile preparations should maintain resource files, including the phone numbers and all correspondence with the medical or clinical affairs departments of pharmaceutical manufacturers. The pharmacy should also have access to a drug information center or the expertise and ability to conduct a literature search for the most up-to-date clinical and pharmaceutical information on parenteral drugs.

GENERAL ABBREVIATIONS

d	day(s)
hr	hour(s)
gm	gram(s)
iso	iso-osmotic
L	liter(s)
m	month(s)
mcg	microgram(s)
mg	milligram(s)
min	minute(s)
mL	milliliter(s)
n/a	not available
RF	refrigeration
RT	room temperature
RTU	ready to use from manufacturer
unspec.	unspecified
wk	week(s)
yr	year(s)

SOLUTION ABBREVIATIONS

BNS	Bacteriostatic Sodium Chloride 0.9%
BWFI	Bacteriostatic Water for Injection
D	Dextrose Solution (percentage unspecified)
D2.5NS	Dextrose 2.5% in Sodium Chloride 0.9%
D2.5½NS	Dextrose 2.5% in Sodium Chloride 0.45%
D3.3⅓NS	Dextrose 3.3% in Sodium Chloride 0.3%
D5LR	Dextrose 5% in Ringer's Injection, Lactated
D5NS	Dextrose 5% in Sodium Chloride 0.9%
D5¼NS	Dextrose 5% in Sodium Chloride 0.225%
D5⅓NS	Dextrose 5% in Sodium Chloride 0.3%
D5½NS	Dextrose 5% in Sodium Chloride 0.45%

DOI 10.37573/9781585286720.FM

D10NS	Dextrose 10% in Sodium Chloride 0.9%
D2.5W	Dextrose 2.5% in Water
D5W	Dextrose 5% in Water
D7W	Dextrose 7% in Water
D10W	Dextrose 10% in Water
D20W	Dextrose 20% in Water
D25W	Dextrose 25% in Water
DXN-6	Dextran 6%
LR	Ringer's Injection, Lactated
M5	Mannitol 5%
M10	Mannitol 10%
M20	Mannitol 20%
NMD5W	Normosol®-M in Dextrose 5%
NRD5W	Normosol®-R in Dextrose 5%
NS	Sodium Chloride 0.9%
R	Ringer's Solution
½NS	Sodium Chloride 0.45%
⅓NS	Sodium Chloride 0.3%
¼NS	Sodium Chloride 0.225%
SWFI	Sterile Water for Injection

TIME CONVERSIONS

Hours (hr)	≤ 72 hours
Days (d)	4-30 days **OR** any number of days not evenly divisible by 7
Weeks (wk)	≥ 35 days **AND** evenly divisible by 7
Months (m)	> 12 weeks **AND** evenly divisible by 4
Years (yr)	> 12 months **AND** evenly divisible by 12

PART I

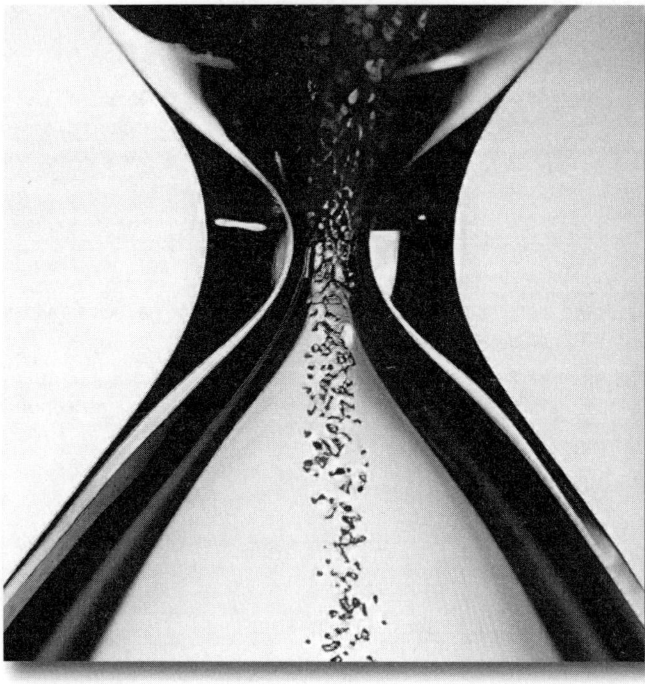

Applying Stability Data in Sterile Compounding

Michelle C. Simpson, Eric G. Schaefer, Rachel V. Marini, Marissa A. Davis

INTRODUCTION

In order to apply stability data in sterile compounding, storage times shown in the drug monographs of this book represent chemical and physical studies of drug stability, container material, and storage conditions. Before the official publication of the United States Pharmacopeia (USP) Chapter <797>, *Pharmaceutical Compounding – Sterile Preparations*, which set enforceable standards related to compounding sterile preparations, beyond-use dates were based primarily on chemical and physical stability, with pharmacies labeling compounded medications for use over several weeks or months. The USP recognizes the risks of microbial contamination as a contributor to patient safety and sets limits on the length of time a compounded sterile preparation (CSP) may be stored before that actual time that clinical administration to the patient starts. Pharmacists responsible for compounding and dispensing parenteral drugs must assign a date to each CSP that represents the date beyond which the preparation should not be stored or used. Assigning an appropriate beyond-use date (BUD) incorporates both chemical and physical factors, plus maintaining a level of quality assurance through the compounding facility's design, equipment, personnel, and procedures.[1] Compiling extended stability information supports pharmacy operations within healthcare organizations by minimizing waste, maximizing product utilization, and managing medication shortages. Additionally, extended stability information allows for the compounding of enough medication to cover a shift at a hospital or a weekly delivery for a home infusion patient.

FACTORS AFFECTING EXTENDED DRUG STABILITY

The stability monographs in the Drug Monographs section of this book show data from studies where at least 90% of the drug is measurable in the container specified under the conditions listed, with the exception of factor products which are required to retain at least 80% activity. Stability involves chemical integrity, physical properties such as appearance and dissolution, as well as microbiological stability by maintaining sterility of the final dosage form. Environmental factors can reduce stability through light exposure or storage temperatures that are higher or lower than recommended. Stability considerations related to the dosage form include particle size, pH, and container material.[2] For more information, refer to Table 1: Conditions Affecting Drug Stability.

When the usage timeframe in the manufacturer product labeling is limited or omitted, published stability studies can potentially support extending the BUD assigned to a CSP. If a referenced study does not match the conditions of a specific CSP's formulation or conditions, assess the individual components based on the diluent used, concentration, container type, storage temperature, and exposure to light to determine if the available stability data may be extrapolated. Predictions of any area of stability impart an element of risk, and the degree of accuracy depends on the extent of the difference between the CSP characteristics.[7]

Extrapolation between diluents is discouraged. For example, stability in sodium chloride 0.9% is not applicable

DOI 10.37573/9781585286720.PT1001

TABLE 1: Conditions Affecting Drug Stability

Stability/Influence	Description	Outcome
Chemical Changes	Active ingredient must remain within labeled amount for the duration of storage and use.[2,8]	• Sub-therapeutic response or toxicity.
Physical Changes	Alteration of the appearance[2,8]	• CSPs with visible changes (eg, color, dissolution, uniformity, turbidity, particles) fail the visual inspection and should not be administered. • Exception: If data are available to support that a visible change (eg, color) does not relate to or affect the stability of the CSP, then the CSP can pass the visual inspection.
Microbiological Contamination	Microbial contamination risk[1]	• Variables affecting microbial risk: ■ Environment (eg, engineering controls) ■ Aseptic processing (eg, personnel aseptic technique) ■ Storage conditions (eg, refrigeration, room temperature) ■ Sterile starting components ■ Sterility testing (eg, air sampling, personnel evaluation) • Controlling these variables ***decreases*** the risk of contaminated CSPs being administered to patients.
Storage Temperature	Heat[2]	• Temperature fluctuations affect chemical reactivity, primarily hydrolysis and oxidation. ■ Heat ***increases*** the rate of hydrolysis. • A fluctuation of 10°C can change the rate of reaction.
	Freezing[2]	• Freezing may either break emulsions or cause a large ***increase*** in the droplet size of emulsions. • Freezing temperatures can denature proteins or cause crystallization or precipitation.
Container	Fluid evaporation[4]	• Evaporation of water through the container material can lead to changes in the concentration of the CSP's active ingredient(s).
	Sorption[4,5]	• Adsorption followed by absorption into the plastic material causing a loss of pharmaceutical activity.
	Leaching[4,5]	• DEHP leaching of lipophilic medications and PVC. • Glass containers have: ■ Relatively ***low*** levels of leachables at pH 4-8. ■ Relatively ***high*** levels of leachables at pH > 9.
Light Exposure	Ultraviolet light (UV)[2]	• Exposure to UV light may cause oxidation. • In susceptible compounds, photochemical energy creates free radicals. ■ Accelerated chemical degradation reactions.
pH	High and low pH extremes[2]	• High and low pH extremes ***increase*** the rate of hydrolysis and oxidation. • Drugs in solution are directly affected by changes in pH. • Small fluctuations can decrease stability by factors of 10. ■ ***Higher*** pH values catalyze and oxidize. ■ ***Lower*** pH values destabilize emulsions and other two-phase systems.
Handling & Transport	Mechanical stress[6]	• Caused by shipping, manipulations, pneumatic tube systems, etc. • Agitation and shearing can affect stability of protein-based or large molecule medications.
	Packing[1]	• Fragile items should be carefully packaged (eg, surrounded by bubble wrap) for delivery and storage.
	Temperature[1,2]	• The delivery process (eg, containers, insulating and packing materials, courier, environmental conditions) should be validated to ensure that the contents of the shipment are maintained at a temperature within established stability parameters. • The pharmacy should be aware of storage and shipping limitations and should take extra precautions when extreme temperature conditions exist (eg, summer heat, winter freezing temperatures) to ensure that preparation stability is not affected throughout the entire shipping process.

to stability in dextrose 5% in water. When several concentrations of a drug are studied with similar stability results, it is reasonable to expect the stability to be the same for concentrations falling within the ones tested.[3] In the absence of stability studies in a specific container, the pharmacist should consider the available container materials and compare them to the materials studied. Comparing data between different containers should consider both the drug degradation mechanism and physical properties of the container.[3] For more information on container material comparison, refer to Table 3: Comparison of Plastics for Compounding and Storage of Parenteral Drugs. Temperature excursion comparisons may widen the options if a medication is studied as stable in another concentration or container at two temperatures. If not explicitly studied, room temperature storage stability data should not be applied to refrigerated storage conditions, and refrigerated storage stability data should not be applied to room temperature storage conditions. Studies performed while the preparation was protected from light cannot be extrapolated to light-exposed conditions. However, stability studies of light-exposed drugs can be extrapolated to light-protected conditions. Time periods reported can only be shortened, not lengthened. For more information, refer to Table 2: Extrapolating Stability Data.

TABLE 2: Extrapolating Stability Data

Comparison of CSP to Studied Conditions	Considerations	Conclusions
Container	Bag Syringe Glass	• Compare available container materials to those studied. • When stability data are available in a wide range of container types, consider documented stability of the drug and diluent in the desired container.[1,3,8,9]
	Elastomeric	• Stability information from Easypump® also applies to SMARTeZ® pumps with reported equivalent drug reservoir and fluid path composition.[9]
Manufacturer	Manufacturer product studied differs from inventory[3]	• Drugs that are generically and chemically identical are expected to have the same results as those studied. • If there are differences in salt form, excipients, or solubilizing agents, the studied stability data may not be applicable.
Concentration	Several concentrations studied with similar stability results[3]	• Prediction of similar stability for a concentration falling within the range of studied concentrations is reasonable. • If there are data available in a container type and diluent with documented stability at two concentrations, concentrations falling within the two data points is acceptable. • Extrapolating stability outside the studied concentrations is not recommended due to increased risk of instability of the final solution. • Drug concentrations studied in differing container types may widen the stability range to specific containers needed for an individualized CSP.
Diluent	Diluent studied is ***different*** in composition to diluent ordered	• Extrapolation of studied stability between diluents with different properties (eg, NS to D5W) is not expected to have similar results and should be avoided.[1,3]
	Diluent studied is ***similar*** in composition to diluent ordered	• Diluents with similar properties (eg, ¼NS to ½NS) are expected to have similar stability to those studied.[1,3]
Temperature	Studied at two temperatures and stable at both vs. studied at only one temperature	• Temperatures should not be extrapolated without studying the drug at the temperature desired.[8]
Light	Light-protected compared to light-exposed	• Do not extrapolate light-protected study results to light-exposed CSPs.[8]
	Light-exposed compared to light-protected	• Stability studies of light-exposed drugs can be extrapolated to light-protected CSPs.
Sterility	Sterility tests from CSP to CSP	• Do not extrapolate sterility studies.[1]
Premix/Ready to Use (RTU)	RTU manufacturer expiration to compounded CSP	• Do not extrapolate RTU manufacturer expiration dates to beyond-use dates for compounded CSPs.

TABLE 3: Comparison of Plastics for Compounding and Storage of Parenteral Drugs

Characteristic	Ethylene Vinyl Acetate (EVA)	Multilayer EVA	Ethylene Propylene Copolymer	Polyethylene (PE)
Brand Names / Examples	• Bag ■ EcoFLX™ DME[25] ■ EcoFLX™ DMP[26] ■ Exactamix®[23]	• Bag ■ Baxa® Multilayer[24]	• Bag ■ Excel®[62] ■ PAB®[63,146]	• Bag ■ Ecoflac® Plus[16,62]
Inert / Nonreactive	Inert[4,20]	Inert[4]	Inert[62,63,146]	Inert[10]
Evaporation	Minimally water permeable[4]	Prevents water loss[4]	Prevents water loss[63,146]	Prevents water loss[20]
Permeation	Oxygen permeable[4,14,20]	Decreases oxidation[14]	Prevents permeation[63,146]	Prevents permeation[4,20]
Sorption	Not affected[4]	Not affected[20]	Not affected[62,63,146]	Not affected[4]
Leaching	No plasticizer[4,14,15]	No plasticizer[14,15]	No plasticizer[62,63,146]	No plasticizer[4,10]
Visibility	Transparent[4]	Clearly visible[4]	Clearly visible	Clearly visible[4]

Characteristic	Multilayer PE	Polypropylene	Polyolefin[a]	Polyvinyl Chloride (PVC)
Brand Names / Examples	• Bag ■ Nexcel®[22]	• Bag ■ AVIVA™[18] ■ Fleboflex®[28] ■ Freeflex®[19] ■ Inerta®[27] ■ IntraCon[29] • Syringe ■ BD Plastipak™[145] ■ Monoject™[144]	• Bag ■ AVIVA™[18] ■ Excel®[16,62] ■ Intravia™[18] ■ PAB®[63,146] ■ Viaflo®[21] ■ VisIV™[12]	• Bag ■ Lifecare®[30] ■ Viaflex™[18] • Cassette ■ CADD® Cassette[11]
Inert / Nonreactive	Inert[10]	Inert[4,20]	Inert[12]	Reactive with surfactants & oils[5,13,20]
Evaporation	Prevents water loss[20]	Prevents water loss[20]	Prevents water loss[20]	Water permeable[4]
Permeation	Decreases oxidation[20]	Prevents permeation[4]	Prevents permeation[20]	Water and oxygen permeable[4,20]
Sorption	Not affected[20]	Not affected[4]	Not affected[12]	Sorption occurs with proteins & susceptible medication[4,5]
Leaching	No plasticizer[10]	May leach additives from syringe plunger[17]	No plasticizer[4,12]	Plasticizer leaching[4,5,17]
Visibility	Clearly visible[4]	Transparent[4]	Clearly visible[4]	Transparent[5]

[a] Polyolefin is a category of polymers made with mixtures of low-density polyethylene, high-density polyethylene, polypropylene, and ethylene vinyl acetate.[4]

PREPARATION STERILITY AND QUALITY ASSURANCE

Individual organizations have to determine their own specific standard operating procedures (SOPs). In order to ensure consistent practices and reproducible results, there should be SOPs for all compounding and related processes. SOPs define the sequence of steps and conditions necessary for compounding CSPs. Consistency in compounding compliance using standardized SOPs can reduce variation among CSPs and decrease the chances of preventable errors occurring. SOPs should be based on applicable laws, regulations, and accreditation standards, and they should be further individualized for the types of compounding performed and equipment used at each facility.[1]

If compounding in batches for more than one patient, a master formulation record provides specific compounding instructions and describes how the CSP was prepared.[57-59] When standardizing compounding records and master formulation records, the names, descriptions, and identifiers of CSPs should be consistent.[59,60] Master formulation records and compounding records should contain sufficient detail to be used on their own without additional verbal explanation.[58]

When CSPs are stored before use, a visual inspection of each CSP should be documented at every stage. A visual inspection should occur during compounding, checking, labeling, dispensing, and before clinical administration to a patient by each individual who handles the CSP. Any visible changes to a CSP should be reported to the pharmacist.[1]

An environmental monitoring program decreases the potential for contamination of CSPs and gives assurance the BUD assigned is appropriate. Maintaining a state of control of the compounding personnel, environment, and equipment is required for quality assurance of sterile preparations. For more information on quality assurance, refer to Table 4: Quality Assurance of Sterile Compounding.

TABLE 4: Quality Assurance of Sterile Compounding[1,31]

Quality Components	Monitoring and Competency	Compliance
Personnel	Garbing, material handling, staging, cleaning	Incorporated into aseptic technique testing
	Gloved fingertip sampling	
	Media fill testing	Proper technique, effective cleaning
	Surface sampling to measure work practices	
Environment	Sampling plan customized for each facility	Create a diagram of locations to be sampled
	Document the number of people in the room during sampling	
	Include surfaces of carts, counters, pass-through windows/doors	Proper technique, effective cleaning
Equipment	Viable air sampling to test the engineering controls	Certification is performed on a schedule by third party
	Automatic compounding devices	Cleaning, calibration, maintenance

ASSIGNING BEYOND-USE DATES TO COMPOUNDED STERILE PREPARATIONS

Assigning a beyond-use date or BUD to a CSP is performed as part of the compounding process and is distinctly different from expiration dates assigned to products during manufacturing. A BUD encompasses the time period starting at the date and time of compounding through the date and time after which the start of clinical administration should not occur. Assigning an appropriate BUD requires the consideration of many factors such as chemical stability, physical properties, component compatibility, sterility, component concentrations, container type, personnel factors, environmental factors, and equipment utilized during the compounding process. BUDs of CSPs are determined using a risk-based approach. The USP limits maximum BUDs to decrease risks posed to patients by requiring a labeled BUD that represents a time span before it is a risk for physical or chemical degradation, microbial contamination and proliferation, and diminished integrity of the container. For more information on container influence on stability, see Table 5: Stability Influence of Containers for Compounding Parenteral Drugs. The date takes into consideration the specific conditions where the CSP was made, the probability for microbial growth, and the time period within which it should be used. In unclassified spaces (eg, home, bedside), shorter BUDs are applied.[1] Extended stability BUDs require aseptic processing, sterile starting components or end sterilization method, sterility testing, and controlled storage conditions. The BUD of a CSP prepared in a small volume container, as defined in USP Chapter <659>, *Packaging and Storage Requirements*, that was packaged by the manufacturer in overwrap should not exceed the BUD of the container after removal from its overwrap unless data on stability and sterility exists for the CSP following guidance provided in USP Chapter <71>, *Sterility Tests*. For more information on dating related to overwrap removal, see Table 7: Manufacturer Storage of Commercial IV Solution Containers after Removal from Protective Overwrap. The BUD of a CSP prepared from another CSP (eg, stock solution, aliquot container) cannot exceed the shortest BUD of the individual starting components.[58]

Labels that specify the storage conditions and BUD of compounded preparations are placed on each parenteral dosage unit. Documentation of the preparation date should be part of the labeling and include the time of compounding, if applicable. If preparation stability varies under different temperature conditions, list the BUD for each anticipated storage condition on the label. If the preparation needs to be warmed to room temperature prior to administration, the label and ancillary instruction material should describe it. If preparations are stable for less than 24 hours at room temperature, the label should be specific about the end-use time.

TABLE 5: Stability Influence of Containers for Compounding Parenteral Drugs

Container	Characteristics
Polyvinyl Chloride (PVC)[5,32]	• Permeability of fluid out of the package: ■ Evaporation leads to ***increased*** concentration of the drug(s) in solution. ■ Small volume containers are most susceptible to permeation. • Drug reactivity to PVC: ■ May cause leaching of plasticizers and chemicals. ■ Sorption of the drug with the container surface may result in ***decreased*** concentration of the drug(s) in solution.
Polyolefins[20]	• May be any of the following types: ■ Low-density polyethylene ■ High-density polyethylene ■ Polypropylene ■ Ethylene
Ethylene Vinyl Acetate (EVA)[17]	• EVA containers are made of a flexible plastic that does not require phthalate plasticizers, such as di(2-ethylhexyl) phthalate (DEHP), in the manufacturing process. • EVA containers can serve as a DEHP-free alternative for preparation of medications when that choice is appropriate for the patient or therapy.
Syringe[4,33,34]	• Plastic syringes are composed of plastic polymers; common types include: ■ Polypropylene ■ Polyethylene ■ Polycarbonate ■ PVC • Medications compounded in a syringe for administration are associated with accuracy, safety, and simplicity. Premeasured doses prepared in syringes reduce medication errors. • Siliconization of rubber closures and lubricants may interact with medication stored in syringes.[a]
Glass[4]	• Used for clarity, inert composition, moisture, and gas barrier. • Storage of drugs with high pH (>9), proteins, and peptides may lead to delamination of the interior surface and contamination of the CSP.
Elastomeric	• It has been determined that stability information for Easypump® also applies to SMARTeZ® pumps.[9]
Ambulatory Infusion System	• CADD® Cassette reservoirs are composed of PVC.[11]
Commercially Prepared Solutions	• Always consult the most current prescribing information/package insert for stability dating of commercially available premixed solutions. • Frozen and post-thaw stability data for each premixed drug applies only to that specific commercial product. • Practitioners must not extrapolate stability data from premixed commercial preparations of drugs in solution to extemporaneously compounded preparations.

[a] In 2015, the FDA provided notice that there were reports of interactions with the rubber stoppers of BD syringes that could cause some drugs stored in them to lose potency when not used immediately. On January 12, 2018, the FDA provided an update related to actions taken by BD. BD informed the FDA that they were no longer using the rubber stopper material that was associated with loss of drug potency in their general use syringes, and that they returned to a rubber stopper they had used previously in syringes.[113,143]

Individuals administering CSPs should be trained to check preparations for current BUDs prior to usage. Practitioners should establish a standardized approach to labeling that is clear, concise, and meets all licensure and regulatory requirements, including USP Chapter <797> general labeling guidelines.[31]

PROFESSIONAL, REGULATORY, AND ACCREDITATION EXPECTATIONS

Pharmacists have professional and legal responsibilities related to all aspects of the medication compounding and dispensing process. In addition to any issues unique to each state's pharmacy practice act, professional standards of practice set the expectations for practitioners in all care settings where pharmaceutical services are provided. Pharmacists should be aware of these expectations, including requirements applicable to their specific practice setting(s).

Professional Associations, Organizations, Standards, and Guidelines

American Society of Health-System Pharmacists (ASHP) *Guidelines on Compounding Sterile Preparations* assist pharmacists in establishing quality assurance procedures for sterile drug preparations based on the risk level associated with the process and preparation.[31] These professional guidelines should be used in conjunction with other best practice resources that address the procedures and quality assurance for compounding sterile preparations.

ASHP *Guidelines on Home Infusion Pharmacy Services* outline the requirements for the operation and management of pharmaceutical services provided by home care pharmacies.[36] These guidelines affirm the pharmacist's responsibility for sterile preparation quality and integrity, including assignment of reliable beyond-use dating.

The Board of Pharmacy Specialties has established a certification for sterile compounding. Board Certified Sterile Compounding Pharmacists (BCSCP) validate their advanced knowledge and experience related to sterile compounding. They specialize in ensuring that compounded sterile preparations meet patients' unique clinical needs while satisfying all quality, safety, and environmental control requirements set by legislative, regulatory, and accreditation bodies. The BCSCP has responsibility in all phases of preparation, storage, transportation, and administration of CSPs and maintain compliance with established standards, regulations, professional guidance, and best practices.[35]

The National Association of Boards of Pharmacy (NABP) is a professional organization that focuses on protecting public health by supporting state boards of pharmacy. The NABP was initially founded in 1904 and had a consultative role in the Drug Quality and Security Act that US Congress enacted in November 2013. The NABP defined the terms *compounding* and *manufacturing* in its Model State Pharmacy Practice Act, which helped distinguish these terms and their differences related to sterile compounding practices.[119]

Regulatory Bodies, Standards, and Guidelines

The United States Pharmacopeia (USP) is an independent, scientific non-profit organization that has set public quality standards for over 200 years. Through rigorous science, USP focuses on setting standards that help build public trust in the supply of safe, quality medications.[118] The standards set by USP are utilized by more than 140 countries around the world. Since the late 1980s, USP has had increased focus on the processes and practices related to CSPs. USP Chapters have been developed to provide guidance for almost all aspects related to sterile and non-sterile compounding. All *USP-NF* chapters numbered under 1,000 are enforceable by state boards of pharmacy, the FDA, and accreditation organizations.[119] Some of the key USP chapters that relate to the assignment of BUDs utilizing extended stability data are summarized below.

- USP General Chapter <71>, *Sterility Tests*, outlines the standards and procedures required to validate sterilization processes or verify that batched products were aseptically compounded. It provides guidance related to culture media selection and use, incubation temperatures, sterility testing methods, method suitability testing, and the quantities that require testing based on batch characteristics (eg, solid vs. liquid, final preparation container volume, parenteral vs. ophthalmic or noninjectable, antibiotic).[114] USP Chapter <71> has become an important part of compounding for facilities that utilize automated compounding devices (ACDs) to compound larger medication batches with extended stability dating applied to prevent waste.
- USP Chapter <659>, *Packaging and Storage Requirements*, provides definitions related to packaging, auxiliary packaging information, and definitions for storage conditions pertinent to the storage and distribution of medications. USP Chapter <659> defines small-volume and large-volume injections, single-dose and multidose containers, and light-resistant containers. It also defines temperature ranges that are important for storing compounded sterile products (eg, controlled room temperature, refrigerator, freezer).[115]
- USP Chapter <797>, *Pharmaceutical Compounding – Sterile Preparations*, outlines the standards and minimum required practices related to CSPs in the United States. It provides the organizational structure, procedures, processes, and resources necessary to ensure predefined quality measures are met by facilities that compound sterile products.[1]
- USP Chapter <800>, *Hazardous Drugs – Handling in Healthcare Settings*, outlines standards and minimum required practices related to handling hazardous drugs. It was developed to ensure that hazardous drugs used within a healthcare setting are handled in a manner that keeps both patients and staff safe while attempting to mitigate any possible negative impacts on the environment. USP Chapter <800> applies to all healthcare personnel who could potentially be exposed to hazardous drugs at any type of healthcare facility that stores, prepares, transports, or administers hazardous drugs. It applies to facilities that treat humans as well as facilities that treat animals. Each facility must ensure that USP Chapter <800> requirements are met for any medication that they store, prepare, transport, or administer that is listed on the National Institute for Occupational Safety and Health's (NIOSH) list of antineoplastic and other hazardous drugs used in healthcare.[116]

- USP Chapter <1163>, *Quality Assurance in Pharmaceutical Compounding*, reinforces the importance of quality assurance systems being implemented by any healthcare facility that prepares compounded preparations, both sterile and nonsterile. It further describes critical components that should be incorporated into quality assurance programs to ensure that compounded preparations are produced with quality attributes appropriate to meet the needs of patients and healthcare professionals. USP Chapter <1163> outlines requirements related to personnel training, standard operating procedures (eg, components, review), compounding documentation and record-keeping, and quality-related testing (eg, analytical, microbial) throughout the entire compounding process as well as the finished products.[117]
- USP Chapter <1191>, *Stability Considerations in Dispensing Practice*, describes different aspects of drug product stability that pharmacists should be concerned with throughout the preparation and dispensing process for medications. Criteria for acceptable levels of stability (eg, chemical, physical, microbiological, therapeutic, toxicological) describe the conditions that must be maintained throughout a drug product's shelf life. Information related to different factors that can affect product stability (eg, hydrolysis, oxidation, photochemical decomposition, pH, temperature) is provided to ensure that healthcare providers have an understanding of reactions that can occur within a dosage form that lead to loss of active drug despite the lack of obvious visual or olfactory evidence of their occurrence.[2]

Accreditation Bodies, Standards, and Guidelines

Accreditation standards are applied to home infusion and hospital pharmacies to ensure that the organization undergoes peer-review and operates using a set of best practices to safeguard patients.[36]

The Centers for Medicare and Medicaid Services (CMS) requires the inclusion of processes related to compounding sterile products in the survey and review process of acute care facilities.[37] Acute care facilities must meet CMS Conditions of Participation to receive reimbursement for services provided to Medicare and Medicaid patients. Surveying and accreditation are generally conducted by CMS-approved accrediting bodies (eg, deeming agencies), which include The Joint Commission (TJC), Accreditation Commission for Health Care (ACHC), The American Osteopathic Association's Healthcare Facilities Accreditation Program (HFAP), Det Norske Veritas (DNV) GL-Healthcare, and the Center for Improvement in Healthcare Quality (CIHQ), that are deemed to have authority by CMS. State agencies confirm that deeming agencies perform to CMS standards by conducting surveys of acute care facilities following the guidance outlined in the interpretive guidelines that CMS maintains.[119,148]

ACHC is a non-profit accreditation organization considered a deeming agency for CMS with authority for home infusion therapy, infusion pharmacy, home health, hospice, renal dialysis, durable medical equipment, prosthetics, orthotics, and supplies. ACHC Infusion Pharmacy Accreditation (IRX) surveys the processes and practices related to the compounding of sterile preparations in compliance with USP Chapters <797> and <800>, and includes standards for dispensing medications, equipment, and supplies to patients receiving home infusion therapy. In addition to accreditation authority, ACHC has distinctions for hazardous drug handling, specialty pharmacy, nutrition support, oncology, infectious diseases, and rare diseases. By achieving ACHC accreditation, pharmacies are able to demonstrate their commitment to providing the highest quality service through compliance with national regulations and industry best practices.[148]

TJC is a non-profit, independent organization considered a deeming agency for CMS. In addition to accreditation of acute care facilities, TJC reviews the processes and practices related to the compounding of sterile products at ambulatory care locations, including ambulatory centers, outpatient surgery centers, physician offices where office-based surgeries are conducted, imaging centers, and urgent care centers. TJC standards exist that connect directly to compliance with USP Chapter <797> and USP Chapter <800>. TJC standards related to sterile compounding span many areas, including human resources (eg, personnel training), medication management, infection control (eg, cleaning and disinfecting, gowning/garbing), environment of care (eg, compounding equipment, hazardous medications), and patient care (eg, patient education).[119]

APPLYING STABILITY DATA USING COMMERCIAL PRODUCTS

Extended stability data does not just apply to preparations manipulated or prepared by an individual healthcare facility. Data are available for intact commercial products stored in a manner that differs from how the product was received from the manufacturer or for products exposed to temperature excursions that differ from the manufacturer's storage requirements as outlined in the official product information. The ability to extend intact commercial products can allow healthcare facilities to utilize medication stock to the greatest extent possible and reduce healthcare spending caused by medication waste.

Commercial Intact Vials and Parenteral Diluents

Many drugs require refrigeration from the time of manufacturing until the time of compounding or administration. Maintaining a controlled refrigerated temperature throughout the supply chain process can pose many challenges due to reliance on a multitude of factors (eg, refrigeration equipment, outside temperature, extreme exposure during transit). Challenges also exist when medications must be stored under refrigeration until use but may be needed urgently in a care location where installation of a refrigerator may not be possible or reasonable (eg, ambulance, operating room). When storage temperature excursions occur, data may be available to support storage outside of the manufacturer's recommendations and provide a BUD for the drug at alternative storage temperatures. See Table 6 for information on BUDs for intact vials stored at room temperature after removal from refrigeration.

Manufacturers of parenteral products packaged in PVC and other non-rigid plastic containers recommend maximum usage times after removal from the overwrap. Table 7 summarizes maximum out-of-overwrap storage times for solution container storage at room temperature. Once additives are placed in these containers, the BUD changes to the shortest date for any of the components, which could be either the drug stability dating or the solution

TABLE 6: Temperature Excursion Stability Data for Refrigerated Intact Vials Stored at Room Temperature

Medication	BUD *AFTER* Removal from Refrigeration
Alprostadil ***(Prostin VR®)***[90]	120 days
Alprostadil ***(Caverject®) (40 mcg/mL vial; Lyophilized Powder)***[74,84]	3 months
Alteplase ***(CathFlo)***[64]	4 months
Ascorbic Acid ***(Ascor®)***[83]	10 days
Atracurium ***(Tracrium™)***[64]	14 days
Bacitracin[65]	14 days
Belimumab ***(Benlysta®)***[93]	21 days [PFL]
Botulinum Toxin[64]	5 days
Bupivacaine Liposome ***(Exparel®)***[71]	30 days [DNR]
Calcitonin ***(Miacalcin®)***[64]	14 days
Carbaprost Tromethamine ***(Hemabate®)***[87]	15 days
Cisatracurium ***(Nimbex®)***[64,75]	21 days [PFL]
Clevidipine ***(Cleviprex®)***[67]	60 days [PFL, DNR]
Dacarbazine ***(DTIC-Dome®)***[64]	3 months
Daptomycin ***(Cubicin®)***[64]	1 year
Darbepoetin Alfa ***(Aranesp®)***[64]	7 days
Desmopressin[84]	21 days
Digoxin Immune fab (Ovine) ***(Digibind®)***[64]	30 days
Diltiazem[72,73]	1 month [DNR]
Diphtheria, Tetanus Toxoids & Acellular Pertussis Vaccine ***(Infanrix®)***[101]	7 days
Diphtheria, Tetanus Toxoids, Acellular Pertussis, Hepatitis B (Recombinant) & Inactivated Poliovirus Vaccine ***(Pediarix®)***[105]	72 hours
Diphtheria, Tetanus Toxoids, Acellular Pertussis & Inactivated Poliovirus Vaccine ***(Kinrix®)***[102]	72 hours
Diphtheria, Tetanus Toxoids, Acellular Pertussis, Inactivated Poliovirus and Haemophilus B Conjugate (Tetanus Toxoid Conjugate) Vaccine Kit ***(Pentacel®)***[123]	≤72 hours [CM] (>8° – ≤25°C)
Epoetin Alfa ***(Procrit®) (multi-dose vial)***[64,84]	7 days
Epoetin Alfa ***(Procrit®) (single-dose vial)***[64,84]	14 days
Epoetin Alfa ***(RETACRIT™)***[91]	30 days
Eptifibatide ***(Integrilin®)***[64]	60 days
Estrogens, Conjugated ***(Premarin® Intravenous)***[88]	1,095 days
Etanercept ***(Enbrel®)***[64]	7 days
Etanercept ***(Enbrel®) (prefilled syringe)***[64]	4 days
Exenatide ***(Byetta®) (vial or prefilled syringe)***[84]	30 days
Famotidine ***(Pepcid®)***[64]	90 days
Filgrastim ***(Neupogen®) (vial or prefilled syringe)***[64]	7 days
Fosphenytoin Sodium ***(Cerebyx®)***[64]	48 hours

TABLE 6: Temperature Excursion Stability Data for Refrigerated Intact Vials Stored at Room Temperature (cont'd)

Medication	BUD *AFTER* Removal from Refrigeration
Gemcitabine[86]	30 days
Glatiramer Acetate ***(Copaxone®)***[84,110]	1 month
Haemophilus B Conjugate Vaccine (Tetanus Toxoid Conjugate) ***(Hiberix®) (Lyophilized Powder)***[100]	7 days
Hepatitis A Vaccine ***(Havrix®)***[99]	72 hours
Hepatitis A Vaccine ***(VAQTA®)***[64]	1 year
Hepatitis A & Hepatitis B Vaccine (Recombinant) ***(Twinrix®)***[107]	7 days
Hepatitis B Vaccine (Recombinant) ***(Engerix-B®)***[96]	7 days
Hepatitis B Vaccine (Recombinant) ***(Recombivax HB®)***[124]	72 hours
Human Papillomavirus 9-valent Vaccine ***(Gardasil®)***[108]	130 months
Hyaluronic Acid ***(Healon)***[64]	14 days
Hyaluronidase (Recombinant) ***(Hylenex®)***[109]	1 year
Influenza Vaccine (Quadrivalent) ***(Fluarix® Quadrivalent)***[97]	72 hours
Influenza Vaccine (Quadrivalent) ***(FluLaval® Quadrivalent)***[98]	72 hours
Influenza Vaccine (Quadrivalent), Live ***(FluMist® Quadrivalent)***[112]	12 hours [SE]
Insulin, Aspart (U-100) ***(Novolog®) (vial or prefilled syringe)***[130]	28 days
Insulin, Aspart Protamine and Insulin, Aspart (U-100) ***(Novolog® Mix 70/30) (vial)***[142]	28 days [PFL]
Insulin, Aspart Protamine and Insulin, Aspart (U-100) ***(Novolog® Mix 70/30) (prefilled syringe)***[142]	14 days [PFL]
Insulin, Degludec (U-100 or U-200) ***(Tresiba®) (vial or prefilled syringe)***[125]	8 weeks [PFL]
Insulin, Detemir (U-100) ***(Levemir®) (vial or prefilled syringe)***[137]	6 weeks [PFL]
Insulin, Glargine (U-100) ***(Lantus®) (vial or prefilled syringe)***[136]	28 days [PFL]
Insulin, Glargine (U-300) ***(Toujeo®) (prefilled syringe)***[143]	8 weeks [PFL]
Insulin, Glulisine (U-100) ***(Apidra®) (vial or prefilled syringe)***[131]	28 days
Insulin, Isophane (U-100) ***(Humulin® N) (vial)***[135]	31 days [PFL]
Insulin, Isophane (U-100) ***(Humulin® N) (prefilled syringe)***[135]	14 days [PFL]
Insulin, Isophane (U-100) ***(Novolin® N) (vial)***[140]	6 weeks
Insulin, Isophane (U-100) ***(Novolin® N) (prefilled syringe)***[140]	28 days
Insulin, Isophane and Insulin, Regular (U-100) ***(Humulin® 70/30) (vial)***[134]	31 days [PFL]
Insulin, Isophane and Insulin, Regular (U-100) ***(Humulin® 70/30) (prefilled syringe)***[134]	10 days [PFL]
Insulin, Isophane and Insulin, Regular (U-100) ***(Novolin® 70/30) (vial)***[139]	6 weeks
Insulin, Isophane and Insulin, Regular (U-100) ***(Novolin® 70/30) (prefilled syringe)***[139]	28 days
Insulin, Lispro-aabc (U-100 or U-200) ***(Lyumjev™) (vial or prefilled syringe)***[138]	28 days
Insulin, Lispro Protamine and Insulin, Lispro (U-100) ***(Humalog® Mix) (vial)***[132,133]	28 days [PFL]
Insulin, Lispro Protamine and Insulin, Lispro (U-100) ***(Humalog® Mix) (prefilled syringe)***[132,133]	10 days [PFL]
Insulin, Regular (U-100) ***(Humulin® R) (vial)***[69]	31 days
Insulin, Regular (U-100) ***(Novolin® R) (vial)***[141]	6 weeks [PFL]
Insulin, Regular (U-100) ***(Novolin® R) (prefilled syringe)***[141]	28 days [PFL]
Insulin, Regular (U-500) ***(Humulin® R U-500) (vial)***[129]	40 days
Insulin, Regular (U-500) ***(Humulin® R U-500) (prefilled syringe)***[129]	28 days
Interferon Beta-1a ***(Avonex®) (vial) (Lyophilized Powder)***[84]	30 days
Interferon Beta-1a ***(Avonex®) (prefilled syringe)***[84]	7 days
Interferon Beta-1a ***(Rebif®) (prefilled syringe)***[84]	30 days
Interferon Gamma-1b ***(Actimmune®)***[84]	12 hours [CM, DNR]
Japanese Encephalitis Inactivated, Adsorbed ***(IXIARO®)***[126]	72 hours

TABLE 6: Temperature Excursion Stability Data for Refrigerated Intact Vials Stored at Room Temperature (cont'd)

Medication	BUD *AFTER* Removal from Refrigeration
Lorazepam[82]	90 days
Meningococcal Groups A, C, Y and W-135 Oligosaccharide Diphtheria CRM_{197} Conjugate Vaccine ***(Menveo®) (Lyophilized Powder)***[103]	2 years
Meningococcal Group B Vaccine ***(Bexsero®)***[94]	48 hours
Meningococcal Group B Vaccine ***(TRUMENBA®)***[92]	7 days
Mepolizumab ***(Nucala®) (autoinjector or prefilled syringe)***[104]	30 days [PFL, CM]
Methylergonovine Maleate ***(Methergine®)***[64]	14 days
Octreotide[79]	14 days [PFL]
Palivizumab ***(Synagis®)***[64,84]	14 days
Pancuronium ***(Pavulon®)***[64,76]	6 months
Peg-interferon Alfa-2a ***(Pegasys®) (vial)***[64]	14 days
Penicillin G Benzathine, Penicillin G Procaine ***(BICILLIN® C-R)***[85]	180 days
Pneumococcal 13-Valent Conjugate Vaccine ***(PREVNAR® 13)***[89]	7 days
Pramlintide Acetate ***(Symlin®) (prefilled syringe)***[84]	30 days
Rabies Immune Globulin (Human) ***(KEDRAB®)***[111]	1 month
Rocuronium[64,77,78]	60 days
Succinylcholine[70,80,81,121]	90 days
Tetanus Toxoid, Reduced Diphtheria Toxoid & Acellular Pertussis Vaccine ***(Boostrix)***[95]	7 days
Vasopressin ***(Vasostrict®)***[68]	1 year
Zoster Vaccine (Recombinant, Adjuvanted) ***(Shingrix™) (Lyophilized Powder)***[106]	72 hours [PFL]

[PFL]Protect from Light, [SE] Single Excursion, [CM] Cumulative, [DNR] Do Not Return to Refrigeration

manufacturer's maximum recommended time for use after removal from the overwrap and storage.

Manufacturers of commercial intravenous solutions place a small amount of excess diluent into each container during the manufacturing process, referred to as *overfill.*

TABLE 7: Manufacturer Storage of Commercial IV Solution Containers after Removal from Protective Overwrap

Brand Name (Manufacturer)	Volume	Maximum Storage Time *(Room Temperature)*
LifeCare™ (HOS) and ADD-Vantage® (PF) PVC containers[66]	25 mL	21 d
	>25 mL	30 d
Viaflex™ (BA) PVC containers[66]	≤50 mL	15 d
	≥100 mL	30 d
	>250 mL	30 d
EXCEL® (BRN) Ethylene propylene copolymer[47]	250 mL	30 d

This overfill amount is required by USP Chapter <1151>, *Pharmaceutical Dosage Forms.* The specifically required volume of excess diluent is based on the labeled size of the solution container and the solution's properties (eg, mobile liquids, viscous liquids). A specifically required volume is noted for labeled container sizes of 0.5 mL, 1 mL, 2 mL, 5 mL, 10 mL, 20 mL, and 30 mL. For any solution with a labeled container size of ≥50 mL, the manufacturer is required to add an additional 2% for mobile liquids or 3% for viscous liquids to the container.[120] Overfill volume of a diluent solution container is essential to consider when preparing CSPs. Suppose the volume of overfill is not considered, and a large amount of drug solution is added to the diluent container. In that case, the final concentration of the CSP may not be the same as the concentration stated on the label. Generally, if the volume of a drug solution that needs to be added to a diluent container is ≥10% of the labeled container size, an equal amount of diluent should be removed from the container before injection of the drug. This "10% rule" helps to ensure that the concentration of the final CSP is as accurate as possible without requiring the exact amount of diluent to be physically measured and transferred to an empty container before injection of the drug. Table 8 provides overfill volumes for select manufacturers of intravenous solutions.

TABLE 8: Overfill Volumes of Commercial IV Solution Containers

Solution	Container Type	Container Size	Average / Target Fill	Fill Range, Minimum	Fill Range, Maximum
Baxter[127]					
Various	Viaflex™	25 mL	31 mL	28 mL	34 mL
		50 mL	58 mL	53 mL	63 mL
		100 mL	110 mL	105 mL	115 mL
		250 mL	275 mL	265 mL	285 mL
		500 mL	547.5 mL	530 mL	565 mL
		1,000 mL	1,050 mL	1,030 mL	1,070 mL
		2,000 mL	2,080 mL	2,055 mL	2,105 mL
B. Braun[46,63,147]					
NS	E3®	1,000 mL	1,027 mL	1,022 mL	1,032 mL
D5W; D10W; LR; ½NS; NS	Excel®	250 mL	270 mL	263 mL	276 mL
		500 mL	532 mL	523 mL	550 mL
		1,000 mL	1,058 mL	1,043 mL	1,088 mL
D5W; NS	PAB®	25 mL	29.5 mL	25.5 mL	33.5 mL
		50 mL	57 mL	53 mL	61 mL
		100 mL	109 mL	105 mL	113 mL
Fresenius Kabi[128]					
D5W	Freeflex®	100 mL	114.5 mL	108 mL	121 mL
		250 mL	270 mL	264 mL	277 mL
		500 mL	529 mL	522 mL	535 mL
		1,000 mL	1,030 mL	1,024 mL	1,035 mL
D10W	Freeflex®	250 mL	-	260 mL	272 mL
		500 mL	-	519 mL	535 mL
		1,000 mL	-	1,023 mL	1,041 mL
LR	Freeflex®	250 mL	270 mL	264 mL	277 mL
		500 mL	529 mL	522 mL	535 mL
		1,000 mL	-	1,024 mL	1,037 mL
½NS; NS	Freeflex®	50 mL	-	57 mL	64 mL
		100 mL	114.5 mL	108 mL	121 mL
		250 mL	-	260 mL	272 mL
		500 mL	-	519 mL	535 mL
		1,000 mL	-	1,023 mL	1,041 mL
ICU Medical[122]					
D5W; NS	Small volume flexible containers	25 mL	29 mL	26 mL	32 mL
D5W; ½NS; NS		50 mL	56 mL	52 mL	62 mL
D5W	Large volume flexible containers	100 mL	107 mL	102 mL	112 mL
½NS; NS		100 mL	107 mL	103 mL	113 mL
D5W; NS		150 mL	175 mL	160 mL	200 mL
D5W; D5¼NS; D5½NS; D10W; M20; LR; ½NS; NS		250 mL	280 mL	260 mL	300 mL
		500 mL	540 mL	520 mL	560 mL
D5⅓NS; D5NS		500 mL	540 mL	520 mL	560 mL
D5W; D5¼NS; D5⅓NS; D5½NS; D5NS; D10W; LR; ½NS; NS; SWFI		1,000 mL	1,040 mL	1,025 mL	1,055 mL
D5W; NS	VisIV™	50 mL	59 mL	56 mL	62 mL
		100 mL	111 mL	107 mL	115 mL
D5W; ½NS; NS		250 mL	272 mL	268 mL	276 mL

TABLE 9: Beyond-Use Dates for Point-of-Care Activated Devices after Assembly

Device	Manufacturer	BUD	Products
ADD-Vantage™	Pfizer	30 d from date diluent removed from overwrap	50 and 100 mL containers[31]
Mini-Bag Plus™	Baxter	15 d from date diluent removed from overwrap	50 and 100 mL containers[31]
		30 d from date diluent removed from overwrap	100 mL containers attached to the following: • Aztreonam 1 gm • Cefazolin 1gm • Ceftriaxone 1 gm • Cefuroxime 750 mg • Piperacillin and tazobactam 3.375 gm
Add-EASE™	Braun	70 d	When connected to 50 or 100 mL PAB® containers[47]
		30 d	When connected to Excel® 250 mL containers[46,47]

Vial-Bag Connectors

Specialized point-of-care activated devices and containers allow for the connection of a vial of medication to a small volume infusion container. Generally, the connection of the vial to the bag is made under aseptic conditions. The actual mixing of the medication with the IV fluid (activation) takes place immediately prior to administration. The bags with attached vials may be stored prior to administration in automated dispensing cabinets or alternate sites to expedite patient access. The pharmacy must consider the specific device manufacturer's guidelines for storage of connected but not activated devices. Table 9 summarizes the manufacturers' BUDs for these devices after assembly in ISO Class 5 PECs and prior to activation.

VASCULAR ACCESS DEVICES AND CATHETERS USED IN MEDICATION ADMINISTRATION

Vascular access devices are flexible catheters inserted into a vein to deliver infusion therapy. Selection criteria for the type of vascular access device (VAD) used should incorporate the length of infusion therapy and physical properties of the medication. The most common types of VADs are peripheral catheter, midline catheter, peripherally inserted central catheter (PICC), central venous catheter (CVC), and implanted port.[38] See Figure 1: Common Types of Vascular Access Devices.

Peripheral catheters are usually 1-1.5 inches in length, with the tip terminating in a peripheral vein. This type of catheter should not be used for continuous infusions of vesicants, parenteral nutrition, or infusates >900 mOsm/L. The anticipated duration of therapy is generally less than 6 days when using a peripheral catheter.[38]

Midline catheters are longer than peripheral catheters, measuring 3-8 inches, with the tip terminating in veins located between the elbow and shoulder.[38] It is inserted similar to a *peripherally inserted central catheter* (PICC) yet terminates in the periphery. Since it is not a central venous catheter, it does not lead to central line-associated bloodstream infections (CLABSI). Hospitals may turn to midlines to avoid CLABSI and related financial penalties.[39] Midline catheter duration of therapy is typically 1 to 4 weeks.[38] This type of catheter is an alternative to PICCs for certain indications, expected length of infusion therapy, and intravenous solutions appropriate for administration into the peripheral vasculature.[39]

The utilization of midlines is increasing in hospitals to improve the rate of appropriate use of PICCs and traditional *central venous catheters* (CVCs). Studies show that midlines are suited for short-term therapy over 6-14 days.[39,40] Properties of the infusion solution should be within the parameters appropriate for peripheral catheters, particularly the osmolarity, irritant, and vesicant characteristics. Each CSP should be assessed for its irritant or vesicant properties prior to administration into the peripheral vasculature, paying attention to excipients added to medications, and verifying the solution is well tolerated by peripheral veins.[38]

A *central venous access device* (CVAD) is a catheter whose tip terminates in the lower segment of the superior vena cava. CVADs may be utilized for the administration of any type of infusion therapy. The large diameter and high blood flow of the superior vena cava permit administration of medications with high osmolality, concentration and/or viscosity, parenteral nutrition, chemotherapy, blood products, and medications with vesicant properties. CVADs may be valved or open-ended. Valved catheters are designed to maintain line patency without the use of an anticoagulant flush.

There are two basic types of CVADs, tunneled and non-tunneled.

FIGURE 1: Common Types of Vascular Access Devices (VADs)

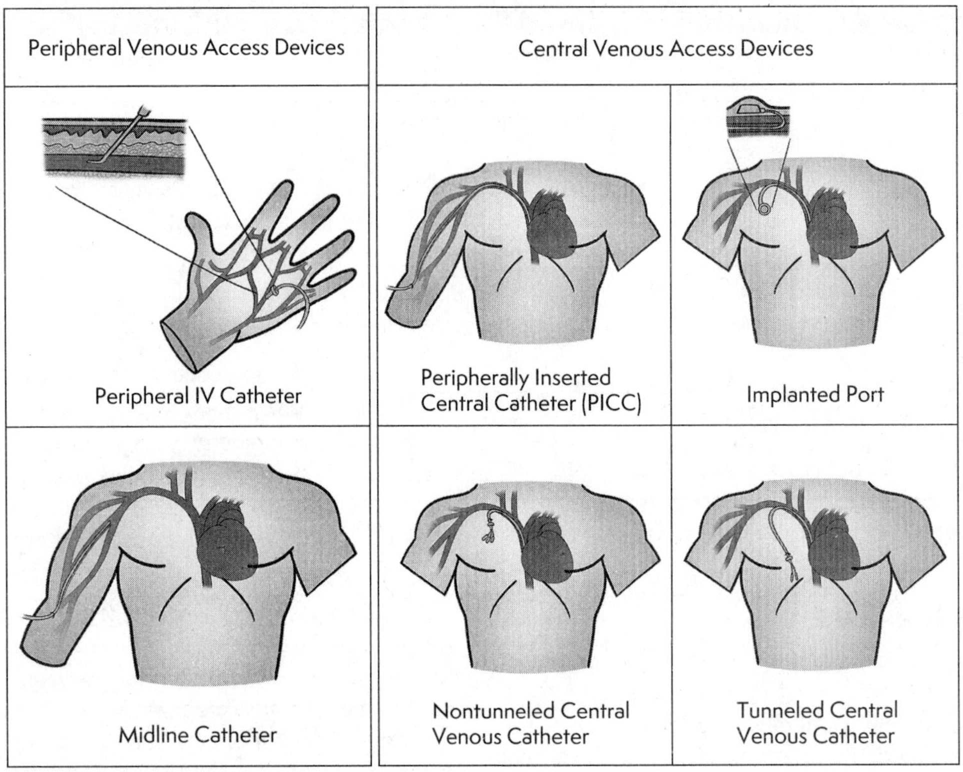

Tunneled CVADs are anchored by tunneling in tissue prior to the insertion into the large blood vessel. They are generally used for permanent or long-term venous access.

- An implanted port is a type of tunneled CVAD that is implanted under skin and tissue with no portion of the catheter externally exposed. Ports must be accessed using a special non-coring needle.

Non-tunneled CVADs are placed via a percutaneous stick into the blood vessel and advanced within the blood vessel. They are not permanently placed.

A PICC is a type of non-tunneled CVAD that is inserted in the antecubital space into the basilic, brachial, or cephalic veins and advanced within the blood vessel to achieve central placement.

Vascular Access Device Complications VAD complications related to the drug concentration, osmolality, and direct contact of irritants include:

- *Infiltration* (leakage of infusate into tissue surrounding a vascular access device) can occur when the VAD tip no longer resides in the blood vessel.
- *Extravasation* (infiltration of vesicant or irritating agents into tissue surrounding a vascular access device) can result in tissue and/or nerve damage.
- *Chemical phlebitis* is an inflammation of the inside of the blood vessel caused by direct contact with an irritant infusate.
- *Catheter occlusion* can cause a complete or partial blockage of the VAD due to incompatibility, resulting in a precipitant in the line.

VASCULAR ACCESS DEVICE FLUSHING AND LOCKING

Flushing with sodium chloride 0.9% (NS) is performed to assess catheter function prior to each infusion and again after each infusion to clear any residual medication from the catheter lumen. Locking of the catheter is a final step to prevent occlusion or infection. Often the two terms are used interchangeably when they are not equal in function and purpose. Nursing standards define the *volume of a flush* as an amount sufficient to clear the medication from the lumen and lock as the minimum volume equal to the internal volume of the catheter and any add-on devices, plus 20%. The catheter lumen volume and add-on devices plus 20% for peripheral and midline catheters are in the range of 1-1.5 mL, and for PICCs and other CVCs, are in the range of 1.5-2.5 mL.[41] These volumes are smaller than the generalized guidance from the nursing standards to administer flushing and locking solutions of 5 mL for

TABLE 10: Vascular Access Device Lumen Volumes[44]

Catheter Type	Lumen Volume
Peripheral catheter	0.03 mL
Midline catheter	0.4 mL
CVAD (4F SL)	0.6 mL
PICC (4F SL)	0.7 mL
Tunneled (small bore)	0.7 mL
Tunneled (large bore)	1.5 mL
Port	1.3 mL

peripheral catheters and 10 mL for central catheters.[38] Flushing with unmedicated NS uses a larger volume for the purpose of clearing the catheter. Considerations for specific flush volumes include the size of the catheter and the type of infusion solution. Viscous solutions, parenteral nutrition, or blood products require a larger volume to remove all of the residual drug.[38,42] When studied with protein-based medication administration, 10 mL of flush did not remove all the proteins from the lumen walls of the catheter, suggesting a larger volume of NS flush for clearing protein-based medications. The method of flushing using a pulsatile push/pause was better at catheter clearance than a single bolus flush.[41,43]

Locking of the VAD using a medicated flush solution is performed to prevent occlusion, maintain patency, and reduce infection risk.[43] Heparin is the most common choice for a catheter lock. It should be administered as a final step after flushing and instilled at the lowest dose for the indication. Based on the internal catheter volume plus add-on device estimations, even though 5-10 mL may be ordered, 50% to 90% of the dose is administered into the patient, and only a small amount remains in the catheter.[44] For information on VAD lumen volumes, refer to Table 10. If the patient is using an antibiotic or ethanol lock, smaller volumes ordered may reflect the internal lumen volume plus a small amount of overfill to account for spillage into the system.

If heparin is contraindicated as a catheter locking medication, there is an option for sodium citrate 4% solution, which had similar efficacy to heparin and fewer incidences of CLABSI.[43] Studies have indicated that sodium chloride 0.9% may be used as a primary agent for maintaining the patency of peripheral catheters in the acute care setting.[61] If locking of the catheter is not feasible, elastomeric infusion devices are available to administer a continuous slow rate of sodium chloride 0.9% to maintain catheter patency in neonates and patients in alternate sites of care.[45,61]

INFUSATE PROPERTIES

Osmolarity is an additive figure for all of the chemical ingredients of a solution, including the diluent. A central VAD is used to administer solutions with high osmolarity (>900 mOsm/L).[38]

ETHANOL AND ANTIBIOTIC LOCK THERAPY

Catheter-related bloodstream infections (CRBSI) and central line-associated bloodstream infections (CLABSI) are complications associated with vascular access devices. Best practice for the management of these infections includes adequate source control (eg, line removal); however, ethanol lock therapy (ELT) and antibiotic lock therapy (ALT) are increasingly used to prevent or manage CRBSIs and CLABSIs. Guidelines recommend line lock therapy for intravenous catheter salvage therapy (Grade B-II recommendation) where line replacement or removal is not feasible.[48] Practitioners must consider the pathogen(s) of interest, available stability data of lock solutions, and catheter compatibility information when utilizing these specialized forms of access device care.[49] The preferred solution and concentration of ELT and ALT have yet to be defined.

Line Lock Therapy Considerations

There are many aspects to consider when selecting a line lock therapy solution, including the antimicrobial spectrum of activity, patient allergies, catheter compatibility, the addition of an anticoagulant, the concentration of the solution, the volume of the solution, dwell time, and the duration of therapy.

The Infectious Diseases Society of America (IDSA) guidelines recommend ELT should be limited to prevention of CRBSIs and CLABSIs[48]; however, additional literature is available describing the use of ELT for treatment.[50-53] Central venous catheter (CVC) removal or replacement is preferred if *Staphylococcus* aureus or Candida *spp.* are isolated.[48] Antifungal lock therapy has been described in the literature for extenuating circumstances, but line removal remains the preferred management in this setting.[54,55]

TABLE 11: Osmolarity and pH of Commercial Infusion Solutions

Solution	Osmolarity (mOsm/L)	pH
Sterile Water for Injection, USP	0	5.5 (5.0-7.0)
Dextrose 5% in Water	252 (calculated)	4.3 (3.2-6.5)
Sodium Chloride 0.9%	308 (calculated)	5.6 (4.5-7.0)
Sodium Chloride 0.45%	154 (calculated)	5.6 (4.5-7.0)
Dextrose 10% in Water	505 (calculated)	4.3 (3.2-6.5)
Dextrose 5% in Lactated Ringers	530 (calculated)	5.0 (4.5-6.0)

Source: accessdata.fda.gov. and dailymed.nlm.nih.gov. Accessed February 2021.

ALT includes a high concentration of antibiotic, usually at least 1,000-times higher than the pathogen minimum inhibitory concentration, as a means to penetrate or disrupt biofilms and eradicate or prevent the growth of bacteria.[48,49] Although the concentration of antibiotic is high at the site of action within the catheter lumen, the concentration of the CSP compounded into a syringe may be low compared to systemic dosages. Extrapolation of concentrations shown in medication monographs may not be applicable to concentrations compounded for ALT. Antibiotic selection for ALT should include an agent with activity against the pathogen(s) of concern and an agent with minimal toxicity concern for the patient (including allergies). Products prepared for lock therapy should be clearly labeled "for line lock therapy" to decrease the risk of inadvertent systemic administration.

Many studies have assessed the stability of various concentrations and drug combinations, but standard recommendations have yet to be defined. ALT and ELT solutions that dwell in the line may be exposed to varying temperatures, including body temperature. When determining BUDs for line lock therapies, professional judgment should be utilized when analyzing stability data of an available product.

Dwell time is the time the ELT or ALT solution sits in the CVC line and lumen. Studies suggest a minimum of 8 hours[49] and should not exceed 48 hours for most scenarios.[48] Dwell time is dependent upon the administration schedule of concomitantly prescribed intravenous medications and available intravenous access. For hemodialysis catheters, ALT dwell time is commonly defined by the time between hemodialysis sessions.

Determining Volume of Line Lock Therapy Solution

Determining the volume of line lock solution can pose a challenge. While there are standard volumes of CVC, patient-specific catheters may be manipulated during placement on a case-by-case basis (eg, lines may need to be shortened, thus decreasing volume for locking). If the volume of a line lumen is unknown, the following procedure can be utilized to determine the volume; this process should be completed for each lumen of the CVC.[56]

1. Prepare the cap of the catheter using aseptic technique.
2. Flush the lumen with 5-10 mL of normal saline.
3. Attach a syringe to the lumen cap and draw back until the blood returns to the inlet of the syringe. The volume in the syringe at this point is the final volume.
4. Re-flush the catheter lumen with 5-10 mL of normal saline.

Most CVCs have multiple lumens, and coordination of locking therapy and administration of intravenous medications/fluids should be completed on a patient-specific basis. If patients do not have alternative intravenous access, coordination with scheduled intravenous medication(s) or fluid administrations should be analyzed. Utilizing separate orders for each lumen to be locked is considered best practice—orders should note the lumen color to be locked for differentiation and include the specific volume of that lumen (lumen volumes on the same line may differ).

SUMMARY

Pharmacists are responsible for dispensing CSPs that meet patients' unique clinical needs while satisfying all quality, safety, and environmental control requirements set by legislative, regulatory, and accreditation bodies. They direct and evaluate all phases of preparation, storage, transportation, and administration of CSPs and maintain compliance with established standards, regulations, professional guidance, and best practices.

REFERENCES

1. USP <797> Pharmaceutical compounding - sterile preparations. In: *2020: USP Compounding Compendium*. Rockville, MD: The United States Pharmacopeial Convention; 2020:40-74.
2. USP <1191> Stability considerations in dispensing practice. In: *2020: USP Compounding Compendium*. Rockville, MD: The United States Pharmacopeial Convention; 2020:435-9.
3. Bing CD. Applying stability and sterility limits to beyond use dating. *Infusion*. 2017; 23(4):39-44.
4. Sacha GA, Saffell-Clemmer W, Abram K, et al. Practical fundamentals of glass, rubber, and plastic sterile packaging systems. *Pharm Dev Technol*. 2010; 15(1):6-34.
5. Tokhadze N, Chennell P, Bernard L, et al. Impact of alternative materials to plasticized PVC infusion tubings on drug sorption and plasticizer release. *Sci Rep*. 2019; 9(1):18917.
6. Le Basle Y, Chennell P, Tokhadze N, et al. Physicochemical stability of monoclonal antibodies: a review. *J Pharm Sci*. 2020; 109(1):169-90.
7. The United States Pharmacopeial Convention. *USP Compounding Standards and Beyond-Use Dates (BUDs) Fact Sheet*; 2019. https://www.usp.org/sites/default/files/usp/document/our-work/compounding/usp-bud-factsheet.pdf (accessed 2020 June).
8. Bing CD. Storage and beyond-use dating. In: Buchanan EC, Schneider PJ, Forrey RA eds. *Compounding Sterile Preparations*. 4th ed. Bethesda, MD: American Society of Health-System Pharmacists; 2017:213-26.
9. *SMARTeZ® - Stability Data for Drugs Using Elastomeric Infusion Pumps*, 2020. Fenton, MO: Progressive Medical, Inc.; Updated May 2020.
10. Favier M, De Cazanove F, Coste A, et al. Stability of carmustine in polyvinyl chloride bags and polyethylene-lined trilayer plastic containers. *Am J Health Syst Pharm*. 2001; 58(3):238-41.
11. *Pharmaceutical report on chemical and physical stability of drugs commonly used with CADD® infusion pumps (IN193109GB-122019)*, 2019. Minneapolis, MN: Smiths Medical ASD, Inc.; Updated December 2019.
12. Trissel LA, Xu QA, Baker M. Drug compatibility with new polyolefin infusion solution containers. *Am J Health Syst Pharm*. 2006; 63(23):2379-82.

13. Cheung JK, Sharma M, Dabbara A, et al. The effect of formulation excipients on leachables for IV-administered products. *Pharmaceutical Outsourcing*. 2012;13.
14. Balet A, Cardona D, Jane S, et al. Effects of multilayered bags vs ethylvinyl-acetate bags on oxidation of parenteral nutrition. *JPEN J Parenter Enteral Nutr*. 2004; 28(2):85-91.
15. Li M, Coursol C, Leclair G. Stability of cyclosporine diluted with 0.9% sodium chloride injection or 5% dextrose injection and stored in ethylene-vinyl acetate containers. *Am J Health Syst Pharm*. 2013; 70(22):1970-2.
16. Ecoflac® Plus IV Container - Compatibility Check. https://www.bbraun.co.uk/en/products-and-therapies/infusion-therapy/ecoflac–plus/compatibility-check.html (accessed 2020 July).
17. Shrewsbury RP. Sterile compounded preparations: types of preparations and devices. *Applied Pharmaceutics in Contemporary Compounding*. 4th ed. Englewood: Morton Publishing; 2020:337-57.
18. Baxter Healthcare Corporation. A Comprehensive Portfolio of Parenteral Solutions (USMP/MG1/13-0127(1)). Round Lake, IL; 2015.
19. 0.9% Sodium Chloride Injection, USP in FreeFlex® Bag [package insert]. Lake Zurich, IL: Fresenius Kabi; August 2016.
20. Akers MJ. Sterile products packaging chemistry. In: Swarbrick J ed. *Sterile Drug Products: Formulation, Packaging, Manufacturing, and Quality*. New York: Informa Healthcare; 2010:86-88.
21. Sodium Chloride Injection, USP in VIAFLO® Plastic Container [package insert]. Deerfield, IL: Baxter Healthcare Corporation; May 2015.
22. NEXCEL® Primary Medical Films: Product Overview. https://www.sealedair.com/products/medical-packaging/medical-films (accessed 2020 August).
23. Product Catalog: EXACTAMIX® Empty EVA Bag - Product Description. https://ecatalog.baxter.com/ecatalog/loadproduct.html?pid=822737&cid=20016&lid=10001&hid=20001 (accessed 2020 August).
24. Product Catalog: Baxa® EVA Multilayer TPN Bags - Product Description. https://ecatalog.baxter.com/ecatalog/loadproduct.html?cid=10001&lid=10011&hid=10000&pid=626435 (accessed 2020 August).
25. EcoFLX™ DME Empty Mixing Containers - Product Information. https://douglasmedicalproducts.com/ecoflx/ (accessed 2020 August).
26. EcoFLX™ DMP Empty Mixing Containers - Product Information. https://douglasmedicalproducts.com/ecoflx/ (accessed 2020 August).
27. Technoflex: Inerta® Flexible Bags - Product Description. https://www.cphi-online.com/inerta-flexible-bags-guaranteeing-drug-prod1234586.html (accessed 2020 August).
28. Sodium Chloride Grifols 0.9% w/v Solution for Infusion in Fleboflex Container [package insert]. Barcelona, Spain: Laboratorios Grifols, S.A.; May 2017.
29. IntraCon IV Containers - Product Description. https://www.medicopack.com/iv-containers#:~:text=Our%20IntraCon%20IV%20containers%20%E2%80%93%20the,-Seal%20(FFS)%20IV%20bags (accessed 2020 August).
30. MedexSupply. Catalog - Description of the Hospira Worldwide Lifecare IV Bag PVC 250mL Sterile Latex Disposable Empty/Flexible (accessed 2021 March).
31. American Society of Health-System Pharmacists. ASHP guidelines on compounding sterile preparations. *Am J Health Syst Pharm.* 2014; 71(2):145-66.
32. USP <1207> Package integrity evaluation - sterile products. In: *2020: USP Compounding Compendium*. Rockville, MD: The United States Pharmacopeial Convention; 2020:459-65.
33. Makwana S, Basu B, Makasana Y, et al. Prefilled syringes: an innovation in parenteral packaging. *Int J Pharm Investig*. 2011; 1(4):200-6.
34. Institute for Safe Medication Practices (ISMP). *ISMP Safe Practice Guidelines for Adult IV Push Medications*. https://www.ismp.org/sites/default/files/attachments/2017-11/ISMP97-Guidelines-071415-3.%20FINAL.pdf (accessed 2021 March).
35. BPS Board of Pharmacy Specialties. Board Certified Sterile Compounding Pharmacist, BCSCP. https://www.bpsweb.org/bps-specialties/compounded-sterile-preparations-pharmacy/ (accessed 2021 February).
36. Petroff B, Johnson C. ASHP guidelines on evaluating and using home or alternate-site infusion service providers. *Am J Health Syst Pharm*. 2016;73(12):922-6.
37. Centers of Medicare & Medicaid Services. S&C: 16-01-Hospital: Revised Hospital Guidance for Pharmaceutical Services and Expanded Guidance Related to Compounding of Medications. https://www.cms.gov/Medicare/Provider-Enrollment-and-Certification/SurveyCertificationGenInfo/Downloads/Survey-and-Cert-Letter-16-01.pdf (accessed 2021 March).
38. Gorski L, Hadaway L, Hagle ME, et al. Infusion therapy standards of practice. *J Infus Nurs.* 2016; 39(1S):S1-159.
39. Chopra V, Kaatz S, Swaminathan L, et al. Variation in use and outcomes related to midline catheters: results from a multicentre pilot study. *BMJ Qual Saf*. 2019; 28(9):714-20.
40. Chopra V, Flanders SA, Saint S, et al. The Michigan Appropriateness Guide for Intravenous Catheters (MAGIC): results from a multispecialty panel using the RAND/UCLA appropriateness method. *Ann Intern Med*. 2015; 163(6 Suppl):S1-40.
41. Guiffant G, Durussel JJ, Merckx J, et al. Flushing of intravascular access devices (IVADs) - efficacy of pulsed and continuous infusions. *J Vasc Access*. 2012; 13(1):75-8.
42. Bard Access Systems. Instructions for Use: BardPort, SlimPort, X-Port (Implantable Ports). Salt Lake City, UT: C.R. Bard, Inc; 2012:24.
43. Siegel M, Arlistico A. Vascular access: maintaining patency and reducing infection risk. *Infusion*. 2019; 25(5):36-46.
44. Goossens GA. Flushing and locking of venous catheters: available evidence and evidence deficit. *Nurs Res Pract.* 2015; 2015: 985686.
45. Heath J, Jones S. Utilization of an elastomeric continuous infusion device to maintain catheter patency. *J Intraven Nurs*. 2001; 24(2):102-6.
46. B. Braun. Product Information: EXCEL® IV Container FAQ. Bethlehem, PA: B. Braun Medical Inc; 2018:4.
47. Storage of Assembled addEASE Binary Connectors Medication Information Letter (Ref#: CKL-3376) [personal communication]. Bethlehem, PA: B. Braun Medical Inc.; 2020:2.
48. Mermel LA, Allon M, Bouza E, et al. Clinical practice guidelines for the diagnosis and management of intravascular catheter-related infection: 2009 Update by the Infectious Diseases Society of America. *Clin Infect Dis*. 2009; 49(1):1-45.
49. Justo JA, Bookstaver PB. Antibiotic lock therapy: review of technique and logistical challenges. *Infect Drug Resist*. 2014; 7:343-63.
50. Tan M, Lau J, Guglielmo BJ. Ethanol locks in the prevention and treatment of catheter-related bloodstream infections. *Ann Pharmacother*. 2014; 48(5):607-15.

51. Maiefski M, Rupp ME, Hermsen ED. Ethanol lock technique: review of the literature. *Infect Control Hosp Epidemiol.* 2009; 30(11):1096-108. Erratum in: *Infect Control Hosp Epidemiol.* 2010; 31(2):202.
52. Wolf J, Connell TG, Allison KJ, et al. Treatment and secondary prophylaxis with ethanol lock therapy for central line-associated bloodstream infection in paediatric cancer: a randomised, double-blind, controlled trial. *Lancet Infect Dis.* 2018; 18(8):854-63.
53. Kubiak DW, Gilmore ET, Buckley MW, et al. Adjunctive management of central line-associated bloodstream infections with 70% ethanol-lock therapy. *J Antimicrob Chemother.* 2014; 69(6):1665-8.
54. Walraven CJ, Lee SA. Antifungal lock therapy. *Antimicrob Agents Chemother.* 2013;57(1):1-8.
55. McGhee W, Michaels MG, Martin JM, et al. Antifungal lock therapy with liposomal amphotericin B: a prospective trial. *J Pediatric Infect Dis Soc.* 2016; 5(1):80-4.
56. Zembles TN, Flannery LS, Huppler AR. Development and implementation of an antimicrobial lock therapy guideline in a pediatric hospital. *Am J Health Syst Pharm.* 2018; 75(5):299-303.
57. Accreditation Commission for Health Care. Items Needed for On-Site Survey: Customized for Pharmacy Compounding Accreditation Board (PCAB). https://www.achc.org/pdf/PCAB_Items_Needed.pdf (accessed 2021 March).
58. The United States Pharmacopeial Convention. United States Pharmacopeia Commentary, *USP 42-NF 37*, Second Supplement: Master Formulation Records and Compounding Records. Rockville, MD; 2019:159-63.
59. California State Board of Pharmacy. Tips for Preparing a Master Formula Document - California Code of Regulations, CCR 1735.2(e). https://www.pharmacy.ca.gov/publications/master_formula_tips.pdf (accessed 2021 February).
60. Institute for Safe Medication Practices (ISMP). *ISMP Guidelines for Safe Preparation of Compounded Sterile Preparations*; 2016. https://www.ismp.org/guidelines/sterile-compounding (accessed 2021 February).
61. Benner K, Lucas AJ. ASHP therapeutic position statement on the institutional use of 0.9% sodium chloride injection to maintain patency of peripheral indwelling intermittent infusion devices. *Am J Health Syst Pharm.* 2012; 69(14):1252-4.
62. Comparison of Ecoflac® Plus and EXCEL® Containers Medication Information Letter (Ref#: N/A) [personal communication]. Bethlehem, PA: B. Braun Medical Inc.; 2016:5.
63. B. Braun. Product Information: PAB® IV Container FAQ. Bethlehem, PA: B. Braun Medical Inc; 2016:2.
64. Cohen V, Jellinek SP, Teperikidis L, et al. Room-temperature storage of medications labeled for refrigeration. *Am J Health Syst Pharm.* 2007; 64(16):1711-5.
65. Pfizer Medical Information. Temperature Stability Calculator: Bacitracin. https://www.pfizermedicalinformation.com/en-us/stability-calculator (accessed 2020 December 7).
66. Troncone M, Rudnick E, Frisolone J. Expiration dates and removal of i.v. bag overwrap. *Am J Health Syst Pharm.* 1995; 52(17):1921.
67. Cleviprex® (Clevidipine) Injection [package insert]. Graz, Austria: Fresenius Kabi Austria GmbH; December 2019.
68. Vasostrict® (Vasopressin) Injection [package insert]. Chestnut Ridge, NY: Par Pharmaceutical, Inc.; April 2020.
69. Humulin® R (Insulin Human) Injection [package insert]. Indianapolis, IN: Eli Lilly and Company; March 2020.
70. Adnet F, Le Moyec L, Smith CE, et al. Stability of succinylcholine solutions stored at room temperature studied by nuclear magnetic resonance spectroscopy. *Emerg Med J.* 2007; 24(3):168-9.
71. Exparel® (Bupivacaine Liposome) Injection, Suspension [package insert]. San Diego, CA: Pacira Pharmaceuticals, Inc.; January 2021.
72. Diltiazem Hydrochloride Injection, Solution [package insert]. Eatontown, NJ: West-Ward Pharmaceuticals Corp.; December 2018.
73. Diltiazem Hydrochloride Injection, Solution [package insert]. Lake Forest, IL: Hospira, Inc.; December 2020.
74. Caverject® (Alprostadil) Injection [package insert]. New York, NY: Pharmacia and Upjohn Company LLC; March 2019.
75. Nimbex® (Cisatracurium Besylate) Injection [package insert]. North Chicago, IL: AbbVie Inc.; April 2020.
76. Pancuronium Bromide Injection [package insert]. Lake Forest, IL: Hospira, Inc.; January 2019.
77. Rocuronium Bromide Injection [package insert]. Rockford, IL: Mylan Institutional LLC; August 2018.
78. Rocuronium Bromide Injection [package insert]. Schaumburg, IL: Sagent Pharmaceuticals; February 2020.
79. Octreotide Acetate Injection [package insert]. Morgantown, WV: Mylan Institutional LLC; January 2021.
80. Roy JJ, Boismenu D, Mamer OA, et al. Room temperature stability of injectable succinylcholine dichloride. *Int J Pharm Compd.* 2008; 12(1):83-5.
81. Schmutz CW, Muhlebach SF. Stability of succinylcholine chloride injection. *Am J Hosp Pharm.* 1991; 48(3):501-6.
82. Jahns BE, Bakst CM. Extension of expiration time for lorazepam injection at room temperature. *Am J Hosp Pharm.* 1993; 50(6):1134.
83. Ascor® Medication Information Letter (Ref#: N/A) [personal communication]. Santa Ana, CA: McGuff Pharmaceuticals, Inc.; 2022:1.
84. Stability of refrigerated and frozen drugs. *Pharmacist's Letter/Prescriber's Letter.* 2008; 24(10):241001.
85. Pfizer Medical Information. Temperature Stability Calculator: BICILLIN® C-R. https://www.pfizermedicalinformation.com/en-us/stability-calculator (accessed 2020 December 7).
86. Pfizer Medical Information. Temperature Stability Calculator: Gemcitabine. https://www.pfizermedicalinformation.com/en-us/stability-calculator (accessed 2020 December 7).
87. Pfizer Medical Information. Temperature Stability Calculator: HEMABATE®. https://www.pfizermedicalinformation.com/en-us/stability-calculator (accessed 2020 December 7).
88. Pfizer Medical Information. Temperature Stability Calculator: PREMARIN® INTRAVENOUS. https://www.pfizermedicalinformation.com/en-us/stability-calculator (accessed 2020 December 7).
89. Pfizer Medical Information. Temperature Stability Calculator: PREVNAR® 13. https://www.pfizermedicalinformation.com/en-us/stability-calculator (accessed 2020 December 7).
90. Pfizer Medical Information. Temperature Stability Calculator: PROSTIN VR®. https://www.pfizermedicalinformation.com/en-us/stability-calculator (accessed 2020 December 7).
91. Pfizer Medical Information. Temperature Stability Calculator: RETACRIT™. https://www.pfizermedicalinformation.com/en-us/stability-calculator (accessed 2020 December 7).
92. Pfizer Medical Information. Temperature Stability Calculator: TRUMENBA®. https://www.pfizermedicalinformation.com/en-us/stability-calculator (accessed 2020 December 7).

93. GSK Medical Information. Stability of Intravenous Benlysta® Under Varying Storage Conditions. https://www.gskus-medicalaffairs.com/docviewer.html?cmd=GSKMedicalIn-formation&token=23108-b6d99299-80ea-40bc-99f2-989 32b3bde8c&dns=gsk-medcomms.veevavault.com&medcom-mid=MED–US-0880 (accessed 2020 December 7).

94. GSK Medical Information. Vaccine Temperature Stability Calculator: Bexsero®. https://www.gskusmedicalaffairs.com/stability-calculator.html# (accessed 2020 December 7).

95. GSK Medical Information. Vaccine Temperature Stability Calculator: Boostrix®. https://www.gskusmedicalaffairs.com/stability-calculator.html# (accessed 2020 December 7).

96. GSK Medical Information. Vaccine Temperature Stability Calculator: Engerix-B®. https://www.gskusmedicalaffairs.com/stability-calculator.html# (accessed 2020 December 7).

97. GSK Medical Information. Vaccine Temperature Stability Calculator: Fluarix® Quadrivalent. https://www.gskusmed-icalaffairs.com/stability-calculator.html# (accessed 2020 December 7).

98. GSK Medical Information. Vaccine Temperature Stability Calculator: FluLaval® Quadrivalent. https://www.gskusmed-icalaffairs.com/stability-calculator.html# (accessed 2020 December 7).

99. GSK Medical Information. Vaccine Temperature Stability Calculator: Havrix®. https://www.gskusmedicalaffairs.com/stability-calculator.html# (accessed 2020 December 7).

100. GSK Medical Information. Stability of Hiberix® When Stored Above Recommended Temperatures. https://www.gskusmedicalaffairs.com/docviewer .html?cmd=GSKMedicalInformation&token=23108-1645c1 8c-b5b5-4f78-8f01-b89d705e7e93&dns=gsk-medcomms.veevavault.com&medcommid=MED–US-1419 (accessed 2020 December 7).

101. GSK Medical Information. Vaccine Temperature Stability Calculator: Infanrix®. https://www.gskusmedicalaffairs.com/stability-calculator.html# (accessed 2020 December 7).

102. GSK Medical Information. Vaccine Temperature Stability Calculator: Kinrix®. https://www.gskusmedicalaffairs.com/stability-calculator.html# (accessed 2020 December 7).

103. Broker M, Cooper B, Detora LM, et al. Critical appraisal of a quadrivalent CRM(197) conjugate vaccine against meningo-coccal serogroups A, C W-135 and Y (Menveo) in the context of treatment and prevention of invasive disease. *Infect Drug Resist*. 2011; 4:137-47.

104. GSK Medical Information. Stability of the Auto-Injector and Pre-Filled Syringe for Nucala® Under Varying Storage Conditions. https://www.gskusmedicalaffairs.com/docviewer.html?cmd=GSKMedicalInformation&token=23108-6854ed 9b-2d9a-4055-99bf-48eb7bbbcb10&dns=gsk-medcomms.veevavault.com&medcommid=MED–US-4948 (accessed 2020 December 7).

105. GSK Medical Information. Vaccine Temperature Stability Calculator: Pediarix®. https://www.gskusmedicalaffairs.com/stability-calculator.html# (accessed 2020 December 7).

106. GSK Medical Information. Vaccine Temperature Stability Calculator: Shingrix™. https://www.gskusmedicalaffairs.com/stability-calculator.html# (accessed 2020 December 7).

107. GSK Medical Information. Vaccine Temperature Stability Calculator: Twinrix®. https://www.gskusmedicalaffairs.com/stability-calculator.html# (accessed 2020 December 7).

108. Shank-Retzlaff ML, Zhao Q, Anderson C, et al. Evaluation of the thermal stability of Gardasil. *Hum Vaccin*. 2006; 2(4):147-54.

109. King M, Convery C, Davies E. This month's guideline: the use of hyaluronidase in aesthetic practice (v2.4). *J Clin Aesthet Dermatol*. 2018; 11(6):E61-E68.

110. Copaxone® (Glatiramer Acetate) Injection [package insert]. Parsippany, NJ: Teva Neuroscience, Inc.; July 2020.

111. KEDRAB® (Rabies Immune Globulin, Human) Injection [package insert]. Fort Lee, NJ: Kedrion Biopharma Inc.; November 2017.

112. FluMist® Quadrivalent (Influenza Vaccine, Live) [package insert]. Gaithersburg, MD: MedImmune, LLC.; August 2020.

113. Food & Drug Administration (FDA). FDA notifies health care professionals that Becton-Dickerson replaced problematic rubber stoppers in its syringes. https://www.fda.gov/drugs/drug-safety-and-availability/fda-notifies-health-care-professionals-becton-dickinson-replaced-problematic-rubber-stoppers-its (accessed 2021 February).

114. USP <71> Sterility Tests. In: *2020: USP Compounding Compendium*. Rockville, MD: The United States Pharmacopeial Convention; 2020:195-202.

115. USP <659> Packaging and Storage Requirements. In: *2020: USP Compounding Compendium*. Rockville, MD: The United States Pharmacopeial Convention; 2020:226-31.

116. USP <800> Hazardous Drugs – Handling in Healthcare Settings. In: *2020: USP Compounding Compendium*. Rockville, MD: The United States Pharmacopeial Convention; 2020:74-92.

117. USP <1163> Quality Assurance in Pharmaceutical Compounding. In: *2020: USP Compounding Compendium*. Rockville, MD: The United States Pharmacopeial Convention; 2020:146-52.

118. The United States Pharmacopeial Convention. About USP. https://www.usp.org/about (accessed 2021 February).

119. Buchanan EC. Standards for compounding sterile prepa-rations. In: Buchanan EC, Schneider PJ, Forrey RA eds. *Compounding Sterile Preparations*. 4th ed. Bethesda, MD: American Society of Health-System Pharmacists; 2017:7-33.

120. USP <1151> Pharmaceutical dosage forms. In: *2020: USP Compounding Compendium*. Rockville, MD: The United States Pharmacopeial Convention; 2020:408-30.

121. Merlin MA, Marques-Baptista A, Yang H, et al. Evaluating degradation with fragment formation of prehospital succi-nylcholine by mass spectrometry. *Acad Emerg Med*. 2010; 17(6):631-7.

122. ICU Medical Overfill Medication Information Letter (Ref#: US2020-02838) [personal communication]. Lake Forest, IL: ICU Medical; 2020:4.

123. Pentacel® Injection Room Temperature Stability Information Response (Ref#: N/A) [personal communication]. 2021.

124. Recombivax HB® (Hepatitis B Vaccine, Recombinant) Injection [package insert]. Whitehouse Station, NJ: Merck Sharp & Dohme Corp.; February 2020.

125. Tresiba® (Insulin Degludec) Injection [package insert]. Plainsboro, NJ: Novo Nordisk; November 2019.

126. IXIARO® (Japanese Encephalitis Vaccine) Injection Room Temperature Stability Information Response (Ref#: N/A) [personal communication]. Valneva Scotland Ltd; 2021.

127. Baxter Overfill Medication Information Letter (Ref#: US2020-05883) [personal communication]. Deerfield, IL: Baxter Healthcare Corporation; 2020:2.

128. Fresenius Kabi Overfill Medication Information Communication (Ref#: N/A) [personal communication]. Lake Zurich, IL: Fresenius Kabi USA, LLC; 2020:4.

129. Humulin® R U-500 (Insulin Human) Injection [package insert]. Indianapolis, IN: Eli Lilly and Company; November 2020.

130. Novolog® (Insulin Aspart) Injection [package insert]. Plainsboro, NJ: Novo Nordisk; November 2019.

131. Apidra® (Insulin Glulisine) Injection [package insert]. Bridgewater, NJ: Sanofi-Aventis U.S. LLC; November 2020.

132. Humalog® 50/50 (Insulin Lispro Protamine and Insulin Lispro) Injection [package insert]. Indianapolis, IN: Eli Lilly and Company; April 2020.

133. Humalog® 75/25 (Insulin Lispro Protamine and Insulin Lispro) Injection [package insert]. Indianapolis, IN: Eli Lilly and Company; July 2020.

134. Humulin® 70/30 (Isophane Insulin Human and Insulin Human) Injection [package insert]. Indianapolis, IN: Eli Lilly and Company; November 2020.

135. Humulin® N (Isophane Insulin Human) Injection [package insert]. Indianapolis, IN: Eli Lilly and Company; November 2020.

136. Lantus® (Insulin Glargine) Injection [package insert]. Bridgewater, NJ: Sanofi-Aventis U.S. LLC; January 2021.

137. Levemir® (Insulin Detemir) Injection [package insert]. Plainsboro, NJ: Novo Nordisk; March 2020.

138. Lyumjev™ (Insulin Lispro-aabc) Injection [package insert]. Indianapolis, IN: Eli Lilly and Company; June 2020.

139. Novolin® 70/30 (Isophane Insulin Human and Insulin Human) Injection [package insert]. Plainsboro, NJ: Novo Nordisk; November 2019.

140. Novolin® N (Isophane Insulin Human) Injection [package insert]. Plainsboro, NJ: Novo Nordisk; November 2019.

141. Novolin® R (Insulin Human) Injection [package insert]. Plainsboro, NJ: Novo Nordisk; November 2019.

142. Novolog® Mix 70/30 (Insulin Aspart Protamine and Insulin Aspart) Injection [package insert]. Plainsboro, NJ: Novo Nordisk; November 2019.

143. Toujeo® (Insulin Glargine) Injection [package insert]. Bridgewater, NJ: Sanofi-Aventis U.S. LLC; December 2020.

144. Monoject™ Syringes - Product Description. https://www.cardinalhealth.com/en/product-solutions/medical/patient-care/sharps-safety/medication-delivery/standard-needles-and-syringes/monoject-syringes/soft-pack-syringes.html (accessed 2021 March).

145. Technical Data Sheet - BD Plastipak™ syringes without needles and BD General Syringes without needle Sterile, Single Use, Latex Free. http://downloads.consumables.com/doc/tds/100-0953_TDS.pdf (accessed 2021 March).

146. 0.9% Sodium Chloride Injection, USP in PAB® IV Containers [package insert]. Bethlehem, PA: B. Braun Medical, Inc.; February 2018.

147. B. Braun. 0.9% Sodium Chloride Injection USP, 1,000 mL in E3® IV Container FAQ. Bethlehem, PA: B. Braun Medical Inc; 2018:3.

148. Accreditation Commission for Health Care. About Accreditation. https://www.achc.org/about-accreditation.html (accessed 2021 March).

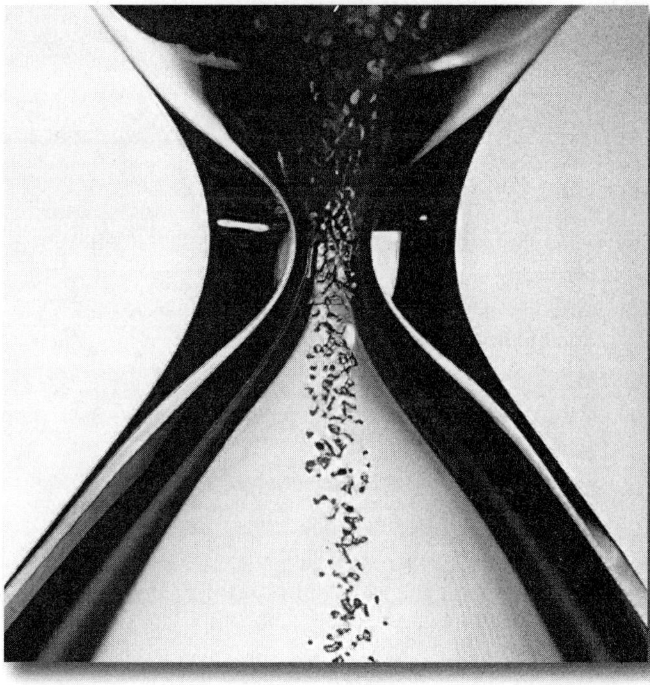

Applying Stability Data in Compounding Parenteral Nutrition

Michelle C. Simpson, Marissa A. Davis

INTRODUCTION

In order to apply stability data in compounding parenteral nutrition, storage times shown in the monographs of this section represent chemical and physical studies of parenteral nutrition components, stability, container material, and storage conditions. Before the official publication of the United States Pharmacopeia (USP) Chapter <797>, *Pharmaceutical Compounding – Sterile Preparations*, which set enforceable standards related to compounding sterile preparations, beyond-use dates were based primarily on chemical and physical stability, often labeling compounded parenteral nutrition for use over several weeks. The USP recognizes the risks of microbial contamination as a contributor to patient safety, and sets limits on the length of time a compounded sterile preparation (CSP) may be stored before the actual time that clinical administration to a patient starts. Pharmacists responsible for compounding and dispensing parenteral nutrition must assign a date representing the date beyond which the preparation should not be stored or used.[1] Assigning an appropriate beyond-use date (BUD) incorporates both chemical and physical factors, plus maintaining a level of quality assurance through the compounding facility's design, equipment, personnel, and processes. The final BUD placed on the CSP container label is determined by applying microbial risk guidance from the USP and data from stability studies of parenteral nutrition. Medication shortages in the United States have led to the importation of international products not previously approved by the FDA. Where applicable, imported products are included in the charts and tables displayed in this chapter.

Stability monographs for single-ingredient CSPs of a parenteral nutrition solution or additive are located in the Drug Monographs section of this book (See: Ascorbic acid, Calcium chloride, Lipid emulsion, Magnesium sulfate).

FACTORS AFFECTING EXTENDED STABILITY OF PARENTERAL NUTRITION

The stability monographs in this chapter provide data from parenteral nutrition studies and indicate the stability of the additive or solution after compounding into the parenteral nutrition formula. Stability studies occasionally assess for changes in a compounded formula's characteristics over time and do not quantify each ingredient. Admixture stability of parenteral nutrition solutions is determined by lack of precipitation, maintenance of pH, visual inspection, and changes to size and distribution of lipid particles. Study data are available for the container specified under the specific conditions noted.[2-4] For more information, refer to Table 1: Conditions Affecting Parenteral Nutrition Stability.

Injectable lipid emulsions have physical and chemical characteristics influencing stability that differ from other intravenous nutrients and fluids. Emulsion stability is included in parenteral nutrition studies to determine the final admixture's stability because emulsions are affected by other ingredients in the parenteral nutrition formula. Droplet size and distribution are essential to parenteral nutrition stability. The USP set a limit to the mean droplet size of not more than 0.5 microns, and the volume-weighted percent of fat droplets greater than 5 microns to be less

DOI 10.37573/9781585286720.PT1002

TABLE 1: Conditions Affecting Parenteral Nutrition Stability

Stability/Influence	Description	Outcome
Chemical Changes	Calcium-phosphate precipitation[3]	• ***Increased*** risk of precipitation with any of the following: ■ High concentrations of calcium and phosphate ■ Less stable salt forms: calcium chloride, mineral form of phosphate ■ Increased pH ■ Low concentration of amino acids and dextrose with increased concentration of lipids ■ Mixing order ■ Storage time ■ Increased temperature
	Lipid peroxidation[3,5,10]	• Soy or fish oil emulsions are more susceptible to peroxidation. • ***Increased*** rate of lipid peroxidation with any of the following: room temperature, incubator temperature, and light. • ***Decreased*** rate of lipid peroxidation with either of the following: multilayered EVA bags and the presence of tocopherol.
Injectable Lipid Emulsion Stability	Formation of large droplets and aggregation[3,5,6]	• Electrolytes and trace elements contribute to aggregation. ■ Concentrations of calcium and magnesium >20 mEq/L leads to instability of the emulsion. • A pH >5 is needed for a stable emulsion. ■ Addition of acidic solutions (eg, dextrose) that decrease pH decreases emulsion stability. ■ Amino acids increase stability.
Compounding	Mixing order[2,6,7]	• For admixtures containing lipids: ■ Transfer the dextrose and amino acids to the container before adding lipid emulsion. ■ Do not inject additives directly into undiluted lipid emulsion.
Microbiological Contamination	Microbial contamination risk[1,5]	• Variables affecting microbial risk: ■ Environment (eg, engineering controls) ■ Aseptic processing (eg, personnel aseptic technique) ■ Storage conditions (eg, refrigeration, room temperature) ■ Sterile starting components ■ Sterility testing (eg, air sampling, personnel evaluation) • Infection risk is ***lower*** when parenteral nutrition is compounded into a single container and ***higher*** when lipids are infused separately.
Storage Temperature	Heat[8]	• Temperature fluctuations affect chemical reactivity, primarily hydrolysis and oxidation. ■ Heat ***increases*** the rate of hydrolysis. • A fluctuation of 10°C can change the rate of reaction.
	Freezing[8,12]	• Freezing may either break emulsions or cause a large ***increase*** in the droplet size of emulsions. • Freezing temperatures can denature proteins or cause crystallization or precipitation.
Container	Oxygen permeable	• ***Increases*** risk of oxidation of lipids and vitamin C.[5]
	Leaching	• DEHP leaching of lipophilic medications and PVC.[10]
Light Exposure	Ultraviolet light (UV)[5,8]	• Exposure to UV light may cause oxidation. • In susceptible compounds, photochemical energy creates free radicals. ■ Accelerated chemical degradation reactions of vitamins. ■ Peroxidation of lipid injectable emulsions.

TABLE 1: Conditions Affecting Parenteral Nutrition Stability (cont'd)

Stability/Influence	Description	Outcome
pH	High and low pH extremes[8]	• High and low pH extremes increase the rate of hydrolysis and oxidation. • ***Higher*** pH: ■ Increases calcium phosphate precipitation. ■ Increases emulsion stability. • ***Lower*** pH: ■ Increases calcium and phosphate solubility. ■ Destabilizes emulsions.

than 0.05%, expressed as $PFAT_5$. Formulations with a $PFAT_5$ exceeding 0.05% are at risk of destabilization over time.[10] The stability of the emulsion is dependent on the zeta potential of the emulsifier. The zeta potential refers to repulsive forces pushing lipid particles apart based on the droplet surface's negative charges. If the zeta potential is neutralized with the addition of cations or the pH decreases below 5, it could lead to coalescence, which causes the droplets to fuse and become larger.[3,10] Physical destabilization occurs in phases, starting with flocculation, creaming, and coalescence, followed by oiling out or cracking. Both flocculation and creaming result from the aggregation of lipid droplets that may or may not be visible; however, the aggregated lipid droplets can be redispersed by gently agitating the container and safely administering to a patient. If yellow or brown oil droplets are found at the surface of the CSP during a visual inspection, it is evidence of coalescence or cracking. Once an emulsion reaches these phases, the lipid droplets cannot be fully redispersed, and the admixture should not be used.[10] For a summary on emulsion instability, refer to Figure 1: Phases of Emulsion Instability.

EXTRAPOLATION CONSIDERATIONS

When the usage timeframe in the manufacturer product labeling is limited or omitted, published stability studies can potentially support extending the BUD assigned to a parenteral nutrition solution. If a referenced study does not match a specific parenteral nutrition formula's conditions, assess the individual components based on the manufacturer, electrolyte salt form, concentration, container type, storage temperature, and exposure to light to determine if the available stability data may be extrapolated. Predictions of any area of stability impart an element of risk, and the degree of accuracy depends on the extent of the difference between the CSP characteristics.[11] When several concentrations of an ingredient are studied with similar stability results, it is reasonable to expect the stability to be the same for concentrations falling within the ones tested.[9] In the absence of stability studies in a specific container, the pharmacist should consider the available container materials and compare them to the materials studied.[9] When compounding parenteral nutrition using a dual-chamber bag, considerations for concentrations of electrolytes and additives should be calculated in the final volume of the container or individual chamber. If compounding software calculates a final volume of both chambers combined, the concentrations of each chamber could exceed limitations and precipitate. If not explicitly studied, room temperature storage stability data should not be applied to refrigerated storage conditions, and refrigerated storage stability data should not be applied to room temperature storage conditions.[1] Studies performed while the preparation was protected from light cannot be extrapolated to light-exposed conditions.[12] However, stability studies of light-exposed preparations can be extrapolated to light-protected conditions. Time periods reported can only be shortened, not lengthened. For more information, refer to Table 2: Extrapolation Considerations for Compounding Parenteral Nutrition.

FIGURE 1: Phases of Emulsion Instability[3]

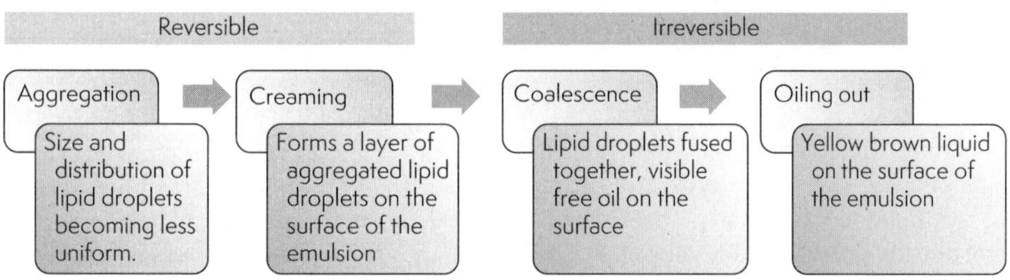

TABLE 2: Extrapolation Considerations for Compounding Parenteral Nutrition

Comparison	Considerations	Conclusions
Manufacturer	Manufacturer product studied differs from inventory[9]	• Drugs that are generically and chemically identical are expected to have the same results as those studied. • If there are differences in salt form, excipients, or solubilizing agents, the studied stability data may not be applicable.
Component	Injectable lipid emulsions[5]	• Lipid products with similar composition are expected to have similar stability to those studied. • Soy and fish oil emulsions are more susceptible to peroxidation than emulsions containing olive oil.
	Calcium gluconate vs. calcium chloride[14]	• Calcium gluconate has a lower degree of dissociation than calcium chloride. • Higher concentrations of calcium gluconate are soluble with phosphate.
	Glycerophosphate/phosphate[14]	• Glycerophosphate ***increases*** calcium phosphate solubility. • Higher concentrations of glycerophosphate are soluble with calcium.
Concentration	Several concentrations studied with similar stability results[9]	• Prediction of similar stability for a concentration falling within the range of studied concentrations is reasonable. • If there are data available in a container type and admixture with documented stability at two concentrations, concentrations falling within the two data points are acceptable. • Extrapolating stability outside the studied concentrations is not recommended due to increased risk of instability of the final solution.
Container	EVA	• Permeable to oxygen.[23]
	Multilayer EVA	• Less permeable to oxygen.[23]
	Polypropylene	• RTU formulas.[13]
	Dual-chamber/single-chamber	• Considerations for concentrations of electrolytes and additives should be calculated in the final volume of the container or individual chamber. ■ If compounding software calculates a final volume of both chambers combined, the concentrations of each chamber could exceed limitations and precipitate.
Light	Light-protected compared to light-exposed	• Do not extrapolate light-protected study results to light-exposed admixtures.[12]
	Light-exposed compared to light-protected	• Stability studies of light-exposed drugs can be extrapolated to light-protected admixtures.
Premix/RTU	RTU manufacturer expiration to compounded admixtures	• Do not extrapolate RTU manufacturer expiration dates to beyond-use dates for compounded admixtures.
Sterility	Sterility tests from CSP to CSP	• Do not extrapolate sterility studies.[1]
Temperature	Studied at two temperatures and stable at both vs. studied at only one temperature	• Temperatures should not be extrapolated without studying the admixture at the temperature desired.[1]

PREPARATION STERILITY AND QUALITY ASSURANCE

Individual organizations have to determine their own specific standard operating procedures (SOPs). In order to ensure consistent practices and reproducible results, there should be SOPs for parenteral nutrition compounding and all related processes. Consistency in compounding compliance using standardized SOPs can reduce variation and decrease the chances of preventable errors occurring. SOPs should be based on applicable laws, regulations, and accreditation standards, and they should be further individualized for the types of compounding performed and equipment used at each facility.[1]

If compounding in batches for more than one patient, a master formulation record provides specific compounding instructions and describes how the CSP was prepared.[15,16] When standardizing compounding records and master formulation records, the names, descriptions, and IDs of CSPs should be consistent.

Automated compounding devices (ACDs) can improve accuracy and efficiency in creating the parenteral nutrition formula, but they can also introduce risk or impact the sterility of a preparation. A pharmacist should ensure tubing in an ACD is not used beyond its labeled timeframe per manufacturer instructions. An appropriate flush should be done between the compounding of incompatible formulations to avoid cross-contamination. Changing or replacing products used by an ACD must be done utilizing proper aseptic techniques, and their hang time should be evaluated to ensure sterility and stability of the product. The mixing order must be considered for high-precipitation risks such as calcium and phosphates, which need to be added separately and into the largest solution volume to avoid forming precipitates during the compounding process.

ASSIGNING BEYOND-USE DATES TO COMPOUNDED PARENTERAL NUTRITION

Assigning a beyond-use date or BUD to a parenteral nutrition admixture is performed as part of the compounding process. A BUD encompasses the time period starting at the date and time of compounding through the date and time after which the start of clinical administration should not occur. Assigning an appropriate BUD requires the consideration of many factors such as chemical stability, physical properties, component compatibility, sterility, component concentrations, container type, personnel factors, environmental factors, and equipment utilized during the compounding process. BUDs are determined using a risk-based approach. The USP limits maximum BUDs to decrease risks posed to patients by requiring a labeled BUD that represents a time span before it is a risk for physical or chemical degradation, microbial contamination and proliferation, and diminished integrity of the container. The date takes into consideration the specific conditions where the parenteral nutrition admixture was compounded, the probability for microbial growth, and the time period within which it should be used.[1]

The clinical guidelines set by the American Society for Parenteral and Enteral Nutrition (ASPEN) recommend compounding parenteral nutrition formulas within macronutrient concentrations that have been studied and report consistent extended stability.[17] For more information, refer to Figure 2: Macronutrient Concentrations Exhibiting Maximum Stability.

Labels that specify the storage conditions and BUD of compounded preparations are placed on each parenteral dosage unit. Documentation of the preparation date should be part of the labeling, and include the time of compounding, if applicable, to any component of the formula. If preparation stability varies under different temperature conditions, list the BUD for each anticipated storage condition on the label. If the preparation needs to be warmed to room temperature prior to administration, the label and ancillary instruction material should describe it. If preparations are stable for less than 24 hours at room temperature, the label should be specific about the end-use time. Individuals administering parenteral nutrition should be trained to check preparations for current BUDs prior to usage. Practitioners should establish a standardized approach to labeling that is clear, concise, and meets all licensure and regulatory requirements, including USP Chapter <797> general labeling guidelines.[18]

PROFESSIONAL, REGULATORY, AND ACCREDITATION GUIDELINES

ASPEN has developed guidance documents related to parenteral nutrition. Following ASPEN guidelines decreases the risk of incompatibility or instability, while outlining in-process and end-product inspections used to confirm compounding accuracy. ASPEN recommendations are aligned with requirements for pharmacies to adhere to USP Chapter <797>, *Pharmaceutical Compounding – Sterile Preparations.*[17,19]

The Centers for Disease Control and Prevention (CDC), in their *Guidelines for the Prevention of Intravascular Catheter-Related Infections,* recommends that lipid emulsions should be infused for no longer than 12 hours when infused alone, and no longer than 24 hours as a component of a lipid containing parenteral nutrition formula. Administration sets for lipids should be changed every 24 hours.[20]

USP Chapter <729>, *Globule Size Distribution in Lipid Injectable Emulsions*, contains the methodology for manufacturers to determine the mean particle size in injectable lipid emulsions. The stability of manufactured injectable lipid emulsions is defined by limiting mean lipid globule size at no greater than 5 microns, and the percent of globules larger than 5 microns should not exceed 0.05%, expressed as $PFAT_5$. When interpreting published stability data on lipid emulsions, similar methodology should be reported and assessed before applying extended stability to a particular admixture.[10]

FIGURE 2: Macronutrient Concentrations Exhibiting Maximum Stability[17]

Container	Admixture Concentration	Room Temperature	Refrigerated Temperature
Ethylene Vinyl Acetate (EVA)	Amino acid ≥4% Dextrose ≥10% Lipid emulsion ≥2%	24 hours	9 days

USP Chapter <797>, *Pharmaceutical Compounding – Sterile Preparations*, outlines the standards and minimum required practices related to compounding sterile preparations in the United States. It provides the organizational structure, procedures, processes, and resources necessary to ensure predefined quality measures are met by facilities that compound sterile preparations. The chapter is enforceable by state boards, the FDA, and accreditation organizations.[1]

APPLYING STABILITY DATA USING COMMERCIAL PRODUCTS

When using premixed or ready-to-use (RTU) products, care must be taken to ensure all calculations and considerations regarding stability include the ingredients of all components. For example, if a concentrated commercial solution of electrolytes is used and additional individual electrolytes are admixed, the total of each component combined should be evaluated for stability. The products should be separated in the compounding process to avoid instability. Similarly, if using a premixed parenteral nutrition product and adding an additive, the pharmacist should review available data to ensure that the final solution containing all components results in a stable solution and that BUDs are appropriately adjusted based on the method of additive addition utilized (eg, pharmacy or bedside addition) and storage conditions.

Many components of parenteral nutrition and premixed solutions come in protective overwrap. If removing this overwrap before the time of compounding, dispensing, or administration, the manufacturer guidelines should be consulted to determine any potential impact on stability. For some products, the overwrap must remain intact for the labeled expiration—once the overwrap is removed, the product may be subject to impacts from hydrolysis, evaporation, or light damage.

SUMMARY

Pharmacists are responsible for dispensing parenteral nutrition admixtures that meet patients' unique clinical needs while satisfying all quality, safety, and environmental control requirements set by legislative, regulatory, and accreditation bodies. They direct all phases of preparation, storage, transportation, and administration of parenteral nutrition and maintain compliance with established standards, regulations, and best practices.

Carnitine *in Parenteral Nutrition*

Container	Formulation/ Concentration	Temperature		Light		Lipids		Refer.
		Refrig	Room	Exposed	Protected	With	Without	
Bag, Ethylene Vinyl Acetate (EVA)	100 mg/L[(a)]	4 d	n/a	n/a	n/a	X	X	(4)

Note

[a] Formulas: Pediatric amino acid (TPH®), dextrose, lipids (Intralipid®, ClinOleic™, Lipofundin®, SMOFlipid®, Lipidem®), electrolytes, trace elements, vitamins, and carnitine.[(4)]

Chromium *in Parenteral Nutrition*

Container	Formulation/ Concentration	Temperature		Light		Lipids		Refer.
		Refrig	Room	Exposed	Protected	With	Without	
Bag, Ethylene Vinyl Acetate (EVA)	(a)	7 d	24 hr	n/a	n/a	X	n/a	(2)
	(b)	7 d	48 hr	n/a	n/a	X	n/a	(22)
	(c)	7 d	48 hr	n/a	X	X	n/a	(23)
	(d)	30 d	24 hr	n/a	n/a	X	n/a	(24)
Bag, Multilayer Polypropylene[(e)]	(e)	7 d	48 hr	n/a	n/a	X	n/a	(13)(25)

Special Considerations: Stability studies assessed changes to characteristics of the admixture over time (pH, precipitation, visual inspection, changes to size and distribution of lipid particles), and did not measure the content of each trace element.

Notes

[a] Formulas: amino acids (Clinisol™, Prosol™, Travasol®), dextrose, lipid (SMOFlipid®), electrolytes, and trace elements (Addamel™: Cr, Cu, F, Fe, I, Mn, Mo, Se, Zn).[(2)]

[b] Formulas: amino acids (Aminosyn®, Plenamine™), dextrose, lipid (SMOFlipid®), electrolytes, and trace elements (Addamel™: Cr, Cu, F, Fe, I, Mn, Mo, Se, Zn).[(22)]

[c] Formulas: amino acids (Aminoplasmal®), dextrose, lipid (Intralipid®, ClinOleic™), electrolytes, and trace elements (Cr, Cu, Mn, Se, Zn).[(23)]

[d] Formulas: amino acids (Neonutrin), dextrose, lipid (SMOFlipid®), electrolytes, and trace elements (Addamel™: Cr, Cu, F, Fe, I, Mn, Mo, Se, Zn).[(24)]

[e] Formulas: Kabiven® (RTU three-chamber bag) (amino acids, dextrose, soy-based lipid), electrolytes, and trace elements (Addamel™: Cr, Cu, F, Fe, I, Mn, Mo, Se, Zn).[(13,25)]

Copper *in Parenteral Nutrition*									
		Temperature			Light		Lipids		
Container	Formulation/ Concentration	Refrig	Room	Body	Exposed	Protected	With	Without	Refer.
Bag, Ethylene Vinyl Acetate (EVA)	[a]	7 d	24 hr	n/a	n/a	n/a	X	n/a	(2)
	[b]	7 d	48 hr	n/a	n/a	n/a	X	n/a	(22)
	[c]	7 d	48 hr	n/a	n/a	X	X	n/a	(23)
	[d]	9 d	24 hr	n/a	n/a	X	X	X	(27)
	[e]	21 d	24 hr	n/a	n/a	X	n/a	X	(29)
	[f]	30 d	24 hr	24 hr	X[i]	X[i]	n/a	X	(14)
	[g]	30 d	24 hr	n/a	n/a	n/a	X	n/a	(24)
Bag, Multilayer Polypropylene[h]	[h]	7 d	48 hr	n/a	n/a	n/a	X	n/a	(13)(25)

Special Considerations: Stability studies assessed changes to characteristics of the admixture over time (pH, precipitation, visual inspection, changes to size and distribution of lipid particles), and did not measure the content of each trace element.

Notes

[a] Formulas: amino acids (Clinisol™, Prosol™, Travasol®), dextrose, lipid (SMOFlipid®), electrolytes, and trace elements (Addamel™: Cr, Cu, F, Fe, I, Mn, Mo, Se, Zn).[2]

[b] Formulas: amino acids (Aminosyn®, Plenamine™), dextrose, lipid (SMOFlipid®), electrolytes, and trace elements (Addamel™: Cr, Cu, F, Fe, I, Mn, Mo, Se, Zn).[22]

[c] Formulas: amino acids (Aminoplasmal®), dextrose, lipid (Intralipid®, ClinOleic™), electrolytes, and trace elements (Cr, Cu, Mn, Se, Zn).[23]

[d] Formulas: amino acid solution, dextrose, lipid, electrolytes, and trace elements (Tralement®: Cu, Mn, Se, Zn).[27]

[e] Formulas: amino acids (Aminoven®, Primene™), dextrose, electrolytes, and trace elements (Peditrace™: Cu. F, I, Mn, Se, Zn).[29]

[f] Formulas: amino acids (Aminoven®, Vaminolact®, Primene™), dextrose electrolytes, and trace elements (Peditrace™: Cu, F, I, Mn, Se, Zn).[14]

[g] Formulas: amino acids (Neonutrin), dextrose, lipid (SMOFlipid®), electrolytes, and trace elements (Addamel™: Cr, Cu, F, Fe, I, Mn, Mo, Se, Zn).[24]

[h] Formulas: Kabiven® (RTU three-chamber bag) (amino acids, dextrose, soy-based lipid), electrolytes, and trace elements (Addamel™: Cr, Cu, F, Fe, I, Mn, Mo, Se, Zn).[13,25]

[i] Light exposed for 30 days RF, light protected for 24 hours at 37°C.[14]

Famotidine *in Parenteral Nutrition*								
		Temperature		Light		Lipids		
Container	Formulation/ Concentration	Refrig	Room	Exposed	Protected	With	Without	Refer.
Bag, Ethylene Vinyl Acetate (EVA)	0.02, 0.05 mg/mL[a]	24 hr[a]	24 hr[a]	n/a	n/a	X	n/a	(41)
	0.02 mg/mL[b]	n/a	24 hr	X	n/a	X	n/a	(42)
	0.02, 0.04 mg/mL[c]	7 d	48 hr	X	n/a	n/a	X	(43)
	0.02 mg/mL[d]	n/a	48 hr	X	n/a	X	X	(44)
	0.02, 0.04 mg/mL[e]	n/a	72 hr	X	n/a	X	n/a	(45)
Bag, Polyvinyl Chloride (PVC)	0.02 mg/mL[f]	5 wk	n/a	n/a	X	n/a	X	(21)

Notes

[a] Stability was 48 hr total (24 hr refrigerated followed by 24 hr at room temp). Formula: amino acids (FreAmine III®), dextrose, lipid emulsion (Intralipid® 20%), electrolytes, and trace elements; no impact on emulsion stability.[41]

[b] Formula: amino acids (Novamine®), dextrose, lipid emulsion, electrolytes, vitamins, and trace elements.[42]

[c] Formula: amino acids (FreAmine III®), dextrose, electrolytes, vitamins, heparin, and trace elements.[43]

[d] Formula: amino acids (Travasol®), dextrose, lipid emulsion (Liposyn II®, Intralipid®), electrolytes, vitamins, and trace elements; no effect on emulsion stability.[44]

[e] Formula: amino acids, glucose, lipid emulsions, electrolytes, vitamins, and trace elements.[45]

[f] Formula: amino acids (Travasol®), dextrose, electrolytes, and trace elements.[21]

Folic Acid *in Parenteral Nutrition*

Container	Formulation/ Concentration	Temperature		Light		Lipids		Refer.
		Refrig	Room	Exposed	Protected	With	Without	
Bag, Ethylene Vinyl Acetate (EVA)	[(a)]	n/a	24 hr	X	n/a	n/a	X	(33)
	[(b)(c)]	48 hr	24 hr	n/a	X	X	n/a	(34)

Notes

a Formula: amino acids, glucose, electrolytes, vitamins, and trace elements (European products).[(33)]

b Formula: amino acids (Viamin), dextrose, lipid (SMOFlipid®), electrolytes, and vitamins.[(34)]

c Stability studies assessed changes to characteristics of the admixture over time (pH, precipitation, visual inspection, changes to size and distribution of lipid particles), and did not measure the content of each vitamin.

Heparin *in Parenteral Nutrition*

Container	Formulation/ Concentration	Temperature		Light		Lipids		Refer.
		Refrig	Room	Exposed	Protected	With	Without	
Bag, Polyvinyl Chloride (PVC)	3, 5, 10, 20 units/mL[(a)]	21 d	n/a	n/a	n/a	n/a	X	(26)
Unspecified	77 units/mL[(b)]	n/a	24 hr	n/a	n/a	n/a	n/a	(28)

Notes

a Formula: amino acids (+/–)[(c)] (Travasol®), dextrose, electrolytes, and trace elements; longer stability with amino acids included in formula.[(26)]

b Neonatal Parenteral Nutrition unspecified.[(28)]

c (+/–) indicates that sample was mixed both with and without the nutrient.

Iron *in Parenteral Nutrition*

Container	Formulation/ Concentration	Temperature		Light		Lipids		Refer.
		Refrig	Room	Exposed	Protected	With	Without	
Bag, Ethylene Vinyl Acetate (EVA)	0.7-1.9 mg/L[(a)(f)(h)]	7 d	24 hr	n/a	n/a	X	n/a	(2)
	0.8 mg/L[(b)(f)(h)]	30 d	24 hr	n/a	n/a	X	n/a	(24)
Bag, Multilayer Polypropylene[(c)]	0.43-1.1 mg/L[(c)(f)(h)]	7 d	48 hr	n/a	n/a	X	n/a	(13)(25)
Unspecified	100 mg/L[(d)(i)]	n/a	18 hr	n/a	n/a	n/a	X	(30)
Vial, Glass	2 mg/L[(e)(i)]	48 hr	48 hr	n/a	n/a	X	n/a	(31)

Notes

a Formulas: amino acids (Clinisol™, Prosol™, Travasol®), dextrose, lipid (SMOFlipid®), electrolytes, and trace elements (Addamel™: Cr, Cu, F, Fe, I, Mn, Mo, Se, Zn).[(2)]

b Formulas: amino acids (Neonutrin), dextrose, lipid (SMOFlipid®), electrolytes, and trace elements (Addamel™: Cr, Cu, F, Fe, I, Mn, Mo, Se, Zn).[(24)]

c Formulas: Kabiven® (RTU three-chamber bag) (amino acids, dextrose, soy-based lipid), electrolytes, and trace elements (Addamel™: Cr, Cu, F, Fe, I, Mn, Mo, Se, Zn).[(13,25)]

d Formulas included amino acids (Travasol®), dextrose, electrolytes, vitamins (+/–)[(g)], and trace elements (+/–)[(g)]. [(30)]

e Formulas included amino acids (Travasol®), dextrose, lipid emulsions (Intralipid®, Liposyn II®), electrolytes, and heparin.[(31)]

f Stability studies assessed changes to characteristics of the admixture over time (pH, precipitation, visual inspection, changes to size and distribution of lipid particles), and did not measure the content of iron.[(2,24,25)]

g (+/–) indicates that sample was mixed both with and without the nutrient.

h Concentration: expressed as mg/L of ferric chloride.

i Concentration: expressed as mg/L of iron dextran.

Manganese *in Parenteral Nutrition*										
	Formulation/	Temperature			Light		Lipids		
Container	Concentration	Refrig	Room	Body	Exposed	Protected	With	Without	Refer.
Bag, Ethylene Vinyl Acetate (EVA)	(a)	7 d	24 hr	n/a	n/a	n/a	X	n/a	(2)
	(b)	7 d	48 hr	n/a	n/a	n/a	X	n/a	(22)
	(c)	7 d	48 hr	n/a	n/a	X	X	n/a	(23)
	(d)	9 d	24 hr	n/a	n/a	X	X	X	(27)
	(e)	21 d	24 hr	n/a	n/a	X	n/a	X	(29)
	(f)	30 d	24 hr	24 hr	X[(i)]	X[(i)]	n/a	X	(14)
	(g)	30 d	24 hr	n/a	n/a	n/a	X	n/a	(24)
Bag, Multilayer Polypropylene[(h)]	(h)	7 d	48 hr	n/a	n/a	n/a	X	n/a	(13)(25)

Special Considerations: Stability studies assessed changes to characteristics of the admixture over time (pH, precipitation, visual inspection, changes to size and distribution of lipid particles), and did not measure the content of each trace element.

Notes

[a] Formulas: amino acids (Clinisol™, Prosol™, Travasol®), dextrose, lipid (SMOFlipid®), electrolytes, and trace elements (Addamel™: Cr, Cu, F, Fe, I, Mn, Mo, Se, Zn).[(2)]

[b] Formulas: amino acids (Aminosyn®, Plenamine™), dextrose, lipid (SMOFlipid®), electrolytes, and trace elements (Addamel™: Cr, Cu, F, Fe, I, Mn, Mo, Se, Zn).[(22)]

[c] Formulas: amino acids (Aminoplasmal®), dextrose, lipid (Intralipid®, ClinOleic™), electrolytes, and trace elements (Cr, Cu, Mn, Se, Zn).[(23)]

[d] Formulas: amino acid solution, dextrose, lipid, electrolytes, and trace elements (Tralement®: Cu, Mn, Se, Zn).[(27)]

[e] Formulas: amino acids (Aminoven®, Primene™), dextrose, electrolytes, and trace elements (Peditrace™: Cu, F, I, Mn, Se, Zn).[(29)]

[f] Formulas: amino acids (Aminoven®, Vaminolact®, Primene™), dextrose electrolytes, and trace elements (Peditrace™: Cu, F, I, Mn, Se, Zn).[(14)]

[g] Formulas: amino acids (Neonutrin), dextrose, lipid (SMOFlipid®), electrolytes, and trace elements (Addamel™: Cr, Cu, F, Fe, I, Mn, Mo, Se, Zn).[(24)]

[h] Formulas: Kabiven® (RTU three-chamber bag) (amino acids, dextrose, soy-based lipid), electrolytes, and trace elements (Addamel™: Cr, Cu, F, Fe, I, Mn, Mo, Se, Zn).[(13,25)]

[i] Light exposed for 30 days RF, light protected for 24 hours at 37°C.[(14)]

Selenium *in Parenteral Nutrition*										
	Formulation/	Temperature			Light		Lipids		
Container	Concentration	Refrig	Room	Body	Exposed	Protected	With	Without	Refer.
Bag, Ethylene Vinyl Acetate (EVA)	(a)	7 d	24 hr	n/a	n/a	n/a	X	n/a	(2)
	(b)	7 d	48 hr	n/a	n/a	n/a	X	n/a	(22)
	(c)	7 d	48 hr	n/a	n/a	X	X	n/a	(23)
	(d)	9 d	24 hr	n/a	n/a	X	X	X	(27)
	(e)	21 d	24 hr	n/a	n/a	X	n/a	X	(29)
	(f)	30 d	24 hr	24 hr	X[(i)]	X[(i)]	n/a	X	(14)
	(g)	30 d	24 hr	n/a	n/a	n/a	X	n/a	(24)
Bag, Multilayer Polypropylene[(h)]	(h)	7 d	48 hr	n/a	n/a	n/a	X	n/a	(13)(25)

Special Considerations: Stability studies assessed changes to characteristics of the admixture over time (pH, precipitation, visual inspection, changes to size and distribution of lipid particles), and did not measure the content of each trace element.

Notes

[a] Formulas: amino acids (Clinisol™, Prosol™, Travasol®), dextrose, lipid (SMOFlipid®), electrolytes, and trace elements (Addamel™: Cr, Cu, F, Fe, I, Mn, Mo, Se, Zn).[(2)]

[b] Formulas: amino acids (Aminosyn®, Plenamine™), dextrose, lipid (SMOFlipid®), electrolytes, and trace elements (Addamel™: Cr, Cu, F, Fe, I, Mn, Mo, Se, Zn).[(22)]

[c] Formulas: amino acids (Aminoplasmal®), dextrose, lipid (Intralipid®, ClinOleic™), electrolytes, and trace elements (Cr, Cu, Mn, Se, Zn).[(23)]

[d] Formulas: amino acid solution, dextrose, lipid, electrolytes, and trace elements (Tralement®: Cu, Mn, Se, Zn).[(27)]

[e] Formulas: amino acids (Aminoven®, Primene™), dextrose, electrolytes, and trace elements (Peditrace™: Cu, F, I, Mn, Se, Zn).[(29)]

[f] Formulas: amino acids (Aminoven®, Vaminolact®, Primene™), dextrose electrolytes, and trace elements (Peditrace™: Cu, F, I, Mn, Se, Zn).[(14)]

[g] Formulas: amino acids (Neonutrin), dextrose, lipid (SMOFlipid®), electrolytes, and trace elements (Addamel™: Cr, Cu, F, Fe, I, Mn, Mo, Se, Zn).[(24)]

[h] Formulas: Kabiven® (RTU three-chamber bag) (amino acids, dextrose, soy-based lipid), electrolytes, and trace elements (Addamel™: Cr, Cu, F, Fe, I, Mn, Mo, Se, Zn).[(13,25)]

[i] Light exposed for 30 days RF, light protected for 24 hours at 37°C.[(14)]

Trace Elements *in Parenteral Nutrition*

Container	Formulation/ Concentration	Temperature			Light		Lipids		Refer.
		Refrig	Room	Body	Exposed	Protected	With	Without	
Bag, Ethylene Vinyl Acetate (EVA)	(a)	7 d	24 hr	n/a	n/a	n/a	X	n/a	(2)
	(b)	7 d	48 hr	n/a	n/a	n/a	X	n/a	(22)
	(c)	7 d	48 hr	n/a	n/a	X	X	n/a	(23)
	(d)	9 d	24 hr	n/a	n/a	X	X	X	(27)
	(e)	21 d	24 hr	n/a	n/a	X	n/a	X	(29)
	(f)	30 d	24 hr	24 hr	X[i]	X[i]	n/a	X	(14)
	(g)	30 d	24 hr	n/a	n/a	n/a	X	n/a	(24)
Bag, Multilayer Polypropylene[h]	(h)	7 d	48 hr	n/a	n/a	n/a	X	n/a	(13)(25)

Special Considerations: Stability studies assessed changes to characteristics of the admixture over time (pH, precipitation, visual inspection, changes to size and distribution of lipid particles), and did not measure the content of each trace element.

Notes

[a] Formulas: amino acids (Clinisol™, Prosol™, Travasol®), dextrose, lipid (SMOFlipid®), electrolytes, and trace elements (Addamel™: Cr, Cu, F, Fe, I, Mn, Mo, Se, Zn).[2]

[b] Formulas: amino acids (Aminosyn®, Plenamine™), dextrose, lipid (SMOFlipid®), electrolytes, and trace elements (Addamel™: Cr, Cu, F, Fe, I, Mn, Mo, Se, Zn).[22]

[c] Formulas: amino acids (Aminoplasmal®), dextrose, lipid (Intralipid®, ClinOleic™), electrolytes, and trace elements (Cr, Cu, Mn, Se, Zn).[23]

[d] Formulas: amino acid solution, dextrose, lipid, electrolytes, and trace elements (Tralement®: Cu, Mn, Se, Zn).[27]

[e] Formulas: amino acids (Aminoven®, Primene™), dextrose, electrolytes, and trace elements (Peditrace™: Cu, F, I, Mn, Se, Zn).[29]

[f] Formulas: amino acids (Aminoven®, Vaminolact®, Primene™), dextrose electrolytes, and trace elements (Peditrace™: Cu, F, I, Mn, Se, Zn).[14]

[g] Formulas: amino acids (Neonutrin), dextrose, lipid (SMOFlipid®), electrolytes, and trace elements (Addamel™: Cr, Cu, F, Fe, I, Mn, Mo, Se, Zn).[24]

[h] Formulas: Kabiven® (RTU three-chamber bag) (amino acids, dextrose, soy-based lipid), electrolytes, and trace elements (Addamel™: Cr, Cu, F, Fe, I, Mn, Mo, Se, Zn).[13,25]

[i] Light exposed for 30 days RF, light protected for 24 hours at 37°C.[14]

Vitamin A *in Parenteral Nutrition*

Container	Formulation/ Concentration	Temperature			Light		Lipids		Refer.
		Refrig	Room	Body	Exposed	Protected	With	Without	
Bag, Ethylene Vinyl Acetate (EVA)	(a)	24 hr	24 hr	24 hr	X	n/a	X	n/a	(35)
	(b)	6 d	24 hr	n/a	X	X	X	n/a	(36)
	(c)	20 d	n/a	n/a	X	X	X	X	(37)
Bag, Polyvinyl Chloride (PVC)	(c)	20 d	n/a	n/a	X	X	X	X	(37)
Vial, Glass	(c)	20 d	n/a	n/a	X	X	X	X	(37)

Notes

[a] Formula: amino acids, glucose, lipid emulsion, electrolytes, vitamins, and trace elements (European products).[35]

[b] Form: Retinyl palmitate. Formula: amino acids, glucose, lipid emulsion (Intralipid®), electrolytes, vitamins, and trace elements (European products); refrigerated samples were protected from light; stability defined as greater than 80% of initial concentration. Room temperature storage followed 6 d refrigeration.[36]

[c] Formula: amino acids, glucose, lipid emulsion, electrolytes, vitamins (MVI-12®), and trace elements (+/–)[d] (European products); stability defined as greater than 80% of initial concentration.[37]

[d] (+/–) indicates that sample was mixed both with and without the nutrient.

Vitamin B1 *in Parenteral Nutrition*

Container	Formulation/ Concentration	Temperature		Light		Lipids		Refer.
		Refrig	Room	Exposed	Protected	With	Without	
Bag, Ethylene Vinyl Acetate (EVA)	(a)	4 d	n/a	n/a	X	X	n/a	(36)
	(b)	n/a	24 hr	X	n/a	n/a	X	(33)
Bag, Multilayer Polypropylene[(d)]	(c)	72 hr	72 hr	X	X	n/a	X	(38)

Notes

[a] Form: thiamine. Formulas: amino acids, glucose, lipid emulsion (Intralipid®), electrolytes, vitamins, and trace elements (European products); stability defined as greater than 80% of initial concentration.[(36)]

[b] Form: thiamine hydrochloride. Formulas: amino acids, glucose, electrolytes, vitamins, and trace elements (European products).[(33)]

[c] Formulas: amino acids, dextrose, electrolytes, trace elements, pediatric multivitamins, high concentration calcium, and organic phosphate (Brazilian products).[(38)]

[d] Polypropylene, polyethylene, polyester multilayer container.[(38)]

Vitamin B2 *in Parenteral Nutrition*

Container	Formulation/ Concentration	Temperature		Light		Lipids		Refer.
		Refrig	Room	Exposed	Protected	With	Without	
Bag, Ethylene Vinyl Acetate (EVA)	(a)	6 d	24 hr	X	X	X	n/a	(36)
Bag, Multilayer Polypropylene[(c)]	(b)	72 hr	72 hr	X	X	n/a	X	(38)

Notes

[a] Form: riboflavin. Formula: amino acids, glucose, lipid emulsion (Intralipid®), electrolytes, vitamins, and trace elements (European products); stability defined as greater than 80% of initial concentration. Room temp studied followed 6 d refrigerated.[(36)]

[b] Formula: amino acids, dextrose, electrolytes, trace elements, pediatric multivitamins, high-concentration calcium, and organic phosphate (Brazilian products).[(38)]

[c] Polypropylene, polyethylene, polyester multilayer container.[(38)]

Vitamin B3 *in Parenteral Nutrition*

Container	Formulation/ Concentration	Temperature		Light		Lipids		Refer.
		Refrig	Room	Exposed	Protected	With	Without	
Bag, Ethylene Vinyl Acetate (EVA)	(a)	4 d	n/a	n/a	X	X	n/a	(36)

Note

[a] Form: nicotinamide. Formulas: amino acids, glucose, lipid emulsion (Intralipid®), electrolytes, vitamins, and trace elements (European products); stability defined as greater than 80% of initial concentration.[(36)]

Vitamin B5 *in Parenteral Nutrition*

Container	Formulation/ Concentration	Temperature		Light		Lipids		Refer.
		Refrig	Room	Exposed	Protected	With	Without	
Bag, Ethylene Vinyl Acetate (EVA)	(a)	4 d	n/a	n/a	X	X	n/a	(36)

Note

[a] Form: pantothenate. Formula: amino acids, glucose, lipid emulsion (Intralipid®), electrolytes, vitamins, and trace elements (European products); stability defined as greater than 80% of initial concentration.[(36)]

Vitamin B6 *in Parenteral Nutrition*								
	Formulation/	Temperature		Light		Lipids		
Container	Concentration	Refrig	Room	Exposed	Protected	With	Without	Refer.
Bag, Ethylene Vinyl Acetate (EVA)	(a)	4 d	n/a	n/a	X	X	n/a	(36)
	(b)	n/a	24 hr	X	n/a	n/a	X	(33)
Bag, Multilayer Polypropylene[(d)]	(c)	72 hr	72 hr	X	X	n/a	X	(38)

Notes

[a] Form: pyridoxine. Formulas: amino acids, glucose, lipid emulsion (Intralipid®), electrolytes, vitamins, and trace elements (European products); stability defined as greater than 80% of initial concentration.[(36)]

[b] Form: pyridoxine hydrochloride. Formulas: amino acids, glucose, electrolytes, vitamins, and trace elements (European products).[(33)]

[c] Formulas: amino acids, dextrose, electrolytes, trace elements, pediatric multivitamins, high-concentration calcium, and organic phosphate (Brazilian products).[(38)]

[d] Polypropylene, polyethylene, polyester multilayer container.[(38)]

Vitamin B12 *in Parenteral Nutrition*								
	Formulation/	Temperature		Light		Lipids		
Container	Concentration	Refrig	Room	Exposed	Protected	With	Without	Refer.
Bag, Ethylene Vinyl Acetate (EVA)	(a)	4 d	n/a	n/a	X	X	n/a	(36)

Note

[a] Form: cyanocobalamin. Formulas: amino acids, glucose, lipid emulsion (Intralipid®), electrolytes, vitamins, and trace elements (European products); stability defined as greater than 80% of initial concentration.[(36)]

Vitamin C *in Parenteral Nutrition*								
	Formulation/	Temperature		Light		Lipids		
Container	Concentration	Refrig	Room	Exposed	Protected	With	Without	Refer.
Bag, Ethylene Vinyl Acetate (EVA)	(a)	24 hr	24 hr	n/a	X	X	n/a	(39)
Bag, Multilayer Polypropylene[(d)]	(c)	72 hr	48 hr	X	X	n/a	X	(38)
Bag, Multilayer Polypropylene[(e)]	(b)	48 hr	48 hr	X	n/a	X	n/a	(40)

Notes

[a] Formulas: amino acids (Aminoplasmal®), dextrose, lipid (Lipofundin®), and electrolytes.[(39)]

[b] Formulas: amino acids, dextrose, lipid, electrolytes, trace elements, and multivitamins.[(40)]

[c] Formulas: amino acids, dextrose, electrolytes, trace elements, pediatric multivitamins, high-concentration calcium, and organic phosphate (Brazilian products).[(38)]

[d] 3-layer container; polypropylene, polyethylene, polyester.[(38)]

[e] 6-layer container with ethylene vinyl acetate gas-impermeable layer.[(40)]

Vitamin D *in Parenteral Nutrition*

Container	Formulation/ Concentration	Temperature		Light		Lipids		Refer.
		Refrig	Room	Exposed	Protected	With	Without	
Bag, Ethylene Vinyl Acetate (EVA)	(a)	24 hr	24 hr	n/a	X	X	n/a	(2)(32)
Bag, Multilayer Polypropylene	(b)	24 hr	24 hr	n/a	X	X	n/a	(13)(25)(32)

Notes

[a] Formulas: amino acids (Clinisol™, Prosol™, Travasol®), dextrose, lipid (SMOFlipid®), electrolytes, trace elements (Addamel™: Cr, Cu, F, Fe, I, Mn, Mo, Se, Zn), and vitamins (Infuvite®).[(2)] After addition of multiple vitamins for injection, use within 24 hours.[(32)]

[b] Formulas: Kabiven® (RTU three-chamber bag) (amino acids, dextrose, soy-based lipid), electrolytes, trace elements (Addamel™: Cr, Cu, F, Fe, I, Mn, Mo, Se, Zn), and vitamins (Vitalipid®).[(13,25)] After addition of multiple vitamins for injection, use within 24 hours.[(25,32)]

Vitamin E *in Parenteral Nutrition*

Container	Formulation/ Concentration	Temperature			Light		Lipids		Refer.
		Refrig	Room	Body	Exposed	Protected	With	Without	
Bag, Ethylene Vinyl Acetate (EVA)	(a)	6 d	24 hr	n/a	X	X	X	n/a	(36)
	(b)	72 hr	72 hr	72 hr	X	n/a	X	n/a	(35)
	(c)	20 d	n/a	n/a	n/a	X	X	X	(37)
Bag, Polyvinyl Chloride (PVC)	(c)	20 d	n/a	n/a	n/a	X	X	X	(37)
Vial, Glass	(c)	20 d	n/a	n/a	n/a	X	X	X	(37)

Notes

[a] Formulas: amino acids, glucose, lipid emulsion (Intralipid®), electrolytes, vitamins, and trace elements (European products); refrigerated samples were protected from light; stability defined as greater than 80% of initial concentration. Room temperature storage followed 6 d refrigeration.[(36)]

[b] Formulas: amino acids, glucose, lipid emulsion, electrolytes, vitamins, and trace elements (European products).[(35)]

[c] Formulas: amino acids, glucose, lipid emulsion, electrolytes, vitamins (MVI-12®), and trace elements (+/–)[(d)] (European products); stability defined as greater than 80% of initial concentration.[(37)]

[d] (+/–) indicates that sample was mixed both with and without the nutrient.

Vitamin K *in Parenteral Nutrition*

Container	Formulation/ Concentration	Temperature		Light		Lipids		Refer.
		Refrig	Room	Exposed	Protected	With	Without	
Bag, Ethylene Vinyl Acetate (EVA)	(a)	20 d	n/a	n/a	X	X	X	(37)
Bag, Polyvinyl Chloride (PVC)	(a)	20 d	n/a	n/a	X	X	X	(37)
Vial, Glass	(a)	20 d	n/a	n/a	X	X	X	(37)

Notes

[a] Vitamin K1; Formula: amino acids, glucose, lipid emulsion, electrolytes, vitamins (MVI-12®), and trace elements (+/–)[(b)] (European products); stability defined as greater than 80% of initial concentration.[(37)]

[b] (+/–) indicates that sample was mixed both with and without the nutrient.

Zinc *in Parenteral Nutrition*									
		Temperature			Light		Lipids		
Container	Formulation/ Concentration	Refrig	Room	Body	Exposed	Protected	With	Without	Refer.
Bag, Ethylene Vinyl Acetate (EVA)	(a)	7 d	24 hr	n/a	n/a	n/a	X	n/a	(2)
	(b)	7 d	48 hr	n/a	n/a	n/a	X	n/a	(22)
	(c)	7 d	48 hr	n/a	n/a	X	X	n/a	(23)
	(d)	9 d	24 hr	n/a	n/a	X	X	X	(27)
	(e)	21 d	24 hr	n/a	n/a	X	n/a	X	(29)
	(f)	30 d	24 hr	24 hr	X[i]	X[i]	n/a	X	(14)
	(g)	30 d	24 hr	n/a	n/a	n/a	X	n/a	(24)
Bag, Multilayer Polypropylene[h]	(h)	7 d	48 hr	n/a	n/a	n/a	X	n/a	(13)(25)

Special Considerations: Stability studies assessed changes to characteristics of the admixture over time (pH, precipitation, visual inspection, changes to size and distribution of lipid particles), and did not measure the content of each trace element.

Notes

[a] Formulas: amino acids (Clinisol™, Prosol™, Travasol®), dextrose, lipid (SMOFlipid®), electrolytes, and trace elements (Addamel™: Cr, Cu, F, Fe, I, Mn, Mo, Se, Zn).(2)

[b] Formulas: amino acids (Aminosyn®, Plenamine™), dextrose, lipid (SMOFlipid®), electrolytes, and trace elements (Addamel™: Cr, Cu, F, Fe, I, Mn, Mo, Se, Zn).(22)

[c] Formulas: amino acids (Aminoplasmal®), dextrose, lipid (Intralipid®, ClinOleic™), electrolytes, and trace elements (Cr, Cu, Mn, Se, Zn).(23)

[d] Formulas: amino acid solution, dextrose, lipid, electrolytes, and trace elements (Tralement®: Cu, Mn, Se, Zn).(27)

[e] Formulas: amino acids (Aminoven®, Primene™), dextrose, electrolytes, and trace elements (Peditrace™: Cu, F, I, Mn, Se, Zn).(29)

[f] Formulas: amino acids (Aminoven®, Vaminolact®, Primene™), dextrose electrolytes, and trace elements (Peditrace™: Cu, F, I, Mn, Se, Zn).(14)

[g] Formulas: amino acids (Neonutrin), dextrose, lipid (SMOFlipid®), electrolytes, and trace elements (Addamel™: Cr, Cu, F, Fe, I, Mn, Mo, Se, Zn).(24)

[h] Formulas: Kabiven® (RTU three-chamber bag) (amino acids, dextrose, soy-based lipid), electrolytes, and trace elements (Addamel™: Cr, Cu, F, Fe, I, Mn, Mo, Se, Zn).(13,25)

[i] Light exposed for 30 days RF, light protected for 24 hours at 37°C.(14)

REFERENCES

1. USP <797> Pharmaceutical compounding - sterile preparations. In: *2020: USP Compounding Compendium*. Rockville, MD: The United States Pharmacopeial Convention; 2020:40-74.
2. SMOFlipid® with Clinisol™ 15%, Prosol™ 20%, or Travasol® 10% All-in-One Parenteral Nutrition Compatibility Information (Ref#: N/A) [personal communication]. Lake Zurich, IL: Fresenius Kabi USA, LLC.; 2020:10.
3. Pertkiewicz M, Cosslett A, Mühlebach S. Basics in clinical nutrition: Stability of parenteral nutrition admixtures. *E-spen, Eur J Clin Nutr Metab*. 2009; 4.
4. Forchielli ML, Bonoli A, Stancari A, et al. Do carnitine and extra trace elements change stability of paediatric parenteral nutrition admixtures? *Clin Nutr*. 2019; 38(5):2369-74.
5. Hardy G, Puzovic M. Formulation, stability, and administration of parenteral nutrition with new lipid emulsions. *Nutr Clin Pract*. 2009; 24(5):616-25.
6. SMOFlipid® with Clinisol™ 15% All-in-One Parenteral Nutrition Compatibility Information (Ref#: N/A) [personal communication]. Lake Zurich, IL: Fresenius Kabi USA, LLC.; 2020:3.
7. Clinolipid™ (Olive Oil and Soybean Oil Lipid Emulsion) Injection [package insert]. Deerfield, IL: Baxter Healthcare Corporation; November 2020.
8. USP <1191> Stability considerations in dispensing practice. In: *2020: USP Compounding Compendium*. Rockville, MD: The United States Pharmacopeial Convention; 2020:435-9.
9. Bing CD. Applying stability and sterility limits to beyond use dating. *Infusion*. 2017; 23(4):39-44.
10. Mirtallo JM, Ayers P, Boullata J, et al. ASPEN Lipid Injectable Emulsion Safety Recommendations, Part 1: background and adult considerations. *Nutr Clin Pract*. 2020; 35(5): 769-82.
11. The United States Pharmacopeial Convention. *USP Compounding Standards and Beyond-Use Dates (BUDs) Fact Sheet*; 2019. https://www.usp.org/sites/default/files/usp/document/our-work/compounding/usp-bud-factsheet.pdf (accessed 2020 June).
12. Bing CD. Storage and beyond-use dating. In: Buchanan EC, Schneider PJ, Forrey RA eds. *Compounding Sterile Preparations*. 4th ed. Bethesda, MD: American Society of Health-System Pharmacists; 2017:213-26.
13. Kabiven® Container Material Information Letter (Ref#: N/A) [personal communication]. Lake Zurich, IL: Fresenius Kabi USA, LLC.; 2020:2.
14. Watrobska-Swietlikowska D. Compatibility of maximum inorganic and organic calcium and phosphate content in neonatal parenteral solutions. *Sci Rep*. 2019; 9(1):10525.
15. The United States Pharmacopeial Convention. United States Pharmacopeia Commentary, *USP 42-NF 37*, Second Supplement: Master Formulation Records and Compounding Records. Rockville, MD; 2019:159-63.
16. Institute for Safe Medication Practices (ISMP). *ISMP Guidelines for Safe Preparation of Compounded Sterile Preparations*; 2016. https://www.ismp.org/guidelines/sterile-compounding (accessed 2021 February).

17. Boullata JI, Gilbert K, Sacks G, et al. A.S.P.E.N. clinical guidelines: parenteral nutrition ordering, order review, compounding, labeling, and dispensing. *JPEN J Parenter Enteral Nutr.* 2014; 38(3):334-77.
18. American Society of Health-System Pharmacists. ASHP guidelines on compounding sterile preparations. *Am J Health Syst Pharm.* 2014; 71(2):145-66.
19. Ayers P, Adams S, Boullata J, et al. A.S.P.E.N. parenteral nutrition safety consensus recommendations. *JPEN J Parenter Enteral Nutr.* 2014; 38(3):296-333.
20. O'Grady NP, Alexander M, Burns LA, et al. Summary of recommendations: guidelines for the prevention of intravascular catheter-related infections. *Clin Infect Dis.* 2011; 52(9):1087-99.
21. DiStefano JE, Mitrano FP, Baptista RJ, et al. Long-term stability of famotidine 20 mg/L in a total parenteral nutrient solution. *Am J Hosp Pharm.* 1989; 46(11):2333-5.
22. SMOFlipid® with Aminosyn® 15% or Plenamine™ 15% All-in-One Parenteral Nutrition Compatibility Information (Ref#: N/A) [personal communication]. Lake Zurich, IL: Fresenius Kabi USA, LLC.; 2020:3.
23. Balet A, Cardona D, Jane S, et al. Effects of multilayered bags vs ethylvinyl-acetate bags on oxidation of parenteral nutrition. *JPEN J Parenter Enteral Nutr.* 2004; 28(2):85-91.
24. Janu M, Brodska H, Vecka M, et al. Comparison of long-term stability of parenteral all-in-one admixtures containing new lipid emulsions prepared under hospital pharmacy conditions. *Medicina (Kaunas).* 2011; 47(6):323-33.
25. Activated Kabiven® with Electrolyte Additions Information (Ref#: N/A) [personal communication]. Lake Zurich, IL: Fresenius Kabi USA, LLC.; 2020:2.
26. Hensrud DD, Burritt MF, Hall LG. Stability of heparin anticoagulant activity over time in parenteral nutrition solutions. *JPEN J Parenter Enteral Nutr.* 1996; 20(3):219-21.
27. Tralement® (trace elements injection 4*, USP) [package insert]. Shirley, NY: American Regent, Inc.; July 2020.
28. Foinard A, Perez M, Décaudin B, et al. Heparin stability in parenteral nutrition bags prepared in a neonatal ICU. *Crit Care.* 2014; 18(Suppl 1):P96-P96.
29. Watrobska-Swietlikowska D, Szlagatys-Sidorkiewicz A, Luszkiewicz K. Evaluation of physical stability of all in one parenteral admixtures for pediatric home care with high electrolytes concentrations. *Nutr Hosp.* 2014; 31(1):236-43.
30. Kwong KW, Tsallas G. Dilute iron dextran formulation for addition to parenteral nutrient solutions. *Am J Hosp Pharm.* 1980; 37(2):206-10.
31. Tu YH, Knox NL, Biringer JM, et al. Compatibility of iron dextran with total nutrient admixtures. *Am J Hosp Pharm.* 1992; 49(9):2233-5.
32. Infuvite® Adult (Multiple Vitamins) Injection [package insert]. Boucherville, Qc, Canada: Sandoz Canada, Inc.; March 2016.
33. van der Horst A, Martens HJ, de Goede PN. Analysis of water-soluble vitamins in total parenteral nutrition solution by high pressure liquid chromatography. *Pharm Weekbl Sci.* 1989; 11(5):169-74.
34. Skouroliakou M, Kountouri A, Hatziantoniou S, et al. Physicochemical stability assessment of all-in-one parenteral emulsion for neonates containing SMOFlipid. *Eur J Hosp Pharm.* 2012; 19:514-18.
35. Dupertuis YM, Morch A, Fathi M, et al. Physical characteristics of total parenteral nutrition bags significantly affect the stability of vitamins C and B1: a controlled prospective study. *JPEN J Parenter Enteral Nutr.* 2002; 26(5):310-6.
36. Dahl GB, Jeppsson RI, Tengborn HJ. Vitamin stability in a TPN mixture stored in an EVA plastic bag. *J Clin Hosp Pharm.* 1986; 11(4):271-9.
37. Billion-Rey F, Guillaumont M, Frederich A, et al. Stability of fat-soluble vitamins A (retinol palmitate), E (tocopherol acetate), and K1 (phylloquinone) in total parenteral nutrition at home. *JPEN J Parenter Enteral Nutr.* 1993; 17(1):56-60.
38. Ribeiro DO, Pinto DC, Lima LM, et al. Chemical stability study of vitamins thiamine, riboflavin, pyridoxine and ascorbic acid in parenteral nutrition for neonatal use. *Nutr J.* 2011;10:47.
39. Stawny M, Gostynska A, Olijarczyk R, et al. Stability studies of parenteral nutrition with a high dose of vitamin C. *J Oncol Pharm Pract.* 2020; 26(8):1894-902.
40. Dupertuis YM, Ramseyer S, Fathi M, et al. Assessment of ascorbic acid stability in different multilayered parenteral nutrition bags: critical influence of the bag wall material. *JPEN J Parenter Enteral Nutr.* 2005; 29(2):125-30.
41. Bullock L, Fitzgerald JF, Glick MR. Stability of famotidine 20 and 50 mg/L in total nutrient admixtures. *Am J Hosp Pharm.* 1989; 46(11):2326-9.
42. Shea BF, Souney PF. Stability of famotidine in a 3-in-1 total nutrient admixture. *DICP.* 1990; 24(3):232-5.
43. Bullock L, Fitzgerald JF, Glick MR, et al. Stability of famotidine 20 and 40 mg/L and amino acids in total parenteral nutrient solutions. *Am J Hosp Pharm.* 1989; 46(11):2321-5.
44. Hatton J, Luer M, Hirsch J, et al. Histamine receptor antagonists and lipid stability in total nutrient admixtures. *JPEN J Parenter Enteral Nutr.* 1994; 18(4):308-12. Erratum in: *JPEN J Parenter Enteral Nutr.* 1994; 18(6):556.
45. Montoro JB, Pou L, Salvador P, et al. Stability of famotidine 20 and 40 mg/L in total nutrient admixtures. *Am J Hosp Pharm.* 1989; 46(11):2329-32.

PART II

DRUG MONOGRAPHS

Acetaminophen

Storage Conditions

						Temperature			Post-thaw Temp			
	Drug Manufacturer	Concentration	Diluents	Osmolality (mOsm/kg)	pH	Room	Refrig	Frozen	Room	Refrig	Body Temp	Refer.
CONTAINER												
Bag, Plastic (Unspecified)	CAD	10 mg/mL	Undiluted	[a]	[b]	6 hr	n/a	n/a	n/a	n/a	n/a	(1)
Syringe, Polypropylene	CAD	10 mg/mL	Undiluted	[a]	5.77	84 hr	n/a	n/a	n/a	n/a	n/a	(5)
Vial, Glass	CAD	10 mg/mL	Undiluted	[a]	[b]	6 hr	n/a	n/a	n/a	n/a	n/a	(1)
	BMS	10 mg/mL[c]	Undiluted[c]	n/a	3.7–6.6	48 hr	n/a	n/a	n/a	n/a	n/a	(3)
	CAD	10 mg/mL	Undiluted	[a]	5.77	84 hr	n/a	n/a	n/a	n/a	n/a	(5)

Flush Compatibility: Sodium chloride 0.9%, heparin.(2)

Special Considerations: Store at room temperature; do not refrigerate or freeze.(2) Acetaminophen is known internationally as paracetamol.(4)

Notes

[a] Osmolality of undiluted solution is approximately 290 mOsm/kg.(1)

[b] pH of undiluted solution is approximately 5.5.(1)

[c] Solution contained ketoprofen (SAA) 100 mg which was diluted and added to the Perfalgan (BMS) 1 gm/100 mL ready-to-use glass vial.(3)

REFERENCES

1. Ofirmev® (Acetaminophen) Injection [package insert]. Hazelwood, MO: Mallinckrodt Hospital Products; March 2018.
2. ASHP's Interactive Handbook on Injectable Drugs, 2020. Bethesda, MD: American Society of Health-System Pharmacists; Accessed May 2020.
3. Kambia NK, Luyckx M, Dine T, et al. Stability and compatibility of paracetamol injection admixed with ketoprofen. *Eur J Hosp Pharm Science*. 2006; 12(4):81–84.
4. Allen LV, Remington JP. Remington, the science and practice of pharmacy. 22nd ed. London; Philadelphia: Pharmaceutical Press; 2013:1193.
5. Kwiatkowski JL, Johnson CE, Wagner DS. Extended stability of intravenous acetaminophen in syringes and opened vials. *Am J Health-Syst Pharm*. 2012; 69:1999–2001.

DOI 10.37573/9781585286720.001

Acyclovir Sodium

Storage Conditions

						Temperature			Post-thaw Temp			
	Drug Manufacturer	Concentration	Diluents	Osmolality (mOsm/kg)	pH	Room	Refrig	Frozen	Room	Refrig	Body Temp	Refer.
CONTAINER												
Bag, Ethylene Vinyl Acetate (EVA)	WEL	2.5, 5 mg/mL	NS	n/a	[h]	28 d	n/a	n/a	n/a	n/a	n/a	(1)
Bag, Polyethylene	GW	5 mg/mL	D5W, NS	289, 316	10.12	24 hr	24 hr	n/a	n/a	n/a	n/a	(1)
Bag, Polyolefin	HOS, GSK	5 mg/mL	NS	[c]	[h]	n/a	21 d[b]	90 d	n/a	21 d[a][b]	n/a	(4)
Bag, Polyvinyl Chloride (PVC)	BW	1 mg/mL	D5W	[c]	[h]	5 wk[d]	5 wk[b]	n/a	n/a	n/a	n/a	(1)
	BW	1, 7, 10 mg/mL	NS	[c]	[h]	7 d[d]	5 wk[b]	n/a	n/a	n/a	n/a	(1)
	BW	5 mg/mL	NS	316	[h]	37 d	37 d[b]	n/a	n/a	n/a	n/a	(1)
	BW	5 mg/mL	D5W	289	[h]	37 d	37 d[b]	n/a	n/a	n/a	n/a	(1)
	BW	7 mg/mL	D5W	278	[h]	28 d[d]	5 wk[b]	n/a	n/a	n/a	n/a	(1)
	BW	10 mg/mL	D5W	[c]	[h]	21 d[d]	5 wk[b]	n/a	n/a	n/a	n/a	(1)
	GW	5 mg/mL	D5W, NS	289, 316	[h]	24 hr	24 hr	n/a	n/a	n/a	n/a	(1)
	WEL	2.5, 5 mg/mL	NS	[c]	[h]	28 d[e]	n/a	n/a	n/a	n/a	n/a	(1)
Syringe, Polypropylene	APP	10 mg/mL	NS	n/a	10.4-10.7	30 d	[i]	n/a	n/a	n/a	n/a	(1)(8)
Vial, Glass	GW	5 mg/mL	D5W, NS	289, 316	[h]	24 hr	24 hr	n/a	n/a	n/a	n/a	(1)
OTHER INFUSION CONTAINERS												
Dosi-Fuser® (Leventon)	WEL	1-10 mg/mL	D5W, NS	n/a	n/a	4 d[f]	n/a	n/a	n/a	n/a	n/a	(7)
	WEL	10 mg/mL	D5W, NS	n/a	n/a	29 d[f]	n/a	n/a	n/a	n/a	n/a	(7)
Easypump® ST/LT (B. Braun)	UN	10 mg/mL	NS	n/a	n/a	5 d	n/a	n/a	n/a	n/a	n/a	(6)
Homepump Eclipse® / Homepump® (Halyard)	UN	10 mg/mL	NS	n/a	[h]	10 d	30 d[b]	n/a	n/a	n/a	n/a	(3)
INTERMATE™ (Baxter)[g]	WEL	1-10 mg/mL	D5W, NS	n/a	[h]	4 d	n/a	n/a	n/a	n/a	n/a	(2)
	WEL	10 mg/mL	D5W, NS	n/a	[h]	29 d	n/a	n/a	n/a	n/a	n/a	(2)
SMARTeZ® (Progressive Medical)	UN	10 mg/mL	NS	n/a	n/a	5 d	n/a	n/a	n/a	n/a	n/a	(5)

DOI 10.37573/9781585286720.002

Flush Compatibility: Sodium chloride 0.9%.[(1)]

Special Considerations: Do not use bacteriostatic water for injection containing parabens or benzyl alcohol for reconstitution. Special attention must be paid to the drug's potential for precipitation. Precipitation depends on preparation, storage conditions, concentration, pH, and diluent.

Notes

[a] Stored under refrigerated conditions after warming in a microwave.

[b] Refrigeration may cause precipitation; product will resolubilize at room temperature but should be used immediately due to reformation of microprecipitates. Physical instability is the principal limitation to long-term storage due to persistent subvisual microprecipitates after as few as 7 d.[(1)]

[c] Acyclovir 10 mg/mL has an osmolality of 342 and 316 mOsm/kg in NS and D5W respectively; at 5 mg/mL osmolality is 316 and 289 mOsm/kg in NS and D5W respectively.[(1)]

[d] Protected from light.[(1)]

[e] Subvisible particulates increase significantly after 7 days due to interaction with PVC containers.[(1)]

[f] Manufacturer(s) extrapolated data from other sources.

[g] INTERMATE™/INFUSOR™ Portable Elastomeric Infusion System devices are no longer available in the United States.

[h] pH of reconstituted solution is approximately 11.[(1)]

[i] Precipitate formed within 5 d stored at 5°C.[(1)]

REFERENCES

1. ASHP's Interactive Handbook on Injectable Drugs, 2020. Bethesda, MD: American Society of Health-System Pharmacists; Accessed May 2020.
2. Stabforum - Stability Database: Acyclovir, Ontario, Canada: Baxter Healthcare; Accessed February 2021.
3. *Stability Data for Drugs Using Homepump Disposable Ambulatory Infusion Systems (MK-00314 rev 3)*, 2015. Alpharetta, GA: Halyard Health; Updated June 2015.
4. Dewulf J, Galanti L, Godet M, et al. Long-term stability of acyclovir in 0.9% NaCl infusion polyolefin bags at 5+/-3 degrees C after freeze-thaw treatment: a generic product versus the brand name. *Ann Pharm Fr*. 2015; 73(2):108–13.
5. *SMARTeZ® - Stability Data for Drugs Using Elastomeric Infusion Pumps*, 2020. Fenton, MO: Progressive Medical, Inc.; Updated May 2020.
6. *Drug Stability for Easypump® ST/LT*, 2020. Bethlehem, PA: B. Braun USA; Updated June 2020.
7. *Drug Stability Table - Dosi-Fuser® Elastomeric Pump (S-CL-00-001v16)*, 2021. Barcelona, Spain: Leventon SAU; Updated May 2021.
8. Ling J, Gupta VD. Stability of acyclovir sodium after reconstitution in 0.9% sodium chloride inection and storage in polypropylene syringes for pediatric use. *Int J Pharm Compd*. 2001 Jan-Feb;5(1):75-7. PMID: 23981803.

ADO-Trastuzumab Emtansine

Storage Conditions

	Drug Manufacturer	Concentration	Diluents	Osmolality (mOsm/kg)	pH	Temperature			Post-thaw Temp			
						Room	Refrig	Frozen	Room	Refrig	Body Temp	Refer.
CONTAINER												
Bag, Polyolefin	GEN	Various[(a)]	NS	n/a	n/a	n/a	24 hr	n/a	n/a	n/a	n/a	(1)(2)
Bag, Polyvinyl Chloride (PVC)	GEN	Various[(a)]	NS	n/a	n/a	n/a	24 hr	n/a	n/a	n/a	n/a	(1)(2)
Vial, Glass	GEN	20 mg/mL	SWFI	n/a	5	n/a	24 hr	n/a	n/a	n/a	n/a	(1)

Flush Compatibility: Sodium chloride 0.9%.[(1)]

Special Considerations: Do not mix or dilute with dextrose 5% solution. Do not shake reconstituted vial or infusion solution. Administer IV only with 0.2 or 0.22 micron in-line polyethersulfone (PES) filter. Do not confuse ADO-Trastuzumab Emtansine with Trastuzumab.[(1)]

Notes

[a] Dose diluted in 250 mL sodium chloride 0.9%.[(1)]

REFERENCES

1. Kadcyla® (ADO-Trastuzumab Emtansine) Injection [package insert]. South San Francisco, CA: Genentech, Inc.; October 2020.
2. Kadcyla® Medication Information Letter (Ref#: 15-015984) [personal communication]. South San Francisco, CA: Genentech, Inc.; 2015:8.

DOI 10.37573/9781585286720.003

Aldesleukin

Storage Conditions

						Temperature			Post-thaw Temp			
	Drug Manufacturer	Concentration	Diluents	Osmolality (mOsm/kg)	pH	Room	Refrig	Frozen	Room	Refrig	Body Temp	Refer.
CONTAINER												
Bag, Polyvinyl Chloride (PVC)	CET	0.005, 0.04 mg/mL[a]	D5W	n/a	[b]	6 d[c]	n/a	n/a	n/a	n/a	n/a	(2)
	CET	0.1-0.5 mg/mL	D5W	n/a	[b]	6 d[c]	n/a	n/a	n/a	n/a	n/a	(2)
Syringe, Plastic (Unspecified)	CET	0.22 mg/mL	D5W	n/a	[b]	n/a	14 d	n/a	n/a	n/a	n/a	(2)
	CET	18 million units/mL	SWFI	n/a	[b]	48 hr	5 d	n/a	n/a	n/a	n/a	(2)
Unspecified	PRO	18 million units/mL (1.1 mg/mL)	SWFI	n/a	[b]	48 hr	48 hr	n/a	n/a	n/a	n/a	(1)
OTHER INFUSION CONTAINERS												
CADD® Cassette (Smiths Medical)	CET	0.005, 0.04 mg/mL[a]	D5W	n/a	[b]	6 d[c]	n/a	n/a	n/a	n/a	n/a	(2)
	CET	0.1-0.5 mg/mL	D5W	n/a	[b]	6 d[c]	n/a	n/a	n/a	n/a	n/a	(2)

Flush Compatibility: D5W.

Special Considerations: Do not mix with sodium chloride 0.9%. Do not use in-line filters. Reconstitution or dilution with NS or BWFI may cause aggregation (deactivation). Do not freeze.[(2)]

Diluted drug concentrations below 0.03 mg/mL or greater than 0.07 mg/mL have shown increased variability in drug delivery and should be avoided. With drug concentration less than 0.03 mg/mL, it is recommended to dilute the dose in D5W that contains albumin human 0.1% to prevent variability in the stability and bioactivity of the drug.[(2)]

Various measurement units have been used and reported for this agent. The International Unit (I.U.) is now the standard measure of activity. Consult current manufacturer's literature for conversion factors.[(2)]

Notes

[a] Albumin human 0.1% added to D5W prior to addition of diluted drug was necessary to maintain physical stability. The albumin human helps keep this agent in its microaggregate state and helps decrease sorption to surfaces.[(2)]

[b] pH of reconstituted product is 7.2-7.8.[(2)]

[c] Solutions stored at 32°C.

DOI 10.37573/9781585286720.004

REFERENCES

1. Proleukin® [package insert]. San Diego, CA: Prometheus Laboratories, Inc.; May 2019.
2. ASHP's Interactive Handbook on Injectable Drugs, 2020. Bethesda, MD: American Society of Health-System Pharmacists; Accessed August 2020.

Alprostadil

Storage Conditions

						Temperature			Post-thaw Temp			
CONTAINER	Drug Manufacturer	Concentration	Diluents	Osmolality (mOsm/kg)	pH	Room	Refrig	Frozen	Room	Refrig	Body Temp	Refer.
Bag, Polyvinyl Chloride (PVC)	PH	11 mcg/mL	NS[a]	n/a	4.6–6.2	n/a	10 d[b]	n/a	n/a	n/a	n/a	(1)
Syringe, Polypropylene	UN	125, 250 mcg/mL	NS	n/a	n/a	n/a	30 d	n/a	n/a	n/a	n/a	(2)
	UN	500 mcg/mL	Undiluted	n/a	n/a	n/a	30 d	n/a	n/a	n/a	n/a	(2)

Flush Compatibility: Sodium chloride 0.9%.

Special Considerations: n/a

Notes

[a] Solution contained 2% ethanol.

[b] Protected from light.

REFERENCES

1. McCluskey SV, Kirkham K, Munson JM. Stability of Alprostadil in 0.9% Sodium Chloride Stored in Polyvinyl Chloride Containers. *Int J Pharm Compd*. 2017; 21(2):150-53.
2. ASHP's Interactive Handbook on Injectable Drugs, 2020. Bethesda, MD: American Society of Health-System Pharmacists; Accessed August 2020.

DOI 10.37573/9781585286720.005

Alteplase

Storage Conditions

						Temperature			Post-thaw Temp			
CONTAINER	Drug Manufacturer	Concentration	Diluents	Osmolality (mOsm/kg)	pH	Room	Refrig	Frozen	Room	Refrig	Body Temp	Refer.
Bag, Polyvinyl Chloride (PVC)	GEN	0.5 mg/mL	D5W, NS	[(b)]	5.0–7.5[(c)]	8 hr	n/a	n/a	n/a	n/a	n/a	(1)(2)
Bag, Unspecified	GEN	0.01 mg/mL	NS	n/a	6.9–7.3[(d)]	24 hr	n/a	n/a	n/a	n/a	n/a	(1)(3)
Syringe, Polypropylene	GEN	0.5, 1, 2 mg/mL	Undiluted	[(b)]	[(a)]	n/a	n/a	14 d[(e)]	n/a	48 hr	n/a	(1)(5)
Unspecified	GEN	0.5 mg/mL[(f)]	D5W, NS	n/a	n/a	24 hr	n/a	n/a	n/a	n/a	n/a	(1)(6)
	GEN	1 mg/mL[(g)]	unspec.	n/a	n/a	24 hr	n/a	n/a	n/a	n/a	n/a	(1)
	GEN	0.5 mg/mL[(h)]	NS	n/a	n/a	24 hr	n/a	n/a	n/a	n/a	n/a	(1)(6)
	GEN	0.5 mg/mL[(i)]	D5W, NS	n/a	n/a	24 hr	n/a	n/a	n/a	n/a	n/a	(1)(6)
Vial, Glass	GEN	0.5 mg/mL	D5W, NS	[(b)]	[(a)]	8 hr	n/a	n/a	n/a	n/a	n/a	(2)
	GEN	1 mg/ml	Undiluted	[(b)]	[(a)]	n/a	n/a	32 d	8 hr	n/a	n/a	(1)(4)

Flush Compatibility: Sodium chloride 0.9%.[(2)]

Special Considerations: Alteplase should be reconstituted with SWFI only; do not use solutions containing preservatives. Use of the accompanying diluent results in a 1-mg/mL concentration.[(1)]

Alteplase may be diluted with an equal volume of sodium chloride 0.9% or dextrose 5% to a 0.5 mg/mL concentration. Dilution to a lower concentration may result in precipitation.[(1)]

Notes

[a] pH of reconstituted solution is 7.3.[(2)]

[b] Osmolality of reconstituted solution is 215 mOsm/kg.[(2)]

[c] Alteplase in solution is stable at pH 5.0 – 7.5.[(1)]

[d] Observed pH remained stable at 6.9 – 7.3 after 24 hours of storage at room temperature.[(3)]

[e] Sample syringes were stored frozen at -70°C and -25°C.[(1,5)]

[f] Solution contained lidocaine HCl 4 mg/mL (AST).

[g] Solution contained eptifibatide 0.75 mg/mL (ME).

[h] Solution contained morphine sulfate 1 mg/mL (WY).

[i] Solution contained nitroglycerin 0.4 mg/mL (ACC).

DOI 10.37573/9781585286720.006

REFERENCES

1. ASHP's Interactive Handbook on Injectable Drugs, 2020. Bethesda, MD: American Society of Health-System Pharmacists; Accessed July 2020.
2. Activase® (Alteplase) Injection [package insert]. South San Francisco, CA: Genentech, Inc.; October 2020.
3. Semba CP, Weck S, Patapoff T. Alteplase: stability and bioactivity after dilution in normal saline solution. *J Vasc Interv Radiol*. 2003; 14:99-102.
4. Generali J, Cada DJ. Alteplase (t-PA) Bolus: Occluded Catheters. *Hosp Pharm*. 2001; 36(1):93-103.
5. Davis SN, Vermeulen L, Banton J, et al. Activity and dosage of alteplase dilution for clearing occlusions of venous-access devices. *Am J Health Syst Pharm*. 2000; 57(11):1039-45.
6. Lam XM, Ward CA. Stability and activity of alteplase with injectable drugs commonly used in cardiac therapy. *Am J Health-Syst Pharm*. 1995; 52:1904-9.

Amikacin Sulfate

Storage Conditions

	Drug Manufacturer	Concentration	Diluents	Osmolality (mOsm/kg)	pH	Temperature			Post-thaw Temp			
						Room	Refrig	Frozen	Room	Refrig	Body Temp	Refer.
CONTAINER												
Bag, Polyvinyl Chloride (PVC)	BR	20 mg/mL	D5W	n/a	[e]	n/a	n/a	30 d	24 hr	n/a	n/a	(1)
Syringe, Polypropylene	BR	187.5 mg/mL	NS	n/a	[e]	48 hr	n/a	n/a	n/a	n/a	n/a	(1)
Unspecified	BR	0.25, 5 mg/mL	NS	[a]	[e]	24 hr	60 d	30 d	n/a	n/a	n/a	(1)
	BR	0.25, 5 mg/mL	D5W	[b]	[e]	24 hr	60 d	30 d	n/a	n/a	n/a	(1)
Vial, Glass	BMS	50 mg/mL	NS	n/a	n/a	n/a	n/a	6 m	n/a	n/a	n/a	(2)
OTHER INFUSION CONTAINERS												
Dosi-Fuser® (Leventon)	UN	10 mg/mL	D5W, NS	n/a	[e]	48 hr	28 d	31 d	n/a	n/a	n/a	(6)
	BMS	20 mg/mL	D5W, NS	n/a	[e]	24 hr	28 d[c]	30 d[c]	n/a	n/a	n/a	(6)
Easypump® ST/LT (B. Braun)	UN	10, 20 mg/mL	NS	n/a	[e]	48 hr	15 d	n/a	n/a	n/a	n/a	(5)
Homepump Eclipse® / Homepump® (Halyard)	UN	10 mg/mL	NS	n/a	[e]	24 hr	10 d	30 d	n/a	n/a	n/a	(4)
	UN	10–20 mg/mL	NS	n/a	[e]	24 hr	28 d	n/a	n/a	n/a	n/a	(4)
INTERMATE™ (Baxter)[g]	BMS	0.25–20 mg/mL	D5W, NS	n/a	[e]	48 hr[f]	28 d	n/a	n/a	n/a	n/a	(3)
	BMS	20 mg/mL	D5W, NS	n/a	[e]	n/a	n/a	30 d	24 hr[d]	n/a	n/a	(3)
SMARTeZ® (Progressive Medical)	UN	10 mg/mL	NS	n/a	[e]	24 hr[c]	7 d[c]	n/a	n/a	n/a	n/a	(7)

Flush Compatibility: Sodium chloride 0.9%. Incompatible with heparin; immediate precipitation occurs.[1]

Special Considerations: n/a

DOI 10.37573/9781585286720.007

Notes

[a] Amikacin sulfate 5 mg/mL in NS has a calculated osmolality of 349 mOsm/kg.[(1)]

[b] Amikacin sulfate 5 mg/mL in D5W has a calculated osmolality of 319 mOsm/kg.[(1)]

[c] Manufacturer(s) extrapolated data from other sources.

[d] Storage for 30 days at -20°C followed by 24 hours at 25°C.[(3)]

[e] pH of undiluted solution is 3.5-5.5.[(1)]

[f] Storage for 28 days at 2-8°C, followed by 48 hours at 25°C.[(3)]

[g] INTERMATE™/INFUSOR™ Portable Elastomeric Infusion System devices are no longer available in the United States.

REFERENCES

1. ASHP's Interactive Handbook on Injectable Drugs, 2020. Bethesda, MD: American Society of Health-System Pharmacists; Accessed May 2020.
2. Chedru-Legros V, Fines-Guyon M, Cherel A, et al. In vitro stability of fortified ophthalmic antibiotics stored at -20 degrees C for 6 months. *Cornea*. 2010; 29(7):807-11.
3. Stabforum - Stability Database: Amikacin, Ontario, Canada: Baxter Healthcare; Accessed December 2020.
4. *Stability Data for Drugs Using Homepump Disposable Ambulatory Infusion Systems (MK-00314 rev 3)*, 2015. Alpharetta, GA: Halyard Health; Updated June 2015.
5. *Drug Stability for Easypump® ST/LT*, 2020. Bethlehem, PA: B. Braun USA; Updated June 2020.
6. *Drug Stability Table - Dosi-Fuser® Elastomeric Pump (S-CL-00-001v16)*, 2021. Barcelona, Spain: Leventon SAU; Updated May 2021.
7. *SMARTeZ® - Stability Data for Drugs Using Elastomeric Infusion Pumps*, 2020. Fenton, MO: Progressive Medical, Inc.; Updated May 2020.

Aminocaproic Acid

Storage Conditions

						Temperature			Post-thaw Temp			
	Drug Manufacturer	Concentration	Diluents	Osmolality (mOsm/kg)	pH	Room	Refrig	Frozen	Room	Refrig	Body Temp	Refer.
CONTAINER												
Bag, Polyvinyl Chloride (PVC)	BA	10, 100 mg/mL	NS, D5W	n/a	6–7.6	7 d	7 d	n/a	n/a	n/a	n/a	(1)

Flush Compatibility: Sodium chloride 0.9%.

Special Considerations: Aminocaproic acid injection is available with benzyl alcohol 0.9% as a preservative and also in preservative-free form.[1]

REFERENCE

1. ASHP's Interactive Handbook on Injectable Drugs, 2020. Bethesda, MD: American Society of Health-System Pharmacists; Accessed August 2020.

DOI 10.37573/9781585286720.008

Amiodarone Hydrochloride

Storage Conditions

						Temperature			Post-thaw Temp			
	Drug Manufacturer	Concentration	Diluents	Osmolality (mOsm/kg)	pH	Room	Refrig	Frozen	Room	Refrig	Body Temp	Refer.
CONTAINER												
Bag, Polyolefin	BED	1 mg/mL	D5W	n/a	[b]	24 hr	n/a	n/a	n/a	n/a	n/a	(3)(2)
Syringe, Polypropylene	SAN	25 mg/mL[d]	D5W	n/a	3.7–4	n/a	28 d[a]	n/a	n/a	n/a	n/a	(1)
Vial, Glass	LZ	0.6 mg/mL	D5W	n/a	n/a	5 d	n/a	n/a	n/a	n/a	n/a	(3)
	WY	2 mg/mL	D5W	n/a	n/a	32 d[c]	32 d[c]	n/a	n/a	n/a	n/a	(3)

Flush Compatibility: D5W.[3]

Special Considerations: Use only glass or polyolefin bags to administer infusions exceeding 2 hours due to adsorption to PVC as well as leaching of plasticizers. The use of evacuated glass containers is not recommended since the buffer in these containers may cause precipitation of amiodarone. Dilute only with D5W due to conflicting stability data in other solutions.[3] Protect from light until time of administration. Preparations do not need to be protected from light during administration. When possible, administer through a central venous catheter. Use an in-line filter during administration.[4]

Notes

[a] Protected from light.

[b] pH of undiluted solution is 4.08.[3]

[c] In amber glass container.

[d] Amiodarone preparations with concentrations greater than 3 mg/mL are associated with a high incidence of peripheral vein phlebitis; however, preparations with concentrations less than or equal to 2.5 mg/mL appear to be less irritating. Amiodarone preparations that will infuse longer than 1 hr should not exceed concentrations greater than 2 mg/mL unless a central venous catheter is used.[4]

REFERENCES

1. Lardinois B, Dimitriou A, Delcave C, et al. Evaluation of the Physicochemical Stability of Amiodarone Hydrochloride in Syringes for the Intensive Care Unit. *Int J Pharm Compd*. 2019; 23(2):163-66.
2. Aloumanis V, Ben M, Kupiec TC, et al. Drug Compatibility with a New Generation of VISIV Polyolefin Infusion Solution Containers. *Int J Pharm Compd*. 2009; 13(2):162-5.
3. ASHP's Interactive Handbook on Injectable Drugs, 2020. Bethesda, MD: American Society of Health-System Pharmacists; Accessed June 2020.
4. Nexterone™ (Amiodarone Hydrochloride) Injection [package insert]. Deerfield, IL: Baxter Healthcare Corporation; November 2016.

DOI 10.37573/9781585286720.009

Amphotericin B (Conventional)

Storage Conditions

						Temperature			Post-thaw Temp			
	Drug Manufacturer	Concentration	Diluents	Osmolality (mOsm/kg)	pH	Room	Refrig	Frozen	Room	Refrig	Body Temp	Refer.
CONTAINER												
Bag, Polyolefin	ERS	0.47, 0.66, 0.75 mg/mL	D5W	n/a	n/a	24 hr	n/a	n/a	n/a	n/a	n/a	(4)
Bag, Polyvinyl Chloride (PVC)	BMS	0.05, 0.5 mg/mL	D5W	n/a	[c]	24 hr	n/a	n/a	n/a	n/a	n/a	(1)
	SQ	0.1 mg/mL	D5W	[a]	[c]	24 hr[d]	n/a	n/a	n/a	n/a	n/a	(1)
	SQ	0.1, 0.25 mg/mL	D5W	[a]	[c]	n/a	5 wk[b]	n/a	n/a	n/a	n/a	(3)
	SQ	0.2, 0.5, 1 mg/mL	D5W	n/a	[c]	5 d	5 d	n/a	n/a	n/a	n/a	(1)
OTHER INFUSION CONTAINERS												
Dosi-Fuser® (Leventon)	SQ	0.2-0.5 mg/mL	D5W	n/a	[c]	n/a	10 d[f]	n/a	n/a	n/a	n/a	(6)
Easypump® ST/LT (B. Braun)	UN	0.1, 0.5, 2 mg/mL	D5W	[a]	[c]	24 hr	4 d[e]	n/a	n/a	n/a	n/a	(5)
INTERMATE™ (Baxter)[g]	SQ	0.2-0.5 mg/mL	D5W	n/a	[c]	n/a	10 d	n/a	n/a	n/a	n/a	(2)

Flush Compatibility: D5W. Incompatible with sodium chloride 0.9% and heparin.[(1)]

Special Considerations: If filtration is necessary, the filter pore size must be 1 micron or larger. Protect from light. Do not interchange amphotericin B (conventional) with other amphotericin product salts or formulations.

Notes

[a] A 0.1 mg/mL solution in D5W is 256 mOsm/kg.[(1)]

[b] Protected from light.[(3)]

[c] pH of 0.1 mg/mL in D5W is 5.7.[(1)]

[d] Stored protected from light and exposed to fluorescent light.[(1)]

[e] Susceptible to crystallization when refrigerated.[(5)]

[f] Manufacturer(s) extrapolated data from other sources.[(6)]

[g] INTERMATE™/INFUSOR™ Portable Elastomeric Infusion System devices are no longer available in the United States.

DOI 10.37573/9781585286720.010

REFERENCES

1. ASHP's Interactive Handbook on Injectable Drugs, 2020. Bethesda, MD: American Society of Health-System Pharmacists; Accessed August 2020.
2. Stabforum - Stability Database: Amphotericin B (Conventional), Ontario, Canada: Baxter Healthcare; Accessed January 2021.
3. Mitrano FP, Outman WR, Baptista RJ, et al. Chemical and visual stability of amphotericin B in 5% dextrose injection stored at 4 degrees C for 35 days. *Am J Hosp Pharm*. 1991; 48(12):2635-7.
4. Kintzel PE, Kennedy PE. Stability of amphotericin B in 5% dextrose injection at 25 degrees C. *Am J Hosp Pharm*. 1991; 48(8):1681.
5. *Drug Stability for Easypump® ST/LT*, 2020. Bethlehem, PA: B. Braun USA; Updated June 2020.
6. *Drug Stability Table - Dosi-Fuser® Elastomeric Pump (S-CL-00-001v16)*, 2021. Barcelona, Spain: Leventon SAU; Updated May 2021.

Amphotericin B (Lipid Complex)

Storage Conditions

						Temperature			Post-thaw Temp			
	Drug Manufacturer	Concentration	Diluents	Osmolality (mOsm/kg)	pH	Room	Refrig	Frozen	Room	Refrig	Body Temp	Refer.
CONTAINER												
Bag, Polyolefin	ZNS	0.4, 0.8, 2 mg/mL	D5W	n/a	[b]	7 d[c]	7 d[c]	n/a	n/a	n/a	n/a	(3)
Bag, Unspecified	LB	1 mg/mL	D5W	n/a	[b]	6 hr[a]	48 hr	n/a	n/a	n/a	n/a	(4)
Unspecified	LB	1 mg/mL	D5W	n/a	[b]	n/a	10 d	n/a	n/a	n/a	n/a	(1)

Flush Compatibility: D5W; incompatible with sodium chloride 0.9% and heparin.(2)

Special Considerations: Use an 18-gauge needle to withdraw required drug amount from drug vial. Use 5-micron filter needle supplied with drug vial to transfer drug from sterile syringe to IV bag containing D5W. Each 5-micron filter needle may be used to filter up to four (4) drug vials. Do not administer with an inline filter. Admixtures of amphotericin B lipid complex in D5W should not be frozen.(2) Do not interchange Amphotericin B Lipid Complex (Abelcet®) with other amphotericin product salts or formulations.

Notes

[a] Stable for 48 hr refrigerated followed by 6 hr at room temperature.

[b] pH of undiluted product is 5-7.(2)

[c] Protected from light.

REFERENCES

1. Abelcet® Medication Information Letter (Ref#: N/A) [personal communication]. Gaithersburg, MD: Sigma-Tau Pharmaceuticals, Inc.; 2012:4.
2. ASHP's Interactive Handbook on Injectable Drugs, 2020. Bethesda, MD: American Society of Health-System Pharmacists; Accessed August 2020.
3. Vanneaux V, Proust V, Cheron M, et al. A physical and chemical stability study of amphotericin B lipid complexes (Abelcet) after dilution in dextrose 5%. *Eur J Hosp Pharm Science*. 2007; 13(1):10-13.
4. Abelcet® (Amphotericin B Lipid Complex Injection) [package insert]. Gaithersburg, MD: Leadiant Biosciences, Inc.; November 2019.

DOI 10.37573/9781585286720.011

Amphotericin B (Liposomal)

Storage Conditions

	Drug Manufacturer	Concentration	Diluents	Osmolality (mOsm/kg)	pH	Temperature Room	Temperature Refrig	Temperature Frozen	Post-thaw Temp Room	Post-thaw Temp Refrig	Body Temp	Refer.
CONTAINER												
Bag, Polyolefin	ASP	0.2 mg/mL	D5W	n/a	[b]	24 hr[c]	11 d[a]	n/a	n/a	n/a	n/a	(2)
	ASP	0.2 mg/mL	D10W	n/a	[b]	n/a	48 hr[a]	n/a	n/a	n/a	n/a	(2)
	ASP	2 mg/mL	D5W	n/a	[b]	24 hr[c]	14 d[a]	n/a	n/a	n/a	n/a	(2)
	ASP	2 mg/mL	D10W, D20W, D25W	n/a	[b]	n/a	48 hr[a]	n/a	n/a	n/a	n/a	(2)
Bag, Polyvinyl Chloride (PVC)	ASP	0.5 mg/mL	D5W	n/a	[b]	n/a	14 d[a]	n/a	n/a	n/a	n/a	(2)
	ASP	2 mg/mL	D5W	n/a	[b]	n/a	14 d[a]	n/a	n/a	n/a	n/a	(2)
Syringe, Polyethylene	ASP	4 mg/mL	SWFI	n/a	[b]	n/a	14 d[a]	n/a	n/a	n/a	n/a	(2)
Syringe, Polypropylene,	ASP	4 mg/mL	SWFI	n/a	[b]	n/a	14 d[a]	n/a	n/a	n/a	n/a	(2)
Vial, Glass	ASP	4 mg/mL	SWFI	n/a	[b]	n/a	14 d[a]	n/a	n/a	n/a	n/a	(1)(2)
OTHER INFUSION CONTAINERS												
Homepump Eclipse® / Homepump® (Halyard)	ASP	0.2 mg/mL	D5W	n/a	[b]	n/a	7 d[a]	n/a	n/a	n/a	n/a	(2)
	ASP	2 mg/mL	D5W	n/a	[b]	n/a	14 d[a]	n/a	n/a	n/a	n/a	(2)

Flush Compatibility: Flush administration line with D5W before and after administration. Sodium chloride 0.9% and bacteriostatic agents may cause precipitation leading to occlusion.[1]

Special Considerations: Do not interchange Amphotericin B Liposome for injection (AmBisome®) with other amphotericin product salts or formulations. Do not freeze.[1]

The volume used to prepare a dose must be filtered through a 5-micron filter as it is added to the final container. Use a new filter with each vial. May administer through an in-line membrane filter with a mean pore diameter not less than 1.0 micron.[1]

Notes

[a] Protected from light.

[b] pH of suspension following reconstitution with SWFI to 4 mg/mL is 5-6.[1]

[c] Exposed to fluorescent light.

DOI 10.37573/9781585286720.012

REFERENCES

1. AmBisome® (Amphotericin B) Liposome for Injection [package insert]. Northbrook, IL: Astellas Pharma US, Inc.; February 2019.
2. AmBisome® Medication Information Letter (Ref#: 00021716) [personal communication]. Northbrook, IL: Astellas Pharma Global Development, Inc.; 3.

Ampicillin Sodium

Storage Conditions

	Drug Manufacturer	Concentration	Diluents	Osmolality (mOsm/kg)	pH	Temperature: Room	Temperature: Refrig	Temperature: Frozen	Post-thaw Temp: Room	Post-thaw Temp: Refrig	Body Temp	Refer.
CONTAINER												
Bag, Polyvinyl Chloride (PVC)	BE	10 mg/mL	NS	[e]	[a]	n/a	48 hr	n/a	n/a	n/a	n/a	(1)
	BE	5 mg/mL	NS	[e]	[a]	n/a	24 hr	n/a	n/a	n/a	n/a	(1)
	BR	20 mg/mL	D5W, NS	[e]	[a]	2 hr[d]	n/a	n/a	n/a	n/a	n/a	(1)
	AY	20 mg/mL	NS	[e]	[a]	24 hr	24 hr	n/a	n/a	n/a	n/a	(1)
	MYL, SZ	12-24 mg/mL	NS	[e]	[a]	24 hr	72 hr[c]	n/a	n/a	n/a	n/a	(2)
Unspecified	SZ	10 mg/mL	D5½NS	[e]	[a]	n/a	1 hr	n/a	n/a	n/a	n/a	(1)
	SZ	2, 10 mg/mL	D5W	[e]	[a]	2 hr	n/a	n/a	n/a	n/a	n/a	(1)
	BR	1 mg/mL	[h]	[e]	[a]	24 hr	24 hr	n/a	n/a	n/a	n/a	(1)
	AY, BAY	2-5 mg/mL	R	[e]	[a]	24 hr	n/a	n/a	n/a	n/a	n/a	(1)
	SZ	30 mg/mL	NS, LR	[e]	[a]	8 hr	24 hr	n/a	n/a	n/a	n/a	(1)
	SZ	20 mg/mL	NS	[e]	[a]	n/a	48 hr	n/a	n/a	n/a	n/a	(1)
	SZ	40 mg/mL	NS	[e]	[a]	6 hr	n/a	n/a	n/a	n/a	n/a	(1)
	SZ	10 mg/mL	NS	[e]	[a]	8 hr	n/a	n/a	n/a	n/a	n/a	(1)
	BAY, BE	2-15 mg/mL	NS	[e]	[a]	24 hr	n/a	n/a	n/a	n/a	n/a	(1)
	BR	1, 6, 10 mg/mL	NS	[e]	[a]	24 hr	24 hr	24 hr[f]	n/a	n/a	n/a	(1)
	AY	2, 30 mg/mL	NS	[e]	[a]	24 hr	n/a	n/a	n/a	n/a	n/a	(1)
	BR	5-40 mg/mL	NS	[e]	[a]	n/a	24 hr	n/a	n/a	n/a	n/a	(1)
OTHER INFUSION CONTAINERS												
CADD® Cassette (Smiths Medical)	WY	60 mg/mL	NS, SWFI	[e]	[a]	24 hr	24 hr[g]	n/a	n/a	n/a	n/a	(7)
Dosi-Fuser® (Leventon)	UN	20 mg/mL	NS	[e]	[a]	8 hr[b]	72 hr[b]	n/a	n/a	n/a	n/a	(3)
Easypump® ST/LT (B. Braun)	UN	20 mg/mL	NS	[e]	[a]	24 hr	72 hr	n/a	n/a	n/a	n/a	(6)
	UN	12 mg/mL	NS	[e]	[a]	6 hr	4 d	n/a	n/a	n/a	n/a	(6)
Homepump Eclipse® / Homepump® (Halyard)	UN	20 mg/mL	NS	[e]	[a]	8 hr	72 hr	n/a	n/a	n/a	n/a	(4)
SMARTeZ® (Progressive Medical)	UN	20 mg/mL	NS	[e]	[a]	24 hr[b]	72 hr[b]	n/a	n/a	n/a	n/a	(5)
	UN	12 mg/mL	NS	[e]	n/a	6 hr[b]	4 d[b]	n/a	n/a	n/a	n/a	(5)

DOI 10.37573/9781585286720.013

Flush Compatibility: Sodium chloride 0.9%, heparin.[(1)]

Special Considerations: Ampicillin stability is concentration dependent; stability decreases as the concentration increases. It is also significantly decreased in D5W. Storage temperature and pH of the solution affect stability. Do not freeze.[(1)]

Notes

[a] pH range of 10 mg/mL in recommended diluents and concentrations is 8-10. pH range of 20-100 mg/mL in SWFI, NS or D5W is 8.7-9.3.[(1)]

[b] Manufacturer extrapolated data from other source(s).

[c] Storage temperature: 72 hours at refrigerated temperature followed by 24 hours at room temperature.[(2)]

[d] Followed by 1 hour simulated infusion.

[e] Osmolality of 40 mg/mL in NS: 444 mOsm/kg, 40 mg/mL in D5W: 418 mOsm/kg; 20 mg/mL in NS: 368 mOsm/kg, 20 mg/mL in D5W: 341 mOsm/kg, 10 mg/mL in NS: 328 mOsm/kg, 10 mg/mL in D5W: 302 mOsm/kg.[(1)]

[f] Only the 10 mg/mL concentration was studied under frozen conditions.

[g] 10% loss in 6 hours and 20% loss in 24 hours during administration at 30°C via portable pump.

[h] Isolyte M or Isolyte P in D5W.[(1)]

REFERENCES

1. ASHP's Interactive Handbook on Injectable Drugs, 2020. Bethesda, MD: American Society of Health-System Pharmacists; Accessed September 2020.
2. Huskey M, Lewis P, Brown SD. Stability of Ampicillin in Normal Saline Following Refrigerated Storage and 24-Hour Pump Recirculation. *Hosp Pharm*. 2020; 0(0):1-6.
3. *Drug Stability Table - Dosi-Fuser® Elastomeric Pump (ES.H.00.73-10)*, 2015. Barcelona, Spain: Leventon SAU; Updated October 2015.
4. *Stability Data for Drugs Using Homepump Disposable Ambulatory Infusion Systems (MK-00314 rev 3)*, 2015. Alpharetta, GA: Halyard Health; Updated June 2015.
5. *SMARTeZ® - Stability Data for Drugs Using Elastomeric Infusion Pumps*, 2020. Fenton, MO: Progressive Medical, Inc.; Updated May 2020.
6. *Drug Stability for Easypump® ST/LT*, 2020. Bethlehem, PA: B. Braun USA; Updated June 2020.
7. *Pharmaceutical report on chemical and physical stability of drugs commonly used with CADD® infusion pumps (IN193109GB-122019)*, 2019. Minneapolis, MN: Smiths Medical ASD, Inc.; Updated December 2019.

Ampicillin Sodium – Sulbactam Sodium

Storage Conditions

						Temperature			Post-thaw Temp			
	Drug Manufacturer	Concentration	Diluents	Osmolality (mOsm/kg)	pH	Room	Refrig	Frozen	Room	Refrig	Body Temp	Refer.
CONTAINER												
Bag, Polyvinyl Chloride (PVC)	PF	20 mg/mL	NS	n/a	[a]	32 hr	68 hr	n/a	n/a	n/a	n/a	(1)
Unspecified	PF	20 mg/mL[b]	NS, SWFI	n/a	[a]	n/a	72 hr	n/a	n/a	n/a	n/a	(1)(3)
	PF	20 mg/mL[b]	D5W	n/a	[a]	2 hr	4 hr	n/a	n/a	n/a	n/a	(1)(3)
	PF	30 mg/mL[b]	NS, SWFI	n/a	[a]	8 hr	48 hr	n/a	n/a	n/a	n/a	(1)(3)
OTHER INFUSION CONTAINERS												
ADD-Vantage® Flexible Container System (Pfizer)	RR	20 mg/mL	NS	n/a	[a]	2 hr[c]	n/a	n/a	n/a	n/a	n/a	(3)
Dosi-Fuser® (Leventon)	UN	20, 45 mg/mL	NS	n/a	[a]	2 hr[d]	72 hr[d]	n/a	n/a	n/a	n/a	(5)
Easypump® ST/LT (B. Braun)	UN	30 mg/mL	NS	n/a	[a]	6 hr	48 hr	n/a	n/a	n/a	n/a	(4)
Homepump Eclipse® / Homepump® (Halyard)	UN	30 mg/mL	NS	n/a	[a]	n/a	72 hr	n/a	n/a	n/a	n/a	(2)
SMARTeZ® (Progressive Medical)	UN	30 mg/mL	NS	n/a	[a]	6 hr[d]	4 d[d]	n/a	n/a	n/a	n/a	(6)

Flush Compatibility: Sodium chloride 0.9%, heparin.[1]

Special Considerations: Stated concentrations represent ampicillin content. Stability applies to both components.

Notes

[a] pH of solutions is 8-10.[1]

[b] Concentration of final dilutions is unspecified. See manufacturer's instructions for preparation. If using bulk pharmacy vials, stability applies to solutions stored for less than one hour at room temperature prior to further dilution.

[c] After activation.

[d] Manufacturer extrapolated data from other source(s).

DOI 10.37573/9781585286720.014

REFERENCES

1. ASHP's Interactive Handbook on Injectable Drugs, 2020. Bethesda, MD: American Society of Health-System Pharmacists; Accessed November 2020.
2. *Stability Data for Drugs Using Homepump Disposable Ambulatory Infusion Systems (MK-00314 rev3)*, 2015. Alpharetta, GA: Halyard Health; Updated June 2015.
3. Unasyn® (Ampicillin Sodium/Sulbactam Sodium) [package insert]. New York, NY: Pfizer; October 2019.
4. *Drug Stability for Easypump® ST/LT*, 2020. Bethlehem, PA: B. Braun USA; Updated June 2020.
5. *Drug Stability Table - Dosi-Fuser® Elastomeric Pump. (ES.H.00.730-10.)*, 2015. Barcleona, Spain: Leventon SAU; Updated October 2015.
6. *SMARTeZ® - Stability Data for Drugs Using Elastomeric Infusion Pumps*, 2020. Fenton, MO: Progressive Medical, Inc.; Updated May 2020.

Ascorbic Acid

Storage Conditions

						Temperature			Post-thaw Temp			
CONTAINER	Drug Manufacturer	Concentration	Diluents	Osmolality (mOsm/kg)	pH	Room	Refrig	Frozen	Room	Refrig	Body Temp	Refer.
Bag, Polyolefin	AMR	10 mg/mL	NS, D5W	n/a	[a]	24 hr[b]	n/a	n/a	n/a	n/a	n/a	(1)(4)
Bag, Polyvinyl Chloride (PVC)	SZ, MYL	37, 40 mg/mL	NS, D5W	n/a	[a]	10 d[b]	14 d[b]	n/a	n/a	n/a	n/a	(2)
	SZ	77 mg/mL	NS, D5W	n/a	[a]	14 d[b]	14 d[b]	n/a	n/a	n/a	n/a	(2)
	MYL	92 mg/mL	NS	n/a	[a]	14 d[b]	14 d[b]	n/a	n/a	n/a	n/a	(2)
	MYL	92 mg/mL	D5W	n/a	[a]	10 d[b]	14 d[b]	n/a	n/a	n/a	n/a	(2)
	MYL	40 mg/mL	NS	n/a	[a]	75 hr	n/a	n/a	n/a	n/a	n/a	(2)
Unspecified	MCG	30 mg/mL	NS	[c]	[a]	4 d	4 d[b]	n/a	n/a	n/a	n/a	(3)(4)
	MCG	50 mg/mL	D5W	[c]	[a]	4 d	4 d[b]	n/a	n/a	n/a	n/a	(3)(4)
	BTK	1.25 mg/mL	D5W, D10W, LR, NS, R, D5½NS	n/a	[a]	24 hr	n/a	n/a	n/a	n/a	n/a	(4)

Flush Compatibility: Sodium chloride 0.9%.[4]

Special Considerations: Pressure may build up during storage of containers of ascorbic acid. To avoid excessive pressure inside unopened ampules, the manufacturer recommends that they should be stored in the refrigerator and not allowed to stand at room temperature before use.[4] However, room temperature stability data is available for unopened vials 4 days (LI); 4 years at temperatures not exceeding 25°C (VI). Protect from light.[4] The final concentration of ascorbic acid admixture solutions for infusion should be in the range of 1 to 25 mg/mL. Each mL of ASCOR® (MCG) contains 0.25 mg of edetate disodium (EDTA). Do not mix formulations that contain EDTA with solutions containing elemental compounds that can be reduced (i.e. copper).[5]

Notes

[a] pH of undiluted solution is 5.5-7.[4]

[b] Protected from light.

[c] Addition of 200 mg of ascorbic acid (MCG) to 7.5 mL of SWFI produces a solution with an approximate osmolarity of 290 mOsmol/L.[5]

DOI 10.37573/9781585286720.015

REFERENCES

1. Chin A, Liu S, Ting-Chan J, et al. Extended stability of ascorbic acid in 5% dextrose injection and 0.9% sodium chloride injection. *Am J Health Syst Pharm*. 2005; 62(10):1073-4.
2. Walker SE, Iazzetta J, Law S, et al. Administration of Intravenous Ascorbic Acid-Practical Considerations for Clinicians. *Nutrients*. 2019; 11(9).
3. Carr A, Wohlrab C, Young P, et al. Stability of intravenous vitamin C solutions: a technical report. *Crit Care Resusc*. 2018; 20(3):180-81.
4. ASHP's Interactive Handbook on Injectable Drugs, 2020. Bethesda, MD: American Society of Health-System Pharmacists; Accessed August 2020.
5. ASCOR® (Ascorbic Acid) Injection [package insert]. Santa Ana, CA: McGuff Pharmaceuticals, Inc.; October 2019.

AzaTHIOprine Sodium

Storage Conditions

						Temperature			Post-thaw Temp			
	Drug Manufacturer	Concentration	Diluents	Osmolality (mOsm/kg)	pH	Room	Refrig	Frozen	Room	Refrig	Body Temp	Refer.
CONTAINER												
Bag, Polyvinyl Chloride (PVC)	BW	2 mg/mL	D5W	n/a	[(a)]	8 d[(c)]	8 d[(b)]	n/a	n/a	n/a	n/a	(1)
	BW	2 mg/mL	NS	n/a	[(a)]	16 d[(c)]	16 d[(b)]	n/a	n/a	n/a	n/a	(1)
	BW	2 mg/mL	½NS	n/a	[(a)]	16 d[(c)]	16 d[(b)]	n/a	n/a	n/a	n/a	(1)
Syringe, Plastic (Unspecified)	BW	10 mg/mL	SWFI	n/a	[(a)]	16 d[(c)]	n/a	n/a	n/a	n/a	n/a	(1)

Flush Compatibility: Sodium chloride 0.9%, heparin.[(2)]

Special Considerations: n/a.

Notes

[a] pH of reconstituted solution: 9.6.[(2)]
[b] Protected from light.[(1)]
[c] Exposed to fluorescent light.[(1)]

REFERENCES

1. Johnson CA, Porter WA. Compatibility of azathioprine sodium with intravenous fluids. *Am J Hosp Pharm*. 1981; 38(6):871-5.
2. Azathioprine Sodium Injection [package insert]. Eatontown, NJ: West-Ward Pharmaceuticals Corp; February 2019.

DOI 10.37573/9781585286720.016

Azithromycin

Storage Conditions

	Drug Manufacturer	Concentration	Diluents	Osmolality (mOsm/kg)	pH	Temperature: Room	Temperature: Refrig	Temperature: Frozen	Post-thaw Temp: Room	Post-thaw Temp: Refrig	Body Temp	Refer.
CONTAINER												
Unspecified	PF, HOS	1-2 mg/mL	D5W, NS[a]	n/a	[c]	24 hr	7 d	n/a	n/a	n/a	n/a	(1)
OTHER INFUSION CONTAINERS												
Easypump® ST/LT (B. Braun)	UN	1-2 mg/mL	NS	n/a	[c]	24 hr	7 d	n/a	n/a	n/a	n/a	(3)
Homepump Eclipse® / Homepump® (Halyard)	UN	1-2 mg/mL	D5W, NS	n/a	[c]	24 hr[b]	7 d[b]	n/a	n/a	n/a	n/a	(4)
SMARTeZ® (Progressive Medical)	UN	1-2 mg/mL	NS	n/a	[c]	24 hr[b]	7 d[b]	n/a	n/a	n/a	n/a	(2)

Flush Compatibility: Sodium chloride 0.9%, D5W, LR, heparin.[5]

Special Considerations: n/a

Notes

[a] Equivalent stability in ½NS, LR, D5½NS, D5LR, D5⅓NS, D5½NS with KCl 20 mEq, Normosol®-M in D5W, Normosol®-R in D5W.[1][5]

[b] Manufacturer extrapolated data from other sources.

[c] pH of reconstituted solution (100 mg/mL) is 6.4-6.8.[6]

REFERENCES

1. ASHP's Interactive Handbook on Injectable Drugs, 2020. Bethesda, MD: American Society of Health-System Pharmacists; Accessed May 2020.
2. *SMARTeZ® - Stability Data for Drugs Using Elastomeric Infusion Pumps*, 2020. Fenton, MO: Progressive Medical, Inc.; Updated May 2020.
3. *Drug Stability for Easypump® ST/LT*, 2020. Bethlehem, PA: B. Braun USA; Updated June 2020.
4. *Stability Data for Drugs Using Homepump Disposable Ambulatory Infusion Systems (MK-00314 rev 3)*, 2015. Alpharetta, GA: Halyard Health; Updated June 2015.
5. Zithromax® (Azithromycin) Injection [package insert]. New York, NY: Pfizer Laboratories Div Pfizer, Inc.; March 2020.
6. Zithromax® (Azithromycin) Injection [safety data sheet]. New York, NY: Pfizer, Inc.; June 26, 2019.

DOI 10.37573/9781585286720.017

Aztreonam

Storage Conditions

	Drug Manufacturer	Concentration	Diluents	Osmolality (mOsm/kg)	pH	Temperature: Room	Temperature: Refrig	Temperature: Frozen	Post-thaw Temp: Room	Post-thaw Temp: Refrig	Body Temp	Refer.
CONTAINER												
Bag, Polyvinyl Chloride (PVC)	SQ	10 mg/mL	NS	n/a	[a]	4 d	4 d	n/a	n/a	n/a	n/a	(1)
	SQ	10, 20 mg/mL	D5W, NS[f]	n/a	[a]	48 hr	7 d	n/a	n/a	n/a	n/a	(1)(2)
Unspecified	BMS	Up to 20 mg/mL	D5W, NS[f]	n/a	[a]	48 hr	7 d	n/a	n/a	n/a	n/a	(1)(2)
	SQ	20 mg/mL	NS	n/a	[a]	37 d	120 d	120 d	n/a	n/a	n/a	(1)
	BMS	> 20 mg/mL	NS, SWFI	n/a	[a]	48 hr	7 d	n/a	n/a	n/a	n/a	(1)(2)
Vial, Glass	SQ	20 mg/mL	D5W, NS	n/a	[a]	48 hr	n/a	n/a	n/a	n/a	n/a	(1)
OTHER INFUSION CONTAINERS												
Dosi-Fuser® (Leventon)	BMS	5-20 mg/mL	D5W, NS	n/a	[a]	24 hr[c]	14 d[c]	30 d[c]	n/a	n/a	n/a	(5)
	SQ	20 mg/mL	NS	n/a	[a]	n/a	28 d	n/a	n/a	n/a	1 hr[d]	(5)
	SQ	20 mg/mL	NS	n/a	[a]	n/a	5 wk	n/a	n/a	n/a	24 hr[g]	(5)
Easypump® ST/LT (B. Braun)	UN	10, 30 mg/mL	NS	n/a	[a]	24 hr	7 d	n/a	n/a	n/a	n/a	(6)
Homepump Eclipse® / Homepump ® (Halyard)	UN	5-20 mg/mL	NS	n/a	[a]	n/a	28 d	n/a	n/a	n/a	n/a	(4)
	UN	20-30 mg/mL	NS	n/a	[a]	n/a	14 d	n/a	n/a	n/a	n/a	(4)
	UN	26.7 mg/mL	NS	n/a	[a]	7 d	7 d	n/a	n/a	n/a	n/a	(4)
	UN	60 mg/mL	NS	n/a	[a]	24 hr	28 d	n/a	n/a	n/a	n/a	(4)
INTERMATE™ (Baxter)[e]	BMS	5 mg/mL	D5W, NS	n/a	[a]	48 hr[d]	28 d	n/a	n/a	n/a	n/a	(3)
	SQ	5-20 mg/mL	D5W, NS	n/a	[a]	24 hr	14 d	30 d	24 hr	n/a	n/a	(3)
	BMS	5-60 mg/mL	D5W, NS	n/a	[a]	24 hr[d]	28 d	n/a	n/a	n/a	n/a	(3)
SMARTeZ® (Progressive Medical)	unspec.	10-30 mg/mL	NS	n/a	[a]	24 hr[c]	7 d[c]	n/a	n/a	n/a	n/a	(7)
COMMERCIAL PREPARATIONS (RTU)												
GALAXY™ Plastic Container (Baxter)	BMS	20, 40 mg/mL	D	iso	4.5-7.5	n/a	n/a	[b]	48 hr[b]	14 d[b]	n/a	(1)

DOI 10.37573/9781585286720.018

Flush Compatibility: Sodium chloride 0.9%, heparin.[(1)]

Special Considerations: Upon addition of diluent to original container, contents should be shaken immediately and vigorously. Reconstituted Azactam® is a colorless to light straw yellow solution which may develop a slight pink tint on standing (potency is not affected).[(2)]

Notes

[a] pH of aqueous solutions is 4.5-7.5.[(1)]

[b] Frozen expiration date per manufacturer's label. Do not extrapolate commercial premix stability data to extemporaneously compounded solutions.

[c] Manufacturer extrapolated data from other source(s).

[d] Following 28 d refrigerated.[(3,5)]

[e] INTERMATE™/INFUSOR™ Portable Elastomeric Infusion System devices are no longer available in the United States.

[f] Equivalent stability in D5LR, D5W, D10W, D5NS, D5½NS, D5¼NS, Ionosol® B with D5W, Isolyte® E, Isolyte® E with D5W, Isolyte® M with D5W, LR, M5, M10, M/6 Sodium Lactate (Sodium Lactate Injection, USP), Normosol®-M, Normosol®-M with D5W, Normosol®-R, Normosol®-R with D5W, NS, Plasma-Lyte M with D5W, R.[(2)]

[g] Following 5 wk refrigerated.[(5)]

REFERENCES

1. ASHP's Interactive Handbook on Injectable Drugs, 2020. Bethesda, MD: American Society of Health-System Pharmacists; Accessed September 2020.
2. Azactam® (Aztreonam) Injection [package insert]. Princeton, NJ: Bristol-Myers Squibb Company; June 2020.
3. Stabforum - Stability Database: Aztreonam, Ontario, Canada: Baxter Healthcare; Accessed January 2021.
4. *Stability Data for Drugs Using Homepump Disposable Ambulatory Infusion Systems (MK-00314 rev 3)*, 2015. Alpharetta, GA: Halyard Health; Updated June 2015.
5. *Drug Stability Table - Dosi-Fuser® Elastomeric Pump (S-CL-00-001v16)*, 2021. Barcelona, Spain: Leventon SAU; Updated May 2021.
6. *Drug Stability for Easypump® ST/LT*, 2020. Bethlehem, PA: B. Braun USA; Updated June 2020.
7. *SMARTeZ® - Stability Data for Drugs Using Elastomeric Infusion Pumps*, 2020. Fenton, MO: Progressive Medical, Inc.; Updated May 2020.

Baclofen

Storage Conditions

	Drug Manufacturer	Concentration	Diluents	Osmolality (mOsm/kg)	pH	Temperature Room	Temperature Refrig	Temperature Frozen	Post-thaw Temp Room	Post-thaw Temp Refrig	Body Temp	Refer.
CONTAINER												
Syringe, Glass	UN[q]	3 mg/mL	NS	n/a	[g]	3 yr	n/a	n/a	n/a	n/a	n/a	(9)
Syringe, Polypropylene	NVA	0.08, 1.6 mg/mL	NS[a]	n/a	[g]	7 d[n]	7 d[n]	n/a	n/a	n/a	n/a	(7)
	NVA	0.08, 1, 1.8 mg/mL	NS[o]	n/a	[g]	7 d[p]	7 d	n/a	n/a	n/a	n/a	(10)
Vial, Glass	CI	0.2 mg/mL	NS[b][c]	n/a	[g]	n/a	n/a	n/a	n/a	n/a	30 d	(1)
	CI	0.2 mg/mL	NS[j]	154-242	[g]	n/a	n/a	n/a	n/a	n/a	30 d	(1)(3)
	CI	0.8 mg/mL	NS[b]	n/a	[g]	n/a	n/a	n/a	n/a	n/a	29 d	(1)
	CI	0.8 mg/mL	NS[c]	n/a	[g]	n/a	n/a	n/a	n/a	n/a	30 d	(1)
	CI	1 mg/mL	NS[d]	154-242	[g]	n/a	n/a	n/a	n/a	n/a	30 d	(1)(3)
	SH	1 mg/mL	NS[e]	n/a	[g]	n/a	n/a	n/a	n/a	n/a	10 wk[n]	(4)
	CI	1.5 mg/mL	NS[i]	154-242	[g]	n/a	n/a	n/a	n/a	n/a	30 d	(1)(3)
	NVA	0.25, 0.5 mg/mL	NS[f]	n/a	[g]	n/a	n/a	n/a	n/a	n/a	4 m	(5)
OTHER INFUSION CONTAINERS												
Codman® MedStream Implantable Pump (Codman-Shurtleff)	UN[q]	3 mg/mL	NS	n/a	n/a	n/a	n/a	n/a	n/a	n/a	180 d	(9)
Implantable Pump (Fresenius Model VIP® 30)	UN	0.5 mg/mL	Undiluted	[l]	[g]	n/a	n/a	n/a	n/a	n/a	8 wk	(1)
Infusaid® Model 400 Implantable Pump (Infusaid)	CI	1 mg/mL	NS[d]	154-242	[g]	n/a	n/a	n/a	n/a	n/a	30 d	(3)
SynchroMed® EL Implantable Pump (Medtronic)	NVA	1 mg/mL	NS[f]	n/a	[g]	n/a	n/a	n/a	n/a	n/a	14 wk	(5)
	NVA	0.5, 2 mg/mL	NS	n/a	[g]	n/a	n/a	n/a	n/a	n/a	90 d	(2)
SynchroMed® II Implantable Pump (Medtronic)	NVA	1.5 mg/mL	[h]	n/a	5.8	n/a	n/a	n/a	n/a	n/a	12 d[m]	(6)
	BB	2 mg/mL	[k]	n/a	6.0	n/a	n/a	n/a	n/a	n/a	20 d[m]	(6)
	NVA	0.5, 2 mg/mL	NS	n/a	[g]	n/a	n/a	n/a	n/a	n/a	180 d	(2)
	UN[q]	3 mg/mL	NS	n/a	n/a	n/a	n/a	n/a	n/a	n/a	219 d	(9)

DOI 10.37573/9781585286720.019

Flush Compatibility: Sodium chloride 0.9%.[1]

Special Considerations: Gablofen® is intended for use by intrathecal route in single bolus test doses (via spinal catheter or lumbar puncture) and for chronic use in the Medtronic SynchroMed® II implanted pump or other pumps specifically labeled for intrathecal administration of Gablofen®.[8] Lioresal® Intrathecal (NVA) is intended only for implantable pumps specifically labeled for its use. Protect from freezing.[1]

Notes

[a] Solution contained: baclofen (NVA) 0.08 mg/mL and morphine sulfate (LAV) 1 mg/mL, or baclofen (NVA) 1.6 mg/mL and morphine sulfate (LAV) 10 mg/mL.[7]

[b] Solution contained: morphine sulfate (DB) 1 mg/mL.[1]

[c] Solution contained: morphine sulfate (DB) 1.5 mg/mL.[1]

[d] Solution contained: morphine sulfate (DB) 15 mg/mL.[3]

[e] Solution compounded with cloNIDine hydrochloride (SH) 0.2 mg/mL. Baclofen (SH) and cloNIDine (SH) were obtained and mixed in powder form.[4]

[f] Combined with cloNIDine 0.25, 0.5 and 1 mg/mL; 1 mg/mL of cloNIDine and baclofen studied in implantable pumps; all three concentration combinations studied in glass vials.[5]

[g] pH of Gablofen® (PCC) is 5.5-7.5. pH of Lioresal® Intrathecal (NVA) is 5-7.[1]

[h] Solution contained: ziconotide (ELN) 25 mcg/mL.[6]

[i] Solution contained: morphine sulfate (DB) 7.5 mg/mL.

[j] Solution contained: morphine sulfate (DB) 21 mg/mL.[3]

[k] Baclofen (BB) powder dissolved in ziconotide (ELN) 25 mcg/mL.[6]

[l] Undiluted baclofen injection is an isotonic solution.[1]

[m] Ziconotide concentration decreased below 90% after this time.[6]

[n] Protected from light.

[o] Solution contained: baclofen (NVA) 0.08 mg/mL and SUFentanil (MLY) 0.045 mg/mL, baclofen (NVA) 0.08 mg/mL and SUFentanil (MLY) 0.003 mg/mL, baclofen (NVA) 1 mg/mL and SUFentanil (MLY) 0.025 mg/mL, or baclofen (NVA) 1.8 mg/mL and SUFentanil (MLY) 0.003 mg/mL.[10]

[p] SUFentanil (MLY) showed degradation over 7 days when stored at 25°C. Stability data only applies to baclofen at the specified concentrations.[10]

[q] Solutions prepared using 5 different lots of baclofen Active Pharmaceutical Ingredient (API) and 1 lot of baclofen United States Pharmacopeial (USP) Convention reference standard.[9]

REFERENCES

1. ASHP's Interactive Handbook on Injectable Drugs, 2020. Bethesda, MD: American Society of Health-System Pharmacists; Accessed June 2020.
2. *Indications, drug stability, and emergency procedures - SynchroMed® and IsoMed® implantable infusion systems (M961293A001 Rev E)*, 2017. Minneapolis, MN: Medtronic, Inc.; Updated December 2017.
3. Sitaram BR, Tsui M, Rawicki HB, et al. Stability and compatibility of intrathecal admixtures containing baclofen and high concentrations of morphine. *Int J Pharm*. 1997; 153(1):13-24
4. Godwin DA, Kim N-H, Zuniga R. Stability of a Baclofen and Clonidine Hydrochloride Admixture for Intrathecal Administration. *Hosp Pharm*. 2001; 36(9):950-54.
5. Alvarez JC, De Mazancourt P, Chartier-Kastler E, et al. Drug stability testing to support clinical feasibility investigations for intrathecal baclofen-clonidine admixture. *J Pain Symptom Manage*. 2004; 28(3):268-72.
6. Shields D, Montenegro R, Aclan J. Chemical stability of admixtures combining ziconotide with baclofen during simulated intrathecal administration. *Neuromodulation*. 2007; 10 Suppl 1:12-7.
7. Robert J, Sorrieul J, Kieffer H, et al. Stability Study of Morphine and Baclofen Solution in Polypropylene Syringes. *Pharmaceutical Technology in Hospital Pharmacy*. 2017; 2(4):173-80.
8. Gablofen® (Baclofen) Injection [package insert]. Bethlehem, PA: Piramal Critical Care, Inc.; October 2020.
9. Yue B, Brendel R, Lukitsch A, et al. Solubility and Stability of Baclofen 3 mg/mL Intrathecal Formulation and Its Compatibility With Implantable Programmable Intrathecal Infusion Systems. *Neuromodulation*. 2017; 20(4):397-404.
10. Sorrieul J, Robert J, Gibory V, et al. Stability of sufentanil and baclofen mixtures for intrathecal analgesia at different concentrations in polypropylene syringes. *Ann Pharm Fr*. 2018; 76(6):444-52.

Bevacizumab

Storage Conditions

	Drug Manufacturer	Concentration	Diluents	Osmolality (mOsm/kg)	pH	Temperature			Post-thaw Temp			
						Room	Refrig	Frozen	Room	Refrig	Body Temp	Refer.
CONTAINER												
Bag, Polyolefin	GEN	unspec.[b]	NS	n/a	[a]	n/a	8 hr	n/a	n/a	n/a	n/a	(1)
	AMG	1.4, 16.5 mg/mL	NS	n/a	n/a	48 hr[c]	5 wk[c]	n/a	n/a	n/a	n/a	(6)
Bag, Polyvinyl Chloride (PVC)	GEN	unspec.[b]	NS	n/a	[a]	n/a	8 hr	n/a	n/a	n/a	n/a	(1)
	AMG	1.4, 16.5 mg/mL	NS	n/a	n/a	48 hr[c]	5 wk[c]	n/a	n/a	n/a	n/a	(6)
Syringe, Plastic (Unspecified)	GEN	25 mg/mL	Undiluted	n/a	[a]	n/a	3 m	n/a	n/a	n/a	n/a	(2)
Syringe, Polycarbonate	GEN	25 mg/mL	Undiluted	n/a	[a]	n/a	6 m	n/a	n/a	n/a	n/a	(4)
Syringe, Polypropylene	GEN	25 mg/mL	Undiluted	n/a	[a]	72 hr	6 m	n/a	n/a	n/a	n/a	(4)(5)
Vial, Glass	GEN	25 mg/mL	Undiluted	n/a	[a]	n/a	3 m[d]	n/a	n/a	n/a	n/a	(2)

Flush Compatibility: Sodium chloride 0.9%.[1]

Special Considerations: Protect vials from light. Do not freeze or shake. Do not administer or mix with dextrose solutions.[1] Storage in syringes for longer than 3 days has resulted in silicone oil microdroplets increasing particle counts that exceed USP standards for ophthalmic administration.[3,5]

Notes

[a] pH of undiluted solution is 6.2.[1]

[b] Concentration of IV dose diluted in 100 mL.[1]

[c] Physically and chemically stable for up to 5 weeks at 2-8°C followed by 48 hours at 30°C storage.[6]

[d] Stability of vial after initial entry.

REFERENCES

1. Avastin® (Bevacizumab) Injection [package insert]. South San Francisco, CA: Genentech, Inc.; December 2020.
2. Bakri SJ, Snyder MR, Pulido JS, et al. Six-month stability of bevacizumab (Avastin) binding to vascular endothelial growth factor after withdrawal into a syringe and refrigeration or freezing. *Retina*. 2006; 26(5):519-22.
3. Pereboom M, Becker ML, Amenchar M, et al. Stability assessment of repackaged bevacizumab for intravitreal administration. *Int J Pharm Compd*. 2015; 19(1):70-2.
4. Khalili H, Sharma G, Froome A, et al. Storage stability of bevacizumab in polycarbonate and polypropylene syringes. *Eye (Lond)*. 2015; 29(6):820-7.
5. Santovena A, Sanchez-Negrin E, Gutierrez F, et al. Assessment of bevacizumab quality and stability in repackaged syringes for clinical use. *Eur J Hosp Pharm*. 2016; 23(6):343-47.
6. Seckute J, Castellanos I, Bane S. 3PC-038 Physicochemical stability of the bevacizumab biosimilar, ABP 215, in intravenous bags after preparation and storage. *GaBI*. 2020; 9(4):A39.2-A39.

DOI 10.37573/9781585286720.020

Bleomycin Sulfate

Storage Conditions

						Temperature			Post-thaw Temp			
	Drug Manufacturer	Concentration	Diluents	Osmolality (mOsm/kg)	pH	Room	Refrig	Frozen	Room	Refrig	Body Temp	Refer.
CONTAINER												
Bag, Polyvinyl Chloride (PVC)	BEL	0.015 units/mL	NS	n/a	[e]	48 hr[b]	n/a	n/a	n/a	n/a	n/a	(1)
	UN	0.15 units/mL	NS	n/a	[e]	28 d[a]	28 d[a]	n/a	n/a	n/a	n/a	(1)(3)
	BR	0.3, 3 units/mL	NS	n/a	[e]	24 hr	n/a	n/a	n/a	n/a	n/a	(1)
	UN	2 units/mL	NS	n/a	[e]	n/a	6 wk[a]	n/a	n/a	n/a	n/a	(3)
Syringe, Polypropylene	UN	0.6 units/mL	NS	n/a	[e]	28 d[a]	28 d[a]	n/a	n/a	n/a	n/a	(3)
Unspecified	UN	unspec.	NS	n/a	[e]	n/a	n/a	n/a	n/a	n/a	10 d	(1)
	BR	0.02, 0.03 units/mL[d]	NS	n/a	[e]	n/a	7 d	n/a	n/a	n/a	n/a	(1)
Vial, Glass	BR	0.3, 3 units/mL	NS	n/a	[e]	24 hr	n/a	n/a	n/a	n/a	n/a	(1)
OTHER INFUSION CONTAINERS												
INTERMATE™ (Baxter)[c]	LUN	0.109 units/mL	NS	n/a	[e]	48 hr[a]	n/a	n/a	n/a	n/a	n/a	(2)

Flush Compatibility: Sodium chloride 0.9%, heparin.[1]

Special Considerations: Do not reconstitute or dilute with D5W.[1]

Notes

[a] Protected from light.

[b] Exposed to light.

[c] INTERMATE™/INFUSOR™ Portable Elastomeric Infusion System devices are no longer available in the United States.

[d] Bleomycin activity was retained after compounding into solution with other medications. Additives were not tested.

[e] pH of reconstituted solution is 4.5-6.[4]

DOI 10.37573/9781585286720.021

REFERENCES

1. ASHP's Interactive Handbook on Injectable Drugs, 2020. Bethesda, MD: American Society of Health-System Pharmacists; Accessed May 2020.
2. Stabforum - Stability Database: Bleomycin, Ontario, Canada: Baxter Healthcare; Accessed May 2020.
3. Allwood M, Stanley A, Wright P. The Cytotoxics Handbook. 4th ed. Abingdon, UK: Radcliffe Medical Press; 2002:273-74.
4. Bleomycin for Injection [product monograph]. Toronto, ON: Fresnius Kabi Canada Ltd.; June 2016.

Blinatumomab

Storage Conditions

CONTAINER	Drug Manufacturer	Concentration	Diluents	Osmolality (mOsm/kg)	pH	Temperature Room	Temperature Refrig	Temperature Frozen	Post-thaw Temp Room	Post-thaw Temp Refrig	Body Temp	Refer.
Bag, Ethylene Vinyl Acetate (EVA)	AMG	0.009–0.2316 mcg/mL[f]	NS[b]	n/a	[a]	48 hr[c]	8 d	n/a	n/a	n/a	n/a	(1)
	AMG	0.9772–1.9091 mcg/mL[d]	BNS[b][e]	n/a	[a]	7 d[c]	14 d	n/a	n/a	n/a	n/a	(1)
	AMG	1.9–4.5 mcg/mL[f]	BNS[b][e]	n/a	[a]	7 d[c]	16 d	n/a	n/a	n/a	4 d	(2)
Bag, Non-DEHP Polyvinyl Chloride (PVC)[h]	AMG	0.009–0.2316 mcg/mL[f]	NS[b]	n/a	[a]	48 hr[c]	8 d	n/a	n/a	n/a	n/a	(1)
	AMG	0.9772–1.9091 mcg/mL[d]	BNS[b][e]	n/a	[a]	7 d[c]	14 d	n/a	n/a	n/a	n/a	(1)
	AMG	1.9–4.5 mcg/mL[f]	BNS[b][e]	n/a	[a]	7 d[c]	16 d	n/a	n/a	n/a	4 d	(2)
Bag, Polyolefin	AMG	0.009–0.2316 mcg/mL[f]	NS[b]	n/a	[a]	48 hr[c]	8 d	n/a	n/a	n/a	n/a	(1)
	AMG	0.9772–1.9091 mcg/mL[d]	BNS[b][e]	n/a	[a]	7 d[c]	14 d	n/a	n/a	n/a	n/a	(1)
	AMG	1.9–4.5 mcg/mL[f]	BNS[b][e]	n/a	[a]	7 d[c]	16 d	n/a	n/a	n/a	4 d	(2)
Vial, Glass[g]	AMG	12.5 mcg/mL	SWFI	n/a	7.0	4 hr	24 hr	n/a	n/a	n/a	n/a	(1)

Flush Compatibility: Do not flush infusion line during bag changing or at the completion of infusion, as this may result in excess dosing and related complications.[1]

Special Considerations: Reconstitute blinatumomab with preservative-free SWFI only. The provided IV Solution Stabilizer is used to coat the prefilled IV bag prior to adding reconstituted blinatumomab, which prevents adhesion of the drug to the bag and administration tubing. The IV Solution Stabilizer should not be used to reconstitute the drug. Strictly follow manufacturer instructions for preparation. Infusion systems require overfill, which is accounted for in the package insert. Do not shake. Remove air from IV bag and prime IV line with prepared solution for infusion. Infuse through dedicated lumen. Administer 24 and 48 hour bags through low protein-binding 0.2 micron in-line filter. Bags formulated with bacteriostatic NS for 7 day infusions do not require a filter. Do not freeze. Protect from light until use.[1]

Notes

[a] pH after reconstitution with SWFI is 7.0.[1]

[b] Containing provided IV Solution Stabilizer, which must be added prior to reconstituted blinatumomab.[1]

[c] Includes storage and infusion time.[1]

[d] Preparation includes blinatumomab diluted in 90 mL BNS and 2.2 mL IV Solution Stabilizer with additional NS as needed to a total volume of 110 mL.[1]

[e] Benzyl alcohol concentrations must be between 0.5% and 0.74% (w/v).[2]

[f] Preparation includes blinatumomab diluted in 270 mL NS with 5.5 mL IV Solution Stabilizer. Total volume is dependent on blinatumomab volume added to NS and Stabilizer preparation.[1]

[g] Stored in original container, protected from light.[1]

[h] Blincyto® is incompatible with di-ethylhexylphthalate (DEHP) due to the possibility of particle formation, leading to a cloudy solution. Use polyolefin, PVC DEHP-Free, or ethyl vinyl acetate (EVA) infusion bags, pump cassettes, and IV tubing sets.[1]

DOI 10.37573/9781585286720.022

REFERENCES

1. Blincyto® (Blinatumomab) Injection [package insert]. Thousand Oaks, CA: Amgen, Inc.; March 2020.
2. Blincyto® Medication Information (Ref#: N/A) [personal communication]. Thousand Oaks, CA: Amgen, Inc.; 2019:8.

Bortezomib

Storage Conditions

CONTAINER	Drug Manufacturer	Concentration	Diluents	Osmolality (mOsm/kg)	pH	Temperature Room	Temperature Refrig	Temperature Frozen	Post-thaw Temp Room	Post-thaw Temp Refrig	Body Temp	Refer.
Syringe, Polypropylene	JC	1 mg/mL	NS	n/a	n/a	5 d[b]	7 d[a]	n/a	n/a	n/a	n/a	(1)(4)
	JC	1 mg/mL	NS	n/a	n/a	5 d[a]	10 d[a]	n/a	n/a	n/a	n/a	(2)
	JN	2.5 mg/mL	NS	n/a	n/a	21 d[b]	21 d[a]	n/a	n/a	n/a	n/a	(4)(6)
Vial, Glass	JC	1 mg/mL	NS	n/a	n/a	n/a	5 d[a]	n/a	n/a	n/a	n/a	(1)(4)
	OB	1 mg/mL	NS	n/a	n/a	6 wk[b]	6 wk[b]	n/a	n/a	n/a	n/a	(4)(5)
	JC	1 mg/mL	NS	n/a	n/a	8 d[a]	10 d[a]	n/a	n/a	n/a	n/a	(2)
	JN	2.5 mg/mL	NS	n/a	n/a	21 d[b]	21 d[a]	n/a	n/a	n/a	n/a	(4)(6)

Flush Compatibility: Sodium chloride 0.9%.[(3)]

Special Considerations: Reconstitute with NS.[(3)] Bortezomib final concentration differs depending on route of administration.[(3)]

Notes

[a] Protected from light.

[b] Exposed to light.

REFERENCES

1. Andre P, Cisternino S, Chiadmi F, et al. Stability of bortezomib 1-mg/mL solution in plastic syringe and glass vial. *Ann Pharmacother*. 2005; 39(9):1462-6.
2. Carati D, Masini C, Minguzzi M, et al. Stability of bortezomib reconstituted under clinical use conditions in original vials and polypropylene syringes at 4°C and room temperature. *Eur J Hosp Pharm: Science and Practice*. 2012; 19(5):428–31.
3. Velcade® (Bortezomib) Injection [package insert]. Cambridge, MA: Millennium Pharmaceuticals, Inc.; May 2020.
4. ASHP's Interactive Handbook on Injectable Drugs, 2020. Bethesda, MD: American Society of Health-System Pharmacists; Accessed June 2020.
5. Walker S, Milliken D, Law S. Stability of Bortezomib Reconstituted with 0.9% Sodium Chloride at 4°C and Room Temperature (23°C). *Can J Hosp Pharm*. 2008; 61(1):14–20.
6. Walker SE, Charbonneau LF, Law S. Stability of Bortezomib 2.5 mg/mL in Vials and Syringes Stored at 4 degrees C and Room Temperature (23 degrees C). *Can J Hosp Pharm*. 2014; 67(2):102–7.

DOI 10.37573/9781585286720.023

Bumetanide

Storage Conditions

	Drug Manufacturer	Concentration	Diluents	Osmolality (mOsm/kg)	pH	Temperature			Post-thaw Temp			
						Room	Refrig	Frozen	Room	Refrig	Body Temp	Refer.
CONTAINER												
Bag, Polyvinyl Chloride (PVC)	RC	0.02 mg/mL	D5W	n/a	n/a	72 hr	n/a	n/a	n/a	n/a	n/a	(2)
	RC	0.2 mg/mL	D5W	n/a	n/a	72 hr	n/a	n/a	n/a	n/a	n/a	(2)
	RC	0.25 mg/mL	Undiluted	n/a	[a]	72 hr	n/a	n/a	n/a	n/a	n/a	(2)
OTHER INFUSION CONTAINERS												
Easypump® ST/LT (B. Braun)	UN	0.016, 0.16 mg/mL	D5W	n/a	n/a	24 hr	n/a	n/a	n/a	n/a	n/a	(3)

Flush Compatibility: Sodium chloride 0.9%.[1]

Special Considerations: n/a

Notes

[a] pH of undiluted solution is ~7.[1]

REFERENCES

1. ASHP's Interactive Handbook on Injectable Drugs, 2020. Bethesda, MD: American Society of Health-System Pharmacists; Accessed June 2020.
2. Cornish LA, Montgomery PA, Johnson CE. Stability of bumetanide in 5% dextrose injection. *Am J Health Syst Pharm*. 1997; 54(4):422–3.
3. *Drug Stability for Easypump® ST/LT*, 2020. Bethlehem, PA: B. Braun USA; Updated June 2020.

DOI 10.37573/9781585286720.024

Bupivacaine Hydrochloride

Storage Conditions

	Drug Manufacturer	Concentration	Diluents	Osmolality (mOsm/kg)	pH[c]	Temperature: Room	Temperature: Refrig	Temperature: Frozen	Post-thaw Temp: Room	Post-thaw Temp: Refrig	Body Temp	Refer.
CONTAINER												
Bag, Polyolefin	HOS	0.01 mg/mL	NS[l]	n/a	3.3–5.9	n/a	28 d[f]	n/a	n/a	n/a	n/a	(7)
	HOS	20 mg/mL	NS[m]	n/a	3.4–4.9	n/a	28 d[f]	n/a	n/a	n/a	n/a	(7)
	HOS	37.5 mg/mL	NS[w]	n/a	4.0–4.9	n/a	28 d[f]	n/a	n/a	n/a	n/a	(7)
Bag, Polyvinyl Chloride (PVC)	UN	0.6 mg/mL	NS[p]	n/a	n/a	30 d	30 d	n/a	n/a	n/a	n/a	(1)
	AB	0.625, 1.25 mg/mL	NS	n/a	[c]	72 hr	n/a	n/a	n/a	n/a	n/a	(1)
	GRI	0.85 mg/mL	NS	n/a	[c]	28 d	28 d	n/a	n/a	n/a	n/a	(1)
	UN	1.25 mg/mL	NS[d]	n/a	n/a	30 d	30 d	n/a	n/a	n/a	n/a	(1)
	AST	4 mg/mL	NS[e]	n/a	4.1–4.3	28 d[f]	n/a	n/a	n/a	n/a	n/a	(4)
Syringe, Polypropylene	HOS	0.01 mg/mL	NS[l]	n/a	3.3–6.0	n/a	28 d[f]	n/a	n/a	n/a	n/a	(7)
	AST	1 mg/mL	NS	n/a	[c]	30 d	30 d	n/a	n/a	n/a	30 d	(1)(5)
	AST	1 mg/mL	NS[g]	n/a	n/a	30 d	30 d	n/a	n/a	n/a	30 d	(5)
	AST	1.25 mg/mL	NS	n/a	[c]	32 d	32 d[f]	n/a	n/a	n/a	n/a	(1)
	AST	2.5 mg/mL	NS[h]	n/a	n/a	13 wk	13 wk[f]	n/a	n/a	n/a	n/a	(6)
	HOS	20 mg/mL	NS[m]	n/a	3.4–5.3	n/a	28 d[f]	n/a	n/a	n/a	n/a	(7)
	HOS	37.5 mg/mL	NS[w]	n/a	4.6–5.0	n/a	28 d[f]	n/a	n/a	n/a	n/a	(7)
OTHER INFUSION CONTAINERS												
CADD® Cassette (Smiths Medical)	WI	0.44 mg/mL	[n]	n/a	n/a	30 d[o]	30 d[o]	n/a	n/a	n/a	48 hr[o]	(1)
	AST	2 mg/mL	NS[a]	n/a	n/a	n/a	30 d	n/a	n/a	n/a	30 d	(1)
	UN	3 mg/mL	NS[b]	n/a	n/a	10 d	10 d	n/a	n/a	n/a	10 d	(1)
	AST	7.5 mg/mL	Undiluted	n/a	n/a	90 d[k]	n/a	n/a	n/a	n/a	n/a	(1)
Dosi-Fuser® (Leventon)	UN	0.6 mg/mL	D5W, NS	n/a	n/a	30 d[x]	n/a	n/a	n/a	n/a	n/a	(2)
	UN	7.5 mg/mL	D5W, NS	n/a	n/a	14 d[x]	180 d[x]	n/a	n/a	n/a	n/a	(2)

DOI 10.37573/9781585286720.025

Storage Conditions

Drug	Manufacturer	Concentration	Diluents	Osmolality (mOsm/kg)	pH[c]	Temperature Room	Temperature Refrig	Temperature Frozen	Post-thaw Temp Room	Post-thaw Temp Refrig	Body Temp	Refer.
OTHER INFUSION CONTAINERS												
Easypump® ST/LT (B. Braun)	UN	5 mg/mL	RTU	n/a	n/a	48 hr	15 d	n/a	n/a	n/a	n/a	(9)
	UN	1.25, 7.5 mg/mL	NS	n/a	n/a	30 d	n/a	n/a	n/a	n/a	n/a	(9)
INFUSOR™ (Baxter)[y]	AST	0.5 mg/mL	D5W[u]	n/a	n/a	n/a	29 d[v]	n/a	n/a	n/a	n/a	(3)
	AST	0.6–7.5 mg/mL	NS, D5W, SWFI	n/a	[c]	30 d	180 d[q]	n/a	n/a	n/a	n/a	(3)
	AST	6.75 mg/mL	NS[s]	n/a	n/a	28 d[r]	93 d[t]	n/a	n/a	n/a	n/a	(3)
SMARTeZ® (Progressive Medical)	UN	5 mg/mL	NS	n/a	n/a	48 hr	15 d	n/a	n/a	n/a	n/a	(8)
		1.25, 7.5 mg/mL	NS	n/a	n/a	30 d	n/a	n/a	n/a	n/a	n/a	(8)
SynchroMed® Implanted Pump (Medtronic)	UN	7.5 mg/mL	[j]	n/a	[c]	n/a	n/a	n/a	n/a	n/a	12 wk	(1)
	UN	25 mg/mL	SWFI[i]	n/a	n/a	n/a	n/a	n/a	n/a	n/a	90 d	(1)

Flush Compatibility: Not used intravenously.

Special Considerations: Do not use products or diluents containing preservatives for intraspinal or epidural administration.

Notes

[a] Solution contained: SUFentanil (JN) 5 mcg/mL at 4°C and at 32°C.[1]

[b] Solution contained: SUFentanil (JN) 20 mcg/mL.[1]

[c] pH range of undiluted product is 4-6.5.[1]

[d] Solution contained: FentaNYL citrate 2 mcg/mL and 20 mcg/mL.[1]

[e] Solution contained: Morphine tartrate (DBL) 1 mg/mL and midazolam hydrochloride (RC) 0.5 mg/mL.[4]

[f] Protected from light.

[g] Solution contained: FentaNYL citrate (JN) 35 mcg/mL and cloNIDine hydrochloride (BI) 9 mcg/mL at 4°C, 21°C, 35°C.[5]

[h] Solution contained: HYDROmorphone (SAB) 0.02 mg/mL or 0.04 mg/mL.[6]

[i] Solution contained: CloNIDine HCl 2 mg/mL and morphine sulfate 50 mg/mL.[1]

[j] In Dextrose 8.25% (Marcaine™ spinal).[1]

[k] Protected from light in 50 mL ambulatory pump cassette reservoirs (Pharmacia Deltec). Drug concentration increased 12% during the observation period, possibly from evaporative loss.[1]

[l] Solution contained: HYDROmorphone (SZ) 0.01 mg/mL or 43 mg/mL; or morphine (SZ) 0.01 mg/mL or 43 mg/mL; or fentaNYL (SZ) 0.15 mcg/mL or 43 mcg/mL.[7]

[m] Solution contained: HYDROmorphone (SZ) 0.01 mg/mL or 25 mg/mL; or morphine (SZ) 0.01 mg/mL or 25 mg/mL; or fentaNYL (SZ) 0.15 mcg/mL or 25 mcg/mL.[7]

[n] Solution contained: FentaNYL citrate (JN) 1.25 mcg/mL and EPINEPHrine hydrochloride (AB) 0.69 mcg/mL.[1]

[o] Followed by 48 hours at 30°C.[1]

[p] Solution contained: FentaNYL 2 mcg/mL.[1]

[q] Followed by 14 days at room temperature.[3]

[r] Followed by 48 hours at 33°C.[3]

[s] Solution contained: SUFentanil citrate (JN) 5 mcg/mL.[3]

[t] Followed by 7 days at 33°C.[3]

[u] Solution contained: FentaNYL citrate (JN) 1-5 mcg/mL.[3]

[v] Followed by 72 hours at room temperature, followed by 5 days at 33°C.[3]

[w] Solution contained: HYDROmorphone (SZ) 0.01 mg/mL; or morphine (SZ) 0.01 mg/mL; or fentaNYL (SZ) 0.15 mcg/mL.

[x] Manufacturer extrapolated data from other sources.

[y] INTERMATE™/INFUSOR™ Portable Elastomeric Infusion System devices are no longer available in the United States.

REFERENCES

1. ASHP's Interactive Handbook on Injectable Drugs, 2020. Bethesda, MD: American Society of Health-System Pharmacists; Accessed July 2020.
2. *Drug Stability Table - Dosi-Fuser® Elastomeric Pump (ES.H.00.73-10)*, 2015. Barcelona, Spain: Leventon SAU; Updated October 2015.
3. Stabforum - Stability Database: Bupivacaine, Ontario, Canada: Baxter Healthcare; Accessed February 2021.
4. La Forgia SP, Sharley NA, Burgess NG, et al. Stability and Compatibility of Morphine, Midazolam and Bupivacaine Combinations for Intravenous Infusion. *J Pharm Pract Res*. 2002; 32(1):65–68.
5. Jappinen AMP, Kokki HM, Naaranlahti TP. pH Stability of Injectable Fentanyl, Bupivacaine, or Clonidine Solution or a Ternary Mixture in 0.9% Sodium Chloride in Two Types of Polypropylene Syringes. *Int J Pharm Compd*. 2002; 6(6):471–4.
6. Donnelly RF. Physical Compatibility and Chemical Stability of Bupivacaine and Hydromorphone in Polypropylene Syringes. *Can J Hosp Pharm*. 2004; 57(4):230–5.
7. Donnelly RF, Wong K, Spencer J. Physical compatibility of high-concentration bupivacaine with hydromorphone, morphine, and fentanyl. *Can J Hosp Pharm*. 2010; 63(2):154–5.
8. *SMARTeZ® - Stability Data for Drugs Using Elastomeric Infusion Pumps*, 2020. Fenton, MO: Progressive Medical, Inc.; Updated May 2020.
9. *Drug Stability for Easypump® ST/LT*, 2020. Bethlehem, PA: B. Braun USA; Updated June 2020.

Calcitriol

Storage Conditions

CONTAINER	Drug Manufacturer	Concentration	Diluents	Osmolality (mOsm/kg)	pH	Temperature: Room	Temperature: Refrig	Temperature: Frozen	Post-thaw Temp: Room	Post-thaw Temp: Refrig	Body Temp	Refer.
Syringe, Polypropylene	UN	0.8, 1, 2 mcg/mL	Undiluted	n/a	[b][c]	n/a	7 d[a]	n/a	n/a	n/a	n/a	(2)
	AB	1, 2 mcg/mL	Undiluted	n/a	[b][c]	8 hr	n/a	n/a	n/a	n/a	n/a	(1)(3)
	AB	0.5 mcg/mL	D5W, NS, SWFI	n/a	[b][c]	8 hr	n/a	n/a	n/a	n/a	n/a	(3)
	AB	2 mcg/mL	Undiluted	iso	[b][c]	20 d[d]	n/a	n/a	n/a	n/a	n/a	(3)

Flush Compatibility: Sodium chloride 0.9%.[1]

Special Considerations: Adsorbs rapidly to polyvinyl chloride (PVC) containers (50% in 2 hr).[1]

Notes

[a] Protected from light.[2]

[b] The pH of undiluted Calcijex® (AB) is 5.9 to 7.0.[1]

[c] The pH of undiluted calcitriol injection (AMR) is 6.7 to 7.7.[1]

[d] 4% loss within 20 d due to sorption.[3]

REFERENCES

1. ASHP's Interactive Handbook on Injectable Drugs, 2020. Bethesda, MD: American Society of Health-System Pharmacists; Accessed August 2020.
2. Vargas-Ruiz M, Bushman LR, Hillegas MS, et al. Stability of parenteral calcitriol in tuberculin syringe. ASHP Midyear Clinical Meeting. Miami Beach, FL; 1994:P-243D. [Abstract]
3. Pecosky DA, Parasrampuria J, Li LC, et al. Stability and sorption of calcitriol in plastic tuberculin syringes. *Am J Hosp Pharm*. 1992; 49(6):1463–6.

DOI 10.37573/9781585286720.026

Calcium Chloride

Storage Conditions

						Temperature			Post-thaw Temp			
	Drug Manufacturer	Concentration	Diluents	Osmolality (mOsm/kg)	pH	Room	Refrig	Frozen	Room	Refrig	Body Temp	Refer.
CONTAINER												
Bag, Polyvinyl Chloride (PVC)	AMR	10, 13.3 mg/mL	NS, D5W	[c]	[b]	7 d[a]	n/a	n/a	n/a	n/a	n/a	(1)

Flush Compatibility: Sodium chloride 0.9%.[2]

Special Considerations: Available in 10-mL single-dose preservative free vials and prefilled syringes containing 1 gm of calcium chloride dihydrate, providing 13.6 mEq (270 mg) of calcium and 13.6 mEq of chloride in water for injection. Severe necrosis and sloughing may result if calcium chloride is injected intramuscularly or subcutaneously or via leakage into the perivascular space.[2]

Notes

[a] Exposed to fluorescent light.

[b] pH may have been adjusted with hydrochloric acid and/or calcium hydroxide, and varies from 5.5 to 7.5 diluted in water to a 5% concentration.[2]

[c] Osmolality of a calcium chloride 10% solution is 1765 mOsm/kg.[2]

REFERENCES

1. Kiser TH, Barber GR, Robinson A. Managing the Intravenous Calcium Shortage: Evaluation of Calcium Chloride Stability in 0.9% Sodium Chloride and Dextrose 5% Water Polyvinyl Chloride Bags. *Hosp Pharm*. 2012; 47(1):27–30.
2. ASHP's Interactive Handbook on Injectable Drugs, 2020. Bethesda, MD: American Society of Health-System Pharmacists; Accessed December 2020.

DOI 10.37573/9781585286720.027

CARBOplatin

Storage Conditions

						Temperature			Post-thaw Temp			
	Drug Manufacturer	Concentration	Diluents	Osmolality (mOsm/kg)	pH	Room	Refrig	Frozen	Room	Refrig	Body Temp	Refer.
CONTAINER												
Bag, Ethylene Vinyl Acetate (EVA)	BR	1 mg/mL	D5W	n/a	4.17–4.9	28 d[b]	28 d[b]	n/a	n/a	n/a	28 d[b][e]	(1)
Bag, Polyolefin	TE	0.7, 2.15 mg/mL	D5W	n/a	4.16–4.67	24 hr	12 wk[b][d]	n/a	n/a	n/a	n/a	(6)(7)
Bag, Polyvinyl Chloride (PVC)	BMS	0.5, 4 mg/mL	D5W	n/a	4.6–4.7	21 d[b]	21 d[b]	n/a	n/a	n/a	n/a	(2)
	TE	0.7, 2.15 mg/mL	D5W	n/a	4.16–4.67	24 hr[a]	12 wk[b][d]	n/a	n/a	n/a	n/a	(6)(7)
	BMS	0.75, 2 mg/mL	D5W	n/a	4.6–4.7	7 d[b]	7 d[b]	n/a	n/a	n/a	n/a	(2)
	TE	0.5 mg/mL	NS	n/a	n/a	72 hr	7 d[b]	n/a	n/a	n/a	n/a	(9)
	TE	2 mg/mL	NS	n/a	n/a	5 d	7 d[b]	n/a	n/a	n/a	n/a	(9)
	TE	4 mg/mL	NS	n/a	n/a	7 d	7 d[b]	n/a	n/a	n/a	n/a	(9)
	BR	1 mg/mL	D5W	n/a	4.39–4.9	28 d[b]	28 d[b]	n/a	n/a	n/a	28 d[b][e]	(1)
	BR	1 mg/mL	SWFI	n/a	n/a	n/a	14 d	n/a	n/a	n/a	14 d	(6)
	BR	2.4 mg/mL	D5W	n/a	n/a	9 d[b]	n/a	n/a	n/a	n/a	n/a	(6)
Syringe, Polypropylene	BR	10 mg/mL	SWFI	n/a	[f]	n/a	5 d[b]	n/a	n/a	n/a	24 hr	(3)
	BMS	10 mg/mL	SWFI	n/a	[f]	8 d[b]	n/a	n/a	n/a	n/a	n/a	(4)
Vial, Glass	BR	1 mg/mL	D5W	n/a	4.39–4.9	28 d[b]	28 d[b]	n/a	n/a	n/a	28 d[b][e]	(1)
	UN	10 mg/mL	SWFI	n/a	[f]	14 d	n/a	n/a	n/a	n/a	n/a	(6)
OTHER INFUSION CONTAINERS												
CADD® Cassette (Smiths Medical)	BR	6, 10 mg/mL	D5W	n/a	[f]	n/a	n/a	n/a	n/a	n/a	28 d[j]	(10)
Dosi-Fuser® (Leventon)	UN	0.5–10 mg/mL	D5W	n/a	[f]	n/a	13 wk[h][i]	n/a	n/a	n/a	7 d[h][i]	(8)
INFUSOR™ (Baxter)[g]	BR	0.5–10 mg/mL	D5W	n/a	n/a	n/a	13 wk[c]	n/a	n/a	n/a	7 d[c]	(5)
	BR	1 mg/mL	D5W	n/a	3.95–4.9	28 d[b]	28 d[b]	n/a	n/a	n/a	7 d[b][e]	(1)

Flush Compatibility: Sodium chloride 0.9%.[6]

DOI 10.37573/9781585286720.028

Special Considerations: Equipment used to prepare or administer CARBOplatin should not contain aluminum because the two interact resulting in a precipitate and loss of CARBOplatin potency.[6]

Notes

[a] Stored at 12 wk refrigerated followed by 24 hr at 25°C.

[b] Protected from light.

[c] Stored 13 wk refrigerated followed by 7 d at 33°C.

[d] Infusions were stored refrigerated for 12 wk, then stored at 25°C for 24 hr, then again refrigerated for another 7 d.

[e] Stored at 35°C.

[f] The pH of a 1% (10 mg/mL) solution is 5-7.[6]

[g] INTERMATE™/INFUSOR™ Portable Elastomeric Infusion System devices are no longer available in the United States.

[h] Stored 13 wk refrigerated followed by 7 d at 37°C.

[i] Manufacturer extrapolated data from other sources.

[j] Degradation reported at 60°C.

REFERENCES

1. Rochard E, Barthes D, Courtois P. Stability and compatibility study of carboplatin with three portable infusion pump reservoirs. *Int J Pharm*. 1994; 101(3):257–62.
2. Diaz Amador F, Sevilla Azzati E, Herreros de Tejada y Lopez-Coterilla A. Stability of carboplatin in polyvinyl chloride bags. *Am J Health Syst Pharm*. 1998; 55(6):602, 04.
3. Sewell GJ, Riley CM, Rowland CG. The stability of carboplatin in ambulatory continuous infusion regimes. *J Clin Pharm Ther*. 1987; 12(6):427–32.
4. Valière C, Arnaud P, Caroff E, et al. Stability and compatibility study of a carboplatin solution in syringes for continuous ambulatory infusion in syringes for continuous ambulatory infusion. *Int J Pharm*. 1996; 138(1):125–28.
5. Stabforum - Stability Database: Carboplatin, Ontario, Canada: Baxter Healthcare; Accessed December 2020.
6. ASHP's Interactive Handbook on Injectable Drugs, 2020. Bethesda, MD: American Society of Health-System Pharmacists; Accessed August 2020.
7. Kaestner S, Sewell G. Dose-banding of carboplatin: rationale and proposed banding scheme. *J Oncol Pharm Pract*. 2007; 13(2):109–17.
8. *Drug Stability Table - Dosi-Fuser® Elastomeric Pump (ES.H.00.73-10)*, 2015. Barcelona, Spain: Leventon SAU; Updated October 2015.
9. Myers AL, Zhang YP, Kawedia JD, et al. Stability study of carboplatin infusion solutions in 0.9% sodium chloride in polyvinyl chloride bags. *J Oncol Pharm Pract*. 2016; 22(1):31–6.
10. *Pharmaceutical report on chemical and physical stability of drugs commonly used with CADD® infusion pumps (IN193109GB-122019)*, 2019. Minneapolis, MN: Smiths Medical ASD, Inc.; Updated December 2019.

Caspofungin Acetate

Storage Conditions

						Temperature			Post-thaw Temp			
	Drug Manufacturer	Concentration	Diluents	Osmolality (mOsm/kg)	pH	Room	Refrig	Frozen	Room	Refrig	Body Temp	Refer.
CONTAINER												
Bag, Plastic (Unspecified)	ME	Up to 0.5 mg/mL	NS, LR, ½NS, ¼NS	n/a	[a]	24 hr	48 hr	n/a	n/a	n/a	n/a	(2)
Bag, Polypropylene	ME	0.5 mg/mL	NS	n/a	[a]	n/a	28 d	n/a	n/a	n/a	n/a	(1)
Vial, Unspecified	ME	Up to 0.5 mg/mL	NS, LR, ½NS, ¼NS	n/a	[a]	24 hr	48 hr	n/a	n/a	n/a	n/a	(2)
OTHER INFUSION CONTAINERS												
Easypump® ST/LT (B. Braun)	UN	0.2, 0.5 mg/mL	NS	n/a	[a]	60 hr	14 d	n/a	n/a	n/a	n/a	(4)
Homepump Eclipse® / Homepump® (Halyard)	ME	0.2, 0.28, 0.5 mg/mL	NS	n/a	[a]	60 hr	14 d	n/a	n/a	n/a	n/a	(3)
SMARTeZ® (Progressive Medical)	UN	0.2–0.5 mg/mL	NS	n/a	[a]	60 hr	14 d	n/a	n/a	n/a	n/a	(5)

Flush Compatibility: Sodium Chloride 0.9%.[2]

Special Considerations: Do not mix with dextrose-containing solutions. Final concentration should not exceed 0.5 mg/mL. The reconstituted solution (vial) may be stored for up to 1 hr at controlled room temperature.[2]

Notes

[a] pH of saturated aqueous solution is approximately 6.6.[2]

REFERENCES

1. Pinder N, Pelzl LH, Walther G, et al. Caspofungin infusion solutions (50 mg/100 mL): chemical stability and antifungal activity against Candida spp. *Pharmazie*. 2017; 72(4):197–99.
2. Cancidas® (Caspofungin Acetate) Injection [package insert]. Whitehouse Station, NJ: Merck Sharp & Dohme Corp.; December 2020.
3. *Stability Data for Drugs Using Homepump Disposable Ambulatory Infusion Systems (MK-00314 rev 3)*, 2015. Alpharetta, GA: Halyard Health; Updated June 2015.
4. *Drug Stability for Easypump® ST/LT*, 2020. Bethlehem, PA: B. Braun USA; Updated June 2020.
5. *SMARTeZ® - Stability Data for Drugs Using Elastomeric Infusion Pumps*, 2020. Fenton, MO: Progressive Medical, Inc.; Updated May 2020.

DOI 10.37573/9781585286720.029

CeFAZolin Sodium

Storage Conditions

	Drug Manufacturer	Concentration	Diluents	Osmolality (mOsm/kg)	pH	Temperature Room	Temperature Refrig	Temperature Frozen	Post-thaw Temp Room	Post-thaw Temp Refrig	Body Temp	Refer.
CONTAINER												
Bag, Polyvinyl Chloride (PVC)	LI	5 mg/mL	D5W	n/a	[e]	4 d[a]	14 d[a]	n/a	n/a	n/a	n/a	(1)
	LI	10 mg/mL	D5W	[p]	[e]	24 hr	n/a	30 d	24 hr	n/a	n/a	(1)
	BR	10 mg/mL	D5W	[p]	[e]	n/a	30 d[a]	n/a	n/a	n/a	n/a	(1)
	LI, SKF	10 mg/mL	D5W, NS	[p]	[e]	n/a	n/a	48 hr	4 hr	n/a	n/a	(1)
	LI	20 mg/mL	NS	[p]	[e]	7 d[a]	15 d[a]	n/a	n/a	n/a	n/a	(1)(4)
	LI	20 mg/mL	D5W	[p]	[e]	5 d[a]	24 d[a]	n/a	n/a	n/a	n/a	(1)(4)
	SKF	20 mg/mL	D5W, NS	[p]	[e]	24 hr	24 hr	30 d	n/a	n/a	n/a	(1)
	APO	20, 40 mg/mL	D5W, NS	[p]	[e]	72 hr[a][q]	30 d[a][q]	n/a	n/a	n/a	n/a	(1)
	SKF	73.2 mg/mL	SWFI	n/a	[e]	n/a	n/a	30 d	n/a	4 d	24 hr	(1)
Syringe, Plastic (Unspecified)	SKF	100, 200 mg/mL	SWFI	n/a	[e]	13 d[a]	28 d[a]	12 wk	n/a	n/a	n/a	(1)
Syringe, Polypropylene	APC	50 mg/mL	NS	n/a	[e]	12 d[a]	22 d[a]	n/a	n/a	n/a	n/a	(1)
	APO	100, 200 mg/mL	SWFI	n/a	[e]	72 hr[a][d]	30 d[a][d]	n/a	n/a	n/a	n/a	(1)
Unspecified	LI	3.33 mg/mL	NS	n/a	n/a	72 hr[a]	7 d	n/a	n/a	n/a	72 hr	(2)
	LI	5 mg/mL	LR	n/a	n/a	7 d[a]	14 d[a]	n/a	n/a	n/a	n/a	(1)
	LI	5 mg/mL	D5W, D5LR	n/a	n/a	4 d[a]	14 d[a]	n/a	n/a	n/a	n/a	(1)
	LI	5 mg/mL	NS	n/a	[e]	4 d[a]	7 d	n/a	n/a	n/a	n/a	(1)
	UN	5, 222.2, 400 mg/mL	SWFI, D5W, NS	n/a	[e]	n/a	n/a	26 wk[c]	n/a	n/a	n/a	(1)
	UN	125, 225, 330 mg/mL	SWFI, NS, BWFI	[o]	[e]	n/a	n/a	12 wk[l]	24 hr	10 d	n/a	(1)
	UN	250 mg/mL	SWFI	n/a	[e]	4 d[a]	14 d[a]	n/a	n/a	n/a	n/a	(1)
	UN	[n]	[n]	n/a	[e]	24 hr	10 d	n/a	n/a	n/a	n/a	(6)

DOI 10.37573/9781585286720.030

Storage Conditions

	Drug Manufacturer	Concentration	Diluents	Osmolality (mOsm/kg)	pH	Temperature: Room	Temperature: Refrig	Temperature: Frozen	Post-thaw Temp: Room	Post-thaw Temp: Refrig	Body Temp	Refer.
CONTAINER												
Vial, Glass	BR	10 mg/mL	D5W	[p]	[e]	n/a	30 d[a]	n/a	n/a	n/a	n/a	(1)
	SKF	10 mg/mL	D5W, NS	[p]	[e]	48 hr[a][m]	n/a	n/a	n/a	n/a	n/a	(1)
	SKF	20 mg/mL	D5W, NS	[p]	[e]	24 hr	24 hr	n/a	n/a	n/a	n/a	(1)
	LI	20 mg/mL	D5W	[p]	[e]	5 d[a]	24 d[a]	n/a	n/a	n/a	n/a	(1)
	SKF	73.2 mg/mL	SWFI	n/a	[e]	n/a	n/a	30 d	n/a	4 d	24 hr	(1)
OTHER INFUSION CONTAINERS												
Dosi-Fuser® (Leventon)	LI	5–40 mg/mL	D5W, NS	n/a	[e]	24 hr[j]	10 d[j]	30d [j]	n/a	n/a	n/a	(8)
	UN	10–40 mg/mL	D5W	n/a	[e]	4 d[a][j]	14 d[a][j]	n/a	n/a	n/a	n/a	(8)
	PF	50 mg/mL	NS	n/a	[e]	4 d[a]	14 d[a]	30 d	24 hr	n/a	n/a	(8)
Easypump® ST/LT (B. Braun)	UN	16.7 mg/mL	NS	n/a	[e]	48 hr[a]	14 d[a]	n/a	n/a	n/a	n/a	(11)
Homepump Eclipse® / Homepump® (Halyard)	UN	20 mg/mL	NS	n/a	[e]	24 hr	7 d	n/a	n/a	n/a	n/a	(5)
INFUSOR™ (Baxter)[k]	SKF	10–40 mg/mL	D5W	n/a	[e]	4 d[a][i]	17 d[a][i]	n/a	n/a	n/a	n/a	(3)
	HOS	5–40 mg/mL	NS	n/a	[e]	n/a	10 d	n/a	n/a	n/a	48 hr	(3)
INTERMATE™ (Baxter)[k]	LI	5–40 mg/mL	D5W, NS	n/a	[e]	24 hr	10 d	30 d	n/a	n/a	n/a	(3)
	LI	20 mg/mL	SWFI	n/a	[e]	n/a	10 d	n/a	n/a	n/a	n/a	(3)
SMARTeZ® (Progressive Medical)	UN	16.7 mg/mL	NS	n/a	[e]	48 hr[a][j]	14 d[a][j]	n/a	n/a	n/a	n/a	(10)
COMMERCIAL PREPARATIONS												
Duplex® Flexible Dual-Chambered Container (B. Braun)[q]	BRN	20, 40 mg/mL	[f]	iso	n/a	24 hr[g]	7 d[g]	n/a	n/a	n/a	n/a	(1)(9)
GALAXY™ Plastic Container (Baxter)[b]	BA	20 mg/mL	D	iso	n/a	n/a	n/a	[b][h]	48 hr[l]	30 d[l]	n/a	(7)

Flush Compatibility: Sodium chloride 0.9%, heparin.[1]

Special Considerations: n/a

Notes

[a] Manufacturer recommends discarding solutions after 24 hr at room temperature and 10 d refrigeration to reduce potential for microbial growth, color change, and pH change.[1]

[b] Frozen expiration date per manufacturer's label. Do not extrapolate commercial premix stability data to extemporaneously compounded solutions.

[c] When frozen within 1 hr of reconstitution.[1]

[d] 30 d at 5°C with light protection, followed by 72 hr at 21–25°C with light exposure.[1]

[e] pH is 4.5-6.0.[1,6]

[f] Diluent in the Duplex® dual-chamber system is iso-osmotic hydrous dextrose USP.[9]

[g] Prior to activation, expiration date is per manufacturer's label. To avoid inadvertent activation, Duplex® container should remain folded until intended activation time. Protect from light after removal of foil strip. Once light-protecting foil strip is removed, product must be activated and used within 7 d.[9]

[h] Thaw at room temperature or under refrigeration. Do not force thaw. Do not re-freeze.

[i] 17 d refrigerated may be followed by 4 d at room temperature.[3]

[j] Manufacturer extrapolated data from other sources.

[k] INTERMATE™/INFUSOR™ Portable Elastomeric Infusion System devices are no longer available in the United States.

[l] In original container. Thawed solution should not be re-frozen.

[m] Exposed to fluorescent light.[1]

[n] Diluted according to manufacturer's instructions.[6]

[o] The osmolality by freezing point depression of ceFAZolin 225 mg/mL in SWFI is 636 mOsm/kg.[1]

[p] The calculated osmolality of ceFAZolin 10 mg/mL (1 gm/100 mL) is 291 mOsm/kg in D5W and 317 mOsm/kg in NS. The calculated osmolality of ceFAZolin 20 mg/mL (1 gm/50 mL) is 321 mOsm/kg in D5W and 344 mOsm/kg in NS. The calculated osmolality of ceFAZolin 40 mg/mL (2 gm/50 mL) is 379 mOsm/kg in D5W and 406 mOsm/kg in NS.[1]

[q] The Duplex® Flexible Dual-Chambered Container is not made with natural rubber latex, PVC or DEHP.[9]

REFERENCES

1. ASHP's Interactive Handbook on Injectable Drugs, 2020. Bethesda, MD: American Society of Health-System Pharmacists; Accessed September 2020.
2. Ahmed I, Day P. Stability of cefazolin sodium in various artificial tear solutions and aqueous vehicles. *Am J Hosp Pharm*. 1987; 44(10):2287-90.
3. Stabforum - Stability Database: Cefazolin, Ontario, Canada: Baxter Healthcare; Accessed February 2021.
4. Gupta VD, Stewart KR. Quantitation of carbenicillin disodium, cefazolin sodium, cephalothin sodium, nafcillin sodium, and ticarcillin disodium by high-pressure liquid chromatography. *J Pharm Sci*. 1980; 69(11):1264-7.
5. *Stability Data for Drugs Using Homepump Disposable Ambulatory Infusion Systems (MK-00314 rev 3)*, 2015. Alpharetta, GA: Halyard Health; Updated June 2015.
6. Cefazolin Injection [package insert]. Weston, FL: Apotex Corp.; December 2019.
7. Cefazolin Injection in GALAXY™ Container [package insert]. Deerfield, IL: Baxter Healthcare Corporation; October 2019.
8. *Drug Stability Table - Dosi-Fuser® Elastomeric Pump (S-CL-00-001v16)*, 2021. Barcelona, Spain: Leventon SAU; Updated May 2021.
9. Cefazolin Injection and Dextrose Injection in Duplex® Container [package insert]. Bethlehem, PA: B. Braun Medical, Inc.; November 2020.
10. *SMARTeZ® - Stability Data for Drugs Using Elastomeric Infusion Pumps*, 2020. Fenton, MO: Progressive Medical, Inc.; Updated May 2020.
11. *Drug Stability for Easypump® ST/LT*, 2020. Bethlehem, PA: B. Braun USA; Updated June 2020.

Cefepime Hydrochloride

Storage Conditions

	Drug Manufacturer	Concentration	Diluents	Osmolality (mOsm/kg)	pH	Temperature: Room	Temperature: Refrig	Temperature: Frozen	Post-thaw Temp: Room	Post-thaw Temp: Refrig	Body Temp	Refer.
CONTAINER												
Bag, Polyvinyl Chloride (PVC)	BMS	1, 40 mg/mL	NS, D5W, D5NS, D5LR, D10W	n/a	[f]	24 hr	7 d	n/a	n/a	n/a	n/a	(1)
	BMS	2.5, 5, 10, 20 mg/mL	D5W, NS[a]	n/a	n/a	48 hr	7 d	n/a	n/a	n/a	n/a	(1)(5)
	BMS	20 mg/mL	NS, D5W	n/a	[f]	48 hr	23 d	n/a	n/a	n/a	n/a	(1)
	BMS	20 mg/mL	D5W	n/a	[f]	n/a	n/a	30 d	n/a	11 d	n/a	(1)
Syringe, Polypropylene	BMS	20 mg/mL	NS	n/a	n/a	48 hr	21 d	n/a	n/a	n/a	n/a	(1)
	BMS	100, 200 mg/mL	SWFI, NS, D5W	n/a	n/a	24 hr[k]	14 d	90 d[e]	24 hr[e]	7 d[e]	n/a	(4)(12)
Unspecified	HOS	1-40 mg/mL	NS, D5W, D5NS, D5LR, D10W	n/a	n/a	24 hr	7 d	n/a	n/a	n/a	n/a	(7)
Vial, Glass	BR	1, 40 mg/mL	NS, D5W	n/a	[f]	24 hr	7 d	n/a	n/a	n/a	n/a	(1)
OTHER INFUSION CONTAINERS												
ADD-Vantage® Flexible Container System (Pfizer)	HOS	10-40 mg/mL	NS, D5W	n/a	n/a	24 hr[h]	7 d[h]	n/a	n/a	n/a	n/a	(7)
Dosi-Fuser® (Leventon)	UN[b]	5-60 mg/mL	NS	n/a	[f]	48 hr	14 d	60 d	24 hr	n/a	n/a	(11)
	BMS	1 mg/mL	NS, D5W	n/a	[f]	48 hr[l]	14 d[l]	9 wk[l]	n/a	n/a	n/a	(11)
	BMS	1-5 mg/mL	NS, D5W	n/a	[f]	48 hr[l]	n/a	n/a	n/a	n/a	n/a	(11)
	BMS	1-60 mg/mL	NS, D5W	n/a	[f]	24 hr[l]	n/a	9 wk[l]	n/a	n/a	n/a	(11)
Easypump® ST/LT (B. Braun)	UN	20 mg/mL	NS	n/a	[f]	24 hr	14 d	n/a	n/a	n/a	n/a	(6)
Homepump Eclipse® / Homepump® (Halyard)	UN	20 mg/mL	NS	n/a	[f]	24 hr	14 d	n/a	n/a	n/a	n/a	(3)
INTERMATE™ (Baxter)[d]	BMS	1-5 mg/mL	D5W	n/a	[f]	48 hr	n/a	n/a	n/a	n/a	n/a	(2)
	BMS	1-5 mg/mL	NS	n/a	[f]	72 hr	n/a	n/a	n/a	n/a	n/a	(2)
	BMS	1 mg/mL	D5W, NS	n/a	[f]	n/a	n/a	9 wk	48 hr	7 d[c]	n/a	(2)
	BMS	1-60 mg/mL	D5W, NS	n/a	[f]	n/a	n/a	9 wk	24 hr	n/a	n/a	(2)
SMARTeZ® (Progressive Medical)	UN	20 mg/ mL	NS	n/a	[f]	24 hr[l]	14 d[l]	n/a	n/a	n/a	n/a	(10)

DOI 10.37573/9781585286720.031

Storage Conditions

	Drug Manufacturer	Concentration	Diluents	Osmolality (mOsm/kg)	pH	Temperature Room	Temperature Refrig	Temperature Frozen	Post-thaw Temp Room	Post-thaw Temp Refrig	Body Temp	Refer.
COMMERCIAL PREPARATIONS (RTU)												
Duplex® Flexible Dual-Chambered Container (B. Braun)	BRN	20, 40 mg/mL	[i]	[i]	n/a	12 hr[j]	5 d[j]	n/a	n/a	n/a	n/a	(9)
GALAXY™ Plastic Container (Baxter)	BA	2 mg/mL	[g]	iso	4.0-6.0	n/a	n/a	[m][n]	24 hr	7 d	n/a	(8)

Flush Compatibility: Sodium chloride 0.9%, heparin.[1]

Special Considerations: n/a

Notes

[a] Solution contained: MetroNIDAZOLE 5 mg/mL (AB, ES, SE).[1,5]

[b] Cepimex formulation, contains cefepime dihydrochloride monohydrate.

[c] Storage temperature: frozen for 9 weeks, followed by 7 days refrigerated, then 48 hours at room temperature.[2]

[d] INTERMATE™/INFUSOR™ Portable Elastomeric Infusion System devices are no longer available in the United States.

[e] Storage temperature: -20°C for 90 days, followed by 7 days at 4°C, followed by 24 hours at 22°C to 24°C.[4]

[f] pH of reconstituted preparation is 4-6.[1]

[g] Diluent is iso-osmotic dextrose hydrous USP, 2.06 gm/100 mL.[8]

[h] Following activation of ADD-Vantage® container, reconstitution and dilution of medication per labeled instructions.[7]

[i] Diluent in the Duplex® dual chamber system is iso-osmotic hydrous dextrose USP. After reconstitution, the drug product in solution is hyper-osmotic and is intended for single IV use.[9]

[j] Prior to activation, expiration date is per manufacturer's label. Protect from light after removal of foil strip. If light-protecting foil strip is removed, product must be activated within 7 d but not beyond the labeled expiration date.[9]

[k] Storage temperature: 4°C for 7 days, followed by 24 hours at 22°C to 24°C.[4]

[l] Manufacturer extrapolated data from other sources.

[m] Thaw at room temperature or under refrigeration. Do not force thaw. Do not re-freeze.[8]

[n] Frozen expiration date per manufacturer's label. Do not extrapolate commercial premix stability data to extemporaneously compounded solutions.[8]

REFERENCES

1. ASHP's Interactive Handbook on Injectable Drugs, 2020. Bethesda, MD: American Society of Health-System Pharmacists; Accessed August 2020.
2. Stabforum - Stability Database: Cefepime, Ontario, Canada: Baxter Healthcare; Accessed February 2021.
3. *Stability Data for Drugs Using Homepump Disposable Ambulatory Infusion Systems (MK-00314 rev 3)*, 2015. Alpharetta, GA: Halyard Health; Updated June 2015.
4. Stewart JT, Warren FW, Maddox FC. Stability of cefepime hydrochloride injection in polypropylene syringes at -20 degrees C, 4 degrees C, and 22-24 degrees C. *Am J Health Syst Pharm*. 1999; 56(5):457-9.

5. Stewart JT, Maddox FC, Warren FW. Stability of Cefepime Hydrochloride Injection and Metronidazole in Polyvinyl Chloride Bags at 4° and 22°–24° C. *Hosp Pharm*. 2000; 35(10):1057-64.
6. *Drug Stability for Easypump® ST/LT*, 2020. Bethlehem, PA: B. Braun USA; Updated June 2020.
7. Maxipime® (Cefepime) Injection [package insert]. Lake Forest, IL: Hospira, Inc.; April 2017.
8. Cefepime Injection in GALAXY™ Container [package insert]. Deerfield, IL: Baxter Healthcare Corporation; May 2020.
9. Cefepime Injection and Dextrose Injection in Duplex® Container [package insert]. Bethlehem, PA: B. Braun Medical, Inc.; November 2018.
10. *SMARTeZ® - Stability Data for Drugs Using Elastomeric Infusion Pumps*, 2020. Fenton, MO: Progressive Medical, Inc.; Updated May 2020.
11. *Drug Stability Table - Dosi-Fuser® Elastomeric Pump (S-CL-00-001v16)*, 2021. Barcelona, Spain: Leventon SAU; Updated May 2021.
12. Stewart JT, Warren FW, Maddox FC. Stability of cefepime hydrochloride injection in polypropylene syringes at -20 degrees C, 4 degrees C, and 22-24 degrees C. *Am J Health Syst Pharm*. 1999;56(5):457-9. Epub 1999/03/30. doi: 10.1093/ajhp/56.5.457. PubMed PMID: 10096708.

Cefotaxime Sodium

Storage Conditions

	Drug Manufacturer	Concentration	Diluents	Osmolality (mOsm/kg)	pH	Temperature Room	Temperature Refrig	Temperature Frozen	Post-thaw Temp Room	Post-thaw Temp Refrig	Body Temp	Refer.
CONTAINER												
Bag, Polyvinyl Chloride (PVC)	UN	[c]	D5W, NS	n/a	[b]	24 hr	5 d	13 wk	n/a	n/a	n/a	(1)
	WW	[c]	D5W, NS	n/a	[b]	24 hr	5 d	n/a	n/a	n/a	n/a	(2)
	UN	[c]	D5W, NS	n/a	[b]	n/a	n/a	13 wk	24 hr	5 d	n/a	(1)
	HO	10 mg/mL	D5W, NS	319, 344	[b]	24 hr	22 d	9 wk	n/a	n/a	n/a	(1)
	HO	20 mg/mL	D5W, NS	327, 351	[b]	24 hr	n/a	n/a	n/a	n/a	n/a	(1)
Syringe, Plastic	UN	[c]	D5W, NS	n/a	[b]	n/a	n/a	13 wk	24 hr	5 d	n/a	(1)
	UN	50, 95 mg/mL	SWFI	[d]	[b]	24 hr	5 d	[e]	n/a	n/a	n/a	(1)
	UN	180, 230, 300, 330 mg/mL	SWFI	[d]	[b]	12 hr	5 d	[e]	n/a	n/a	n/a	(1)
Syringe, Polypropylene	AVE	50 mg/mL	NS	n/a	[b]	48 hr	18 d	n/a	n/a	n/a	n/a	(1)
Vial, Glass[g]	WW	10-40 mg/mL	D5W, NS	n/a	n/a	24 hr	10 d	[e]	n/a	n/a	n/a	(2)
	WW	50, 95 mg/mL	SWFI	[d]	[b]	24 hr	7 d	[e]	n/a	n/a	n/a	(2)
	WW	180, 230, 300, 330 mg/mL	SWFI	[d]	[b]	12 hr	7 d	[e]	n/a	n/a	n/a	(2)
OTHER INFUSION CONTAINERS												
Dosi-Fuser® (Leventon)	HO	40 mg/mL	NS	n/a	n/a	24 hr[a]	10 d[a]	n/a	n/a	n/a	n/a	(3)
	HO	5-40 mg/mL	D5W, NS	n/a	n/a	24 hr[a]	n/a	30 d[a]	24 hr[a]	n/a	n/a	(3)
Easypump® ST/LT (B. Braun)	UN	16.66 mg/mL	NS	n/a	n/a	24 hr	72 hr	n/a	n/a	n/a	n/a	(5)
	UN	10, 15 mg/mL	NS	n/a	n/a	24 hr	14 d	n/a	n/a	n/a	n/a	(5)
Homepump Eclipse® / Homepump® (Halyard)	UN	16.66 mg/mL	NS	n/a	n/a	24 hr	n/a	n/a	n/a	n/a	n/a	(4)
INTERMATE™ (Baxter)[f]	HO	5-40 mg/mL	D5W, NS	n/a	n/a	24 hr	n/a	30 d	24 hr	n/a	n/a	(7)
	HO	40 mg/mL	NS	n/a	n/a	24 hr	10 d	n/a	n/a	n/a	n/a	(7)
SMARTeZ® (Progressive Medical)	UN	20 mg/mL	NS	n/a	n/a	24 hr[a]	14 d[a]	n/a	n/a	n/a	n/a	(6)

DOI 10.37573/9781585286720.032

Flush Compatibility: Sodium chloride 0.9%, heparin.[1]

Special Considerations: n/a

Notes

[a] Manufacturer extrapolated data from other sources.
[b] pH of injectable solutions is 5-7.5.[1]
[c] Concentrations of dilutions based on reconstitution and/or dilution per manufacturer's labeling. Refer to current package insert for instructions.
[d] A solution of 71 mg/mL in SWFI is isotonic.[1]
[e] Reconstituted solutions stored in original containers and plastic syringes remain stable for 13 wk frozen.[2]
[f] INTERMATE™/INFUSOR™ Portable Elastomeric Infusion System devices are no longer available in the United States.
[g] In original container.[2]

REFERENCES

1. ASHP's Interactive Handbook on Injectable Drugs, 2020. Bethesda, MD: American Society of Health-System Pharmacists; Accessed June 2020.
2. Cefotaxime Injection [package insert]. Eatontown, NJ: West-Ward Pharmaceuticals Corp; December 2018.
3. *Drug Stability Table - Dosi-Fuser® Elastomeric Pump (S-CL-00-001v16)*, 2021. Barcelona, Spain: Leventon SAU; Updated May 2021.
4. *Stability Data for Drugs Using Homepump Disposable Ambulatory Infusion Systems (MK-00314 rev 3)*, 2015. Alpharetta, GA: Halyard Health; Updated June 2015.
5. *Drug Stability for Easypump® ST/LT*, 2020. Bethlehem, PA: B. Braun USA; Updated June 2020.
6. *SMARTeZ® - Stability Data for Drugs Using Elastomeric Infusion Pumps*, 2020. Fenton, MO: Progressive Medical, Inc.; Updated May 2020.
7. Stabforum - Stability Database: Cefotaxime, Ontario, Canada: Baxter Healthcare; Accessed January 2021.

CefoTEtan Disodium

Storage Conditions

	Drug Manufacturer	Concentration	Diluents	Osmolality[g] (mOsm/kg)	pH	Temperature Room	Temperature Refrig	Temperature Frozen	Post-thaw Temp Room	Post-thaw Temp Refrig	Body Temp	Refer.
CONTAINER												
Bag, Polyvinyl Chloride (PVC)	STU	2 mg/mL	D5W	n/a	[b]	14 d	14 d	14 d	n/a	n/a	n/a	(1)
	STU	20 mg/mL	NS, D5W	n/a	[b]	48 hr	41 d	60 d	n/a	n/a	n/a	(1)
	AY	20, 40 mg/mL	NS	n/a	[b]	84 hr	14 d	n/a	n/a	n/a	n/a	(1)
	AY	20, 40 mg/mL	D5W	n/a	[b]	84 hr	13 d	n/a	n/a	n/a	n/a	(1)
Syringe, Polypropylene	ZEN	60 mg/mL	NS	n/a	[b]	6 d	24 d	n/a	n/a	n/a	n/a	(3)
OTHER INFUSION CONTAINERS												
Dosi-Fuser® (Leventon)	STU	60 mg/mL	NS, D5W	n/a	[b]	24 hr[a]	n/a	30 d[a]	n/a	n/a	n/a	(2)
	STU	5-60 mg/mL	NS	n/a	[b]	n/a	10 d[a]	n/a	n/a	n/a	n/a	(2)
	STU	5-60 mg/mL	D5W	n/a	[b]	24 hr[a]	10 d[a]	n/a	n/a	n/a	n/a	(2)
Homepump Eclipse® / Homepump® (Halyard)	UN	10-40 mg/mL	NS, D5W	n/a	[b]	24 hr[a]	4 d[a]	7 d[a]	n/a	n/a	n/a	(5)
	UN	20 mg/mL	NS, D5W	n/a	[b]	n/a	n/a	60 d[a]	n/a	n/a	n/a	(5)
INTERMATE™ (Baxter)[f]	STU	5-60 mg/mL	D5W	n/a	[b]	24 hr	10 d	n/a	n/a	n/a	n/a	(4)
	STU	5-60 mg/mL	NS	n/a	[b]	n/a	10 d	n/a	n/a	n/a	n/a	(4)
	STU	30 mg/mL	SWFI	n/a	[b]	n/a	10 d	n/a	n/a	n/a	n/a	(4)
	STU	60 mg/mL	NS, D5W	n/a	[b]	24 hr	10 d	30 d	24 hr	n/a	n/a	(4)
COMMERCIAL PREPARATIONS (RTU)												
Duplex® Flexible Dual-Chambered Container (B. Braun)	BRN	20, 40 mg/mL	[c]	290[c]	4-6.5	12 hr[d]	5 d[d]	[e]	n/a	n/a	n/a	(1)(6)

Flush Compatibility: Sodium chloride 0.9%, heparin.[1]

Special Considerations: n/a

DOI 10.37573/9781585286720.033

Notes

[a] Manufacturer extrapolated data from other sources.

[b] pH of reconstituted solutions is 4.5-6.5.[1]

[c] Diluent in the Duplex® dual chamber system is Hydrous Dextrose in Water for Injection at a concentration that renders the reconstituted solution iso-osmotic.[6]

[d] Prior to activation, expiration date is per manufacturer's label. To avoid inadvertent activation, Duplex® container should remain folded until intended activation time. Protect from light after removal of foil strip. If light-protecting foil strip is removed, product must be activated within 7 d but not beyond the labeled expiration date.[6]

[e] Do not freeze Duplex® container.[6]

[f] INTERMATE™/INFUSOR™ Portable Elastomeric Infusion System devices are no longer available in the United States.

[g] CefoTEtan disodium solution 100-200 mg/mL in SWFI is 400-800 mOsm/L.

REFERENCES

1. ASHP's Interactive Handbook on Injectable Drugs, 2020. Bethesda, MD: American Society of Health-System Pharmacists; Accessed July 2020.
2. *Drug Stability Table - Dosi-Fuser® Elastomeric Pump (S-CL-00-001v16)*, 2021. Barcelona, Spain: Leventon SAU; Updated May 2021.
3. Zaid AN. Chemical Stability of Cefotetan Disodium in 0.9% Sodium Chloride Sterile Saline Solutions and Storage in Polypropylene Syringe. *J Al-Aqsa Unv*. 2007:22-31.
4. Stabforum - Stability Database: Cefotetan, Ontario, Canada: Baxter Healthcare; Accessed December 2020.
5. *Stability Data for Drugs Using Homepump Disposable Ambulatory Infusion Systems (MK-00314 rev 3)*, 2015. Alpharetta, GA: Halyard Health; Updated June 2015.
6. Cefotetan and Dextrose Injection in Duplex® Drug Delivery System [package insert]. Bethlehem, PA: B. Braun Medical, Inc.; January 2020.

CefOXitin Sodium

Storage Conditions

Container	Drug Manufacturer	Concentration	Diluents	Osmolality (mOsm/kg)	pH	Temperature: Room	Temperature: Refrig	Temperature: Frozen	Post-thaw Temp: Room	Post-thaw Temp: Refrig	Body Temp	Refer.
CONTAINER												
Bag, Polyvinyl Chloride (PVC)	MSD	1 mg/mL	NS	n/a	[c]	48 hr	n/a	n/a	n/a	n/a	n/a	(1)
	MSD	1 mg/mL	D5W	n/a	[c]	24 hr	n/a	n/a	n/a	n/a	n/a	(1)
	UN	10, 20 mg/mL	D5W, NS	[f]	[c]	n/a	n/a	72 hr	6 hr	n/a	n/a	(1)(2)
	MSD	20 mg/mL	NS	352	[c]	24 hr	13 d	n/a	n/a	n/a	n/a	(1)
	MSD	20 mg/mL	D5W	326	[c]	24 hr	13 d	30 d	n/a	n/a	n/a	(1)
	MSD	40 mg/mL	SWFI	n/a	[c]	n/a	n/a	30 d[a]	n/a	4 d[a]	24 hr[a]	(1)
	MSD	1 mg/mL	LR	n/a	[c]	48 hr	n/a	n/a	n/a	n/a	n/a	(1)
Syringe, Plastic (Unspecified)	MSD	100 mg/mL	SWFI	[f]	[c]	48 hr	23 d	12 wk	n/a	n/a	n/a	(1)
	MSD	200 mg/mL	SWFI	n/a	[c]	48 hr	23 d	12 wk	n/a	n/a	n/a	(1)
Unspecified	UN	100 mg/mL	SWFI	[f]	n/a	48 hr	7 d	30 wk	24 hr	7 d	n/a	(1)
	UN	250 mg/mL	SWFI	n/a	n/a	48 hr	7 d	13 wk	n/a	n/a	n/a	(1)
	UN	500 mg/mL	SWFI	n/a	n/a	48 hr	30 d	n/a	n/a	n/a	n/a	(1)
Vial, Glass	MSD	1 mg/mL	NS	n/a	[c]	24 hr	n/a	n/a	n/a	n/a	n/a	(1)
	MSD	10, 20 mg/mL	NS	[f]	[c]	24 hr	48 hr	n/a	n/a	n/a	n/a	(1)
	MSD	20 mg/mL	D5W	[f]	[c]	24 hr	7 d	13 wk	n/a	n/a	n/a	(1)
	MSD	1, 2, 10 mg/mL	D5W	[f]	[c]	24 hr	7 d	n/a	n/a	n/a	n/a	(1)
	MSD	1, 2, 10, 20 mg/mL	D5LR, LR	n/a	[c]	24 hr	7 d	n/a	n/a	n/a	n/a	(1)
	MSD	1, 2, 10 mg/mL	[i]	n/a	[c]	24 hr	7 d	n/a	n/a	n/a	n/a	(1)
	MSD	1, 2, 10, 20 mg/mL	[j]	n/a	[c]	24 hr	7 d	n/a	n/a	n/a	n/a	(1)
	MSD	40 mg/mL	SWFI	[f]	[c]	n/a	n/a	30 d[a]	n/a	4 d[a]	24 hr[a]	(1)
OTHER INFUSION CONTAINERS												
Dosi-Fuser® (Leventon)	MSD	5-60 mg/mL	NS, D5W	[f]	[c]	n/a	10 d[b]	30 d[b]	n/a	n/a	n/a	(8)
	MSD	10 mg/mL	NS, D5W	[f]	[c]	54 hr[b]	7 d[b]	n/a	n/a	n/a	n/a	(8)
	UN	20 mg/mL	NS, D5W	[f]	[c]	24 hr[b]	48 hr[b]	26 wk[b]	n/a	n/a	n/a	(8)
	UN	100 mg/mL	NS, D5W	[f]	[c]	48 hr[b]	7 d[b]	30 wk[b]	n/a	n/a	n/a	(8)

DOI 10.37573/9781585286720.034

Storage Conditions

	Drug Manufacturer	Concentration	Diluents	Osmolality (mOsm/kg)	pH	Temperature: Room	Temperature: Refrig	Temperature: Frozen	Post-thaw Temp: Room	Post-thaw Temp: Refrig	Body Temp	Refer.
OTHER INFUSION CONTAINERS												
Easypump® ST/LT (B. Braun)	UN	1 mg/mL	NS	[f]	[c]	48 hr[b]	7 d[b]	n/a	n/a	n/a	n/a	(3)
	UN	10 mg/mL	NS	[f]	[c]	48 hr[b]	7 d[b]	n/a	n/a	n/a	n/a	(3)
Homepump Eclipse® / Homepump® (Halyard)	UN	20 mg/mL	NS, D5W	[f]	[c]	24 hr[b]	13 d[b]	n/a	n/a	n/a	n/a	(5)
INTERMATE™ (Baxter)[h]	MSD	5 mg/mL	NS	n/a	[c]	n/a	n/a	30 d	n/a	n/a	n/a	(4)
	MSD	5-60 mg/mL	D5W	[f]	[c]	n/a	10 d	30 d	n/a	n/a	n/a	(4)
	MSD	30 mg/mL	SWFI	n/a	[c]	n/a	10 d	n/a	n/a	n/a	n/a	(4)
	MSD	60 mg/mL	NS	[f]	[c]	n/a	10 d	n/a	n/a	n/a	n/a	(4)
SMARTeZ® (Progressive Medical)	UN	1 mg/mL	NS	[f]	[c]	48 hr[b]	7 d[b]	n/a	n/a	n/a	n/a	(7)
	UN	10 mg/mL	NS	[f]	[c]	48 hr[b]	7 d[b]	n/a	n/a	n/a	n/a	(7)
COMMERCIAL PREPARATIONS (RTU)												
Duplex® Flexible Dual-Chambered Container (B. Braun)	BRN	20, 40 mg/mL	D[d]	290	6.5	12 hr[e]	7 d[e]	[g]	n/a	n/a	n/a	(6)

Flush Compatibility: Sodium chloride 0.9%, heparin.[1]

Special Considerations: n/a

Notes

[a] Storage temperature: Frozen for 30 days, followed by 4 days refrigerated, followed by 24 hours at 37°C.

[b] Manufacturer(s) extrapolated data from other sources.

[c] pH of reconstituted solution is 4.2-7.[1]

[d] Diluent chamber of the DUPLEX® container has 50 mL Dextrose Injection (4.4% for 1 gm dose and 2.2% for 2 gm dose) such that the reconstituted solutions are iso-osmotic.[6]

[e] Prior to activation, expiration date is per manufacturer's label. To avoid inadvertent activation, DUPLEX® container should remain folded until intended activation time. Protect from light after removal of foil strip. If light-protecting, foil strip is removed; product must be activated within 7 d. Allow refrigerated reconstituted DUPLEX® bag to equilibrate to room temperature before administration.[6]

[f] Osmolality of 10, 20, 40, and 62 mg/mL in D5W is 290, 326-329, 388, and 531 mOsm/kg; solutions of 10, 20, 40, and 56 mg/mL in NS is 319, 352-355, 415, and 508 mOsm/kg. At 112 mg/mL in SWFI, osmolality is 437 mOsm/kg.[1]

[g] Do not freeze DUPLEX® containers.[6]

[h] INTERMATE™/INFUSOR™ Portable Elastomeric Infusion System devices are no longer available in the United States.

[i] Solution tested in: Ionosol® B in D5W.[1]

[j] Solution tested in: Normosol® M in D5W.[1]

REFERENCES

1. ASHP's Interactive Handbook on Injectable Drugs, 2020. Bethesda, MD: American Society of Health-System Pharmacists; Accessed August 2020.
2. Stiles ML. Effect of microwave radiation on the stability of frozen cefoxitin sodium solution in plastic bags. *Am J Hosp Pharm*. 1981; 38(11):1743-5.
3. *Drug Stability for Easypump® ST/LT*, 2020. Bethlehem, PA: B. Braun USA; Updated June 2020.
4. Stabforum - Stability Database: Cefoxitin, Ontario, Canada: Baxter Healthcare; Accessed February 2021.
5. *Stability Data for Drugs Using Homepump Disposable Ambulatory Infusion Systems (MK-00314 rev 3)*, 2015. Alpharetta, GA: Halyard Health; Updated June 2015.
6. Cefoxitin Injection and Dextrose Injection [package insert]. Bethlehem, PA: B. Braun Medical, Inc.; July 2019.
7. *SMARTeZ® - Stability Data for Drugs Using Elastomeric Infusion Pumps*, 2020. Fenton, MO: Progressive Medical, Inc.; Updated May 2020.
8. *Drug Stability Table - Dosi-Fuser® Elastomeric Pump (ES.H.00.73-10)*, 2015. Barcelona, Spain: Leventon SAU; Updated October 2015.

Ceftaroline Fosamil

Storage Conditions

	Drug Manufacturer	Concentration	Diluents	Osmolality (mOsm/kg)	pH	Temperature			Post-thaw Temp			
						Room	Refrig	Frozen	Room	Refrig	Body Temp	Refer.
CONTAINER												
Bag, Unspecified	FOR	8-12 mg/mL[c]	NS, D5W, D2.5W, ½NS, LR	n/a	[a]	6 hr	24 hr	n/a	n/a	n/a	n/a	(1)
OTHER INFUSION CONTAINERS												
Homepump Eclipse® / Homepump® (Halyard)	FOR	12 mg/mL	D5W	n/a		6 hr	24 hr	n/a	n/a	n/a	n/a	(2)
INFUSOR™ (Baxter)[d]	ASZ	6 mg/mL	NS	n/a	[e]	24 hr	6 d	n/a	n/a	n/a	[f]	(2)(3)
	ASZ	6 mg/mL	D5W	n/a	[e]	24 hr	6 d	n/a	n/a	n/a	[g]	(2)(3)
Mini-Bag Plus™ (Baxter)	FOR	4-12 mg/mL[c]	NS	n/a	[a]	6 hr[b]	24 hr[b]	n/a	n/a	n/a	n/a	(1)

Flush Compatibility: Sodium chloride 0.9%, heparin.[2]

Special Considerations: Store un-reconstituted vials at 25°C; excursions are permitted to 15-30°C. Infusion solution concentration should not exceed 12 mg/mL; for dilution in 50 mL bags, withdraw 20 mL of solution from bag prior to addition of the reconstituted drug.[1]

Notes

[a] pH of constituted solution (20-30 mg/mL) is 4.8-6.5.[1]

[b] After activation/reconstitution in 50 or 100 mL containers.[1]

[c] Reconstituted and diluted according to package insert.[1]

[d] INTERMATE™/INFUSOR™ Portable Elastomeric Infusion System devices are no longer available in the United States.

[e] pH of diluted (NS) solution 5.27 and D5W 5.42.[3]

[f] Physically compatible with less than 10% loss in 12 hr at 30°C and 12 hr at 35°C.[3]

[g] Physically compatible with less than 10% loss in 12 hr at 30°C and 6 hr at 35°C.[3]

REFERENCES

1. Teflaro® (Cefaroline Fosamil) Injection [package insert]. Madison, NJ: Allergan USA, Inc.; November 2020.
2. ASHP's Interactive Handbook on Injectable Drugs, 2020. Bethesda, MD: American Society of Health-System Pharmacists; Accessed August 2020.
3. Al Madfai F, Zaidi STR, Ming LC, et al. Physical and chemical stability of ceftaroline in an elastomeric infusion device. *Eur J Hosp Pharm*. 2018; 25(e2):e115-e19.

DOI 10.37573/9781585286720.035

CefTAZidime

Storage Conditions

	Drug Manufacturer	Concentration	Diluents	Osmolality (mOsm/kg)	pH	Temperature: Room	Temperature: Refrig	Temperature: Frozen	Post-thaw Temp: Room	Post-thaw Temp: Refrig	Body Temp	Refer.
CONTAINER												
Bag, Polyvinyl Chloride (PVC)	GL	2, 6 mg/mL	D5W, NS	n/a	[a]	24 hr	n/a	n/a	n/a	n/a	n/a	(1)
	UN	4 mg/mL	D5W, NS	n/a	[a]	24 hr	24 hr	n/a	n/a	n/a	n/a	(1)
	GW	10 mg/mL	D5W, NS	n/a	[a]	24 hr	24 hr	n/a	n/a	n/a	n/a	(1)
	GL	40 mg/mL	NS	n/a	[a]	24 hr	14 d	n/a	n/a	n/a	n/a	(1)
	GL	40 mg/mL	D5W	n/a	[a]	24 hr	10 d	n/a	n/a	n/a	n/a	(1)
	GL	36.6 mg/mL	SWFI	n/a	[a]	n/a	n/a	30 d	n/a	4 d	24 hr	(1)
Syringe, Plastic (Unspecified)	HOS	1 mg/mL	NS[b]	n/a	[a]	72 hr	17 d	60 d	n/a	n/a	n/a	(1)
Syringe, Polypropylene	GL	100, 200 mg/mL	SWFI[b]	n/a	[a]	8 hr	4 d	13 wk	8 hr	4 d	n/a	(1)
Unspecified	COV, SAG	1-40 mg/mL	D5W, NS, D5NS, D5¼NS, D5½NS, D10W, LR	n/a	[a]	12 hr	72 hr	n/a	n/a	n/a	n/a	(8)(9)
	HOS	1-40 mg/mL	D5W, NS, D5NS, D5¼NS, D5½NS, D10W, LR	n/a	5.0-7.5	24 hr	7 d	n/a	n/a	n/a	n/a	(2)
	GL	20 mg/mL	NS	n/a	[a]	n/a	n/a	97 d	24 hr	4 d	n/a	(1)
	GL	20 mg/mL	D5W, D5NS, NS	n/a	[a]	24 hr	48 hr	n/a	n/a	n/a	n/a	(1)
	UN	95-280 mg/mL	SWFI	n/a	[a]	24 hr	7 d	n/a	n/a	n/a	n/a	(1)
	GSK	100-180 mg/mL	NS, SWFI	n/a	[a]	n/a	n/a	6 m	24 hr	7 d	n/a	(1)
	HOS	100-180 mg/mL	NS, D5W	n/a	[a]	n/a	n/a	3 m	8 hr	4 d	n/a	(1)
	UN	280 mg/mL	BWFI[e]	n/a	[a]	24 hr	7 d	n/a	n/a	n/a	n/a	(1)
	GSK, HOS	280 mg/mL	SWFI	n/a	[a]	n/a	n/a	3 m	8 hr	4 d	n/a	(1)
Vial, Glass	UN	40 mg/mL	D5W	n/a	[a]	48 hr	21 d	90 d	n/a	n/a	n/a	(1)
	UN	40 mg/mL	NS	n/a	[a]	48 hr	28 d	90 d	n/a	n/a	n/a	(1)
	GL	100, 200 mg/mL	SWFI[b]	n/a	[a]	8 hr	4 d	13 wk	8 hr	4 d	n/a	(1)
	GL	36.6 mg/mL	SWFI	n/a	[a]	n/a	n/a	30 d	n/a	4 d	24 hr	(1)
OTHER INFUSION CONTAINERS												
CADD® Cassette (Smiths Medical)	UN	30, 60 mg/mL	SWFI	n/a	[a]	n/a	10 d	30 d	n/a	4 d	n/a	(11)

DOI 10.37573/9781585286720.036

Storage Conditions

						Temperature			Post-thaw Temp			
	Drug Manufacturer	Concentration	Diluents	Osmolality (mOsm/kg)	pH	Room	Refrig	Frozen	Room	Refrig	Body Temp	Refer.
OTHER INFUSION CONTAINERS												
Dosi-Fuser® (Leventon)	GSK	5-40 mg/mL	NS, D5W	n/a	[a]	24 hr[c]	7 d[c]	n/a	n/a	n/a	n/a	(3)
	GSK	5-60 mg/mL	NS	n/a	[a]	n/a	7 d[c]	8 wk[c]	n/a	n/a	n/a	(3)
	GSK	20 mg/mL	NS	n/a	[a]	n/a	10 d	n/a	n/a	n/a	n/a	(3)
	UN	30 mg/mL	NS	n/a	[a]	n/a	40 d	n/a	n/a	n/a	n/a	(3)
	GSK	60 mg/mL	NS, D5W	n/a	[a]	7 d	28 d	3 m	n/a	n/a	n/a	(3)
Easypump® ST/LT (B. Braun)	UN	40 mg/mL	NS	n/a	[a]	24 hr	14 d	n/a	n/a	n/a	n/a	(4)
	UN	1 mg/mL	NS	n/a	[a]	24 hr	48 hr	n/a	n/a	n/a	n/a	(4)
Homepump Eclipse® / Homepump® (Halyard)	UN	5-30 mg/mL	NS	n/a	[a]	n/a	28 d	n/a	n/a	n/a	n/a	(5)
	UN	5-40 mg/mL	NS	n/a	[a]	24 hr	14 d	n/a	n/a	n/a	n/a	(5)
	UN	20 mg/mL	NS	n/a	[a]	18 hr	7 d	3 m	n/a	n/a	n/a	(5)
	UN	60 mg/mL	NS	n/a	[a]	n/a	14 d	14 d	n/a	n/a	n/a	(5)
INFUSOR™ (Baxter)[d]	GL	10-40 mg/mL	D5W	n/a	[a]	18 hr	4 d	n/a	n/a	n/a	n/a	(6)
INTERMATE™ (Baxter)[d]	VB	1-60 mg/mL	NS	n/a	[a]	6 hr	6 d	n/a	n/a	n/a	n/a	(6)
	GL	5-40 mg/mL	NS, D5W	n/a	[a]	24 hr	10 d	30 d	24 hr	n/a	n/a	(6)
	GL	5-60 mg/mL	NS	n/a	[a]	n/a	n/a	8 w	n/a	7 d	n/a	(6)
	GL	20 mg/mL	SWFI	n/a	[a]	n/a	10 d	n/a	n/a	n/a	n/a	(6)
SMARTeZ® (Progressive Medical)	UN	40 mg/mL	NS	n/a	[a]	24 hr[c]	14 d[c]	n/a	n/a	n/a	n/a	(7)
COMMERCIAL PREPARTIONS (RTU)												
ADD-Vantage® (Hospira)	HOS	unspec.	D5W, NS, ½NS	n/a	5.0-7.5	24 hr[i]	n/a	n/a	n/a	n/a	n/a	(12)
Duplex® Flexible Dual-Chambered Container (B. Braun)	BRN	20, 40 mg/mL	D5W	340, 400	5.0-7.5	12 hr[f]	72 hr[f]	n/a	n/a	n/a	n/a	(10)
GALAXY™ Plastic Container (Baxter)	COV	20, 40 mg/mL	[g]	300	5.0-7.5	n/a	n/a	[h][i]	8 hr	72 hr	n/a	(8)

Flush Compatibility: Sodium chloride 0.9%, heparin.[2]

Special Considerations: n/a

Notes

[a] The pH of reconstituted solutions is 5-8.[(1)]

[b] CefTAZidime produces gas bubbles after reconstitution; allow the gas to disperse before placing in syringes.

[c] Manufacturer extrapolated data from other sources.

[d] INTERMATE™/INFUSOR™ Portable Elastomeric Infusion System devices are no longer available in the United States.

[e] Solutions contained lidocaine HCl 0.5% and 1%.[(1)]

[f] After activation. Protect from light after removal of foil strip. If light-protecting foil strip is removed, product must be activated within 7 d.

[g] Dextrose added to adjust osmolarity.

[h] Frozen expiration date per manufacturer's label. Do not extrapolate commercial premix stability data to extemporaneously compounded solutions.

[i] Thaw at room temperature or under refrigeration. Do not force thaw. Do not re-freeze.

[j] Solutions of Tazicef® in D5W or NS are stable for at least 6 hr at room temperature in plastic tubing, drip chambers, and volume control devices of common IV infusion sets.[(12)]

REFERENCES

1. ASHP's Interactive Handbook on Injectable Drugs, 2020. Bethesda, MD: American Society of Health-System Pharmacists; Accessed November 2020.
2. Tazicef® (Ceftazidime) Injection [package insert]. Lake Forest, IL: Hospira; December 2020.
3. *Drug Stability Table - Dosi-Fuser® Elastomeric Pump (S-CL-00-001v16)*, 2021. Barcelona, Spain: Leventon SAU; Updated May 2021.
4. *Drug Stability for Easypump® ST/LT*, 2020. Bethlehem, PA: B. Braun USA; Updated June 2020.
5. *Stability Data for Drugs Using Homepump Disposable Ambulatory Infusion Systems (MK-00314 rev 3)*, 2015. Alpharetta, GA: Halyard Health; Updated June 2015.
6. Stabforum - Stability Database: Ceftazidime, Ontario, Canada: Baxter Healthcare; Accessed January 2021.
7. *SMARTeZ® - Stability Data for Drugs Using Elastomeric Infusion Pumps*, 2020. Fenton, MO: Progressive Medical, Inc.; Updated May 2020.
8. Fortaz® (Ceftazidime) Injection [package insert]. Buena, NJ: Teligent Pharma, Inc.; February 2019.
9. Ceftazidime Injection [package insert]. Schaumburg, IL: Sagent Pharmaceuticals; October 2020.
10. Ceftazidime and Dextrose Injection in Duplex® Drug Delivery System [package insert]. Bethlehem, PA: B. Braun Medical Inc.; August 2019.
11. *Pharmaceutical report on chemical and physical stability of drugs commonly used with CADD® infusion pumps (IN193109GB-122019)*, 2019. Minneapolis, MN: Smiths Medical ASD, Inc.; Updated December 2019.
12. Tazicef® (Ceftazidime) Injection for Intravenous Use in ADD-Vantage® Vials [package insert]. Lake Forest, IL: Hospira; December 2020.

Ceftolozane – Tazobactam

Storage Conditions

						Temperature			Post-thaw Temp			
	Drug Manufacturer	Concentration[c]	Diluents	Osmolality (mOsm/kg)	pH	Room	Refrig	Frozen	Room	Refrig	Body Temp	Refer.
CONTAINER												
Bag, Polyvinyl Chloride (PVC)	MSD	1-20 mg/mL	D5W, NS	[b]	[a]	24 hr	7 d	n/a	n/a	n/a	n/a	(1)(4)
	CUB	2.4, 23.1 mg/mL	D5W, NS	[b]	[a]	24 hr	7 d[d]	n/a	n/a	n/a	n/a	(5)
Vial, Glass	MSD	87.7 mg/mL	NS, SWFI	n/a	n/a	1 hr	n/a	n/a	n/a	n/a	n/a	(1)(4)
OTHER INFUSION CONTAINERS												
Easypump® ST/LT (B. Braun)	MSD	1, 2, 30 mg/mL	NS	n/a	n/a	24 hr	14 d[d]	n/a	n/a	n/a	n/a	(6)
Homepump Eclipse® / Homepump® (Halyard)	MSD	9.86 mg/mL	D5W, NS	[b]	[a]	24 hr	7 d	n/a	n/a	n/a	n/a	(3)
	MSD	1.21 mg/mL	D5W, NS	[b]	[a]	24 hr	7 d	n/a	n/a	n/a	n/a	(3)
SMARTeZ® (Progressive Medical)	MSD	1 mg/mL	NS	n/a	n/a	24 hr	14 d[d]	n/a	n/a	n/a	n/a	(7)
	MSD	2 mg/mL	NS	n/a	n/a	24 hr	14 d[d]	n/a	n/a	n/a	n/a	(7)

Flush Compatibility: Sodium chloride 0.9%, heparin.[1]

Special Considerations: Reconstituted solution is not suitable for direct injection. Refrigerate intact vials protected from light. Slight color variations (colorless to slightly yellow) do not affect potency. Do not freeze reconstituted or diluted solutions.[1]

Notes

[a] pH when reconstituted with NS or SWFI and diluted in D5W or NS 100 mL is 5.9-6.0.[2]

[b] Osmolality of 1000/500 mg ceftolozane/tazobactam reconstituted with 10 mL NS and diluted in D5W or NS 100 mL is approximately 500 mOsm/kg.[2]

[c] Concentrations are reported as the ceftolozane sulfate component, which is in a 2:1 fixed ratio with the tazobactam sodium component.[1]

[d] Tested over 14 days refrigerated temperature and 48 hours at room temperature. Drug concentrations remained above 90% during the test period. Due to the appearance of degradation compounds, the manufacturer recommends that IV bags stored under refrigeration be used within 7 days, and within 24 hours if stored at room temperatures.[5]

REFERENCES

1. ASHP's Interactive Handbook on Injectable Drugs, 2020. Bethesda, MD: American Society of Health-System Pharmacists; Accessed September 2020.
2. Zerbaxa® pH & Osmolality Information Letter (Ref#: US15-045829) [personal communication]. North Wales, PA: Merck & Co., Inc.; 2015:2.

DOI 10.37573/9781585286720.037

3. Zerbaxa® Stability in Elastomeric Pumps Information Letter (Ref#: US15-053880) [personal communication]. North Wales, PA: Merck & Co., Inc.; 2015:2.
4. Zerbaxa® (Ceftolozane & Tazobactam) Injection, Lyophilized [package insert]. Whitehouse Station, NJ: Merck Sharp & Dohme Corp.; September 2020.
5. Zerbaxa® Stability Medication Information Letter (Ref#: 2015-013418) [personal communication]. Lexington, MA: Cubist Pharmaceuticals; 2015:10.
6. *Drug Stability for Easypump® ST/LT*, 2020. Bethlehem, PA: B. Braun USA; Updated June 2020.
7. *SMARTeZ® - Stability Data for Drugs Using Elastomeric Infusion Pumps*, 2020. Fenton, MO: Progressive Medical, Inc.; Updated May 2020.

CefTRIAXone Sodium

Storage Conditions

	Drug Manufacturer	Concentration	Diluents	Osmolality (mOsm/kg)	pH	Temperature Room	Temperature Refrig	Temperature Frozen	Post-thaw Temp Room	Post-thaw Temp Refrig	Body Temp	Refer.
CONTAINER												
Bag, Polyethylene	RC	1 mg/mL	NS	n/a	[a]	10 d	n/a	n/a	n/a	n/a	n/a	(1)
Bag, Polyolefin	RC	10-40 mg/mL	D5W, NS	n/a	[a]	n/a	n/a	26 wk	n/a	n/a	n/a	(1)(2)
	RC	20 mg/mL	D5W	n/a	[a]	n/a	n/a	14 wk	44 d	n/a	n/a	(1)
Bag, Polyvinyl Chloride (PVC)	RC	1 mg/mL	NS	n/a	[a]	10 d	n/a	n/a	n/a	n/a	n/a	(1)
	RC	2 mg/mL	D5W	n/a	[a]	14 d	14 d	14 d	n/a	n/a	n/a	(1)
	RC	10-40 mg/mL	D5W, NS	n/a	[a]	n/a	n/a	26 wk	n/a	n/a	n/a	(1)(2)
	RC	10, 20, 40 mg/mL	D5½NS, D5NS	n/a	[a]	48 hr	n/a	n/a	n/a	n/a	n/a	(2)
	RC	10, 20, 40 mg/mL	D5W, NS, SWFI	n/a	[a]	48 hr	10 d	n/a	n/a	n/a	n/a	(2)
	RC	40 mg/mL	D5W	n/a	[a]	n/a	14 d	n/a	n/a	n/a	n/a	(1)
	RC	40 mg/mL	NS	n/a	[a]	72 hr	30 d	n/a	n/a	n/a	n/a	(1)
Syringe, Polypropylene	RC	10, 40 mg/mL	D5W, NS	n/a	[a]	48 hr	48 hr	10 d	n/a	n/a	n/a	(1)
	RC	100 mg/mL	SWFI	n/a	[a]	72 hr	40 d	180 d	n/a	n/a	n/a	(1)
	RC	250, 450 mg/mL	D5W, BWFI[b]	n/a	[a]	n/a	10 d	8 wk	n/a	n/a	n/a	(1)
Unspecified	UN	5, 40 mg/mL	D5W, NS	n/a	[a]	n/a	20 d	n/a	n/a	n/a	n/a	(1)
	RC	10 mg/mL	D5½NS	n/a	[a]	48 hr	4 d	n/a	n/a	n/a	n/a	(1)
	RC	10 mg/mL	D5W	n/a	[a]	7 d	12 wk	12 wk	n/a	n/a	n/a	(1)
	RC	50 mg/mL	NS	364	[a]	7 d	5 wk	n/a	n/a	n/a	n/a	(1)
	RC	50 mg/mL	D5W	351	[a]	24 hr	12 wk	12 wk	n/a	n/a	n/a	(1)
	RC	100 mg/mL	D5W, NS, SWFI	n/a	[a]	48 hr	10 d	n/a	n/a	n/a	n/a	(1)(2)
	RC	100 mg/mL	BWFI[b][f]	n/a	[a]	24 hr	10 d	n/a	n/a	n/a	n/a	(1)(2)
	RC	250, 350 mg/mL	D5W, NS, SWFI, BWFI[b][f]	n/a	[a]	24 hr	72 hr	n/a	n/a	n/a	n/a	(1)(2)
OTHER INFUSION CONTAINERS												
Dosi-Fuser® (Leventon)	RC	5-40 mg/mL	D5W, NS	n/a	[a]	24 hr[c]	21 d[c]	30 d[c]	n/a	n/a	n/a	(3)
Easypump® ST/LT (B. Braun)	UN	10 mg/mL	D5W	n/a	[a]	24 hr	6 d[d]	n/a	n/a	n/a	n/a	(4)
	UN	10, 50 mg/mL	NS	n/a	[a]	48 hr	14 d	n/a	n/a	n/a	n/a	(4)

DOI 10.37573/9781585286720.038

Storage Conditions

	Drug Manufacturer	Concentration	Diluents	Osmolality (mOsm/kg)	pH	Temperature: Room	Temperature: Refrig	Temperature: Frozen	Post-thaw Temp: Room	Post-thaw Temp: Refrig	Body Temp	Refer.
OTHER INFUSION CONTAINERS												
Homepump Eclipse® / Homepump® (Halyard)	UN	10, 20, 40 mg/mL	D5W, NS	n/a	[a]	72 hr[c]	10 d[c]	26 wk[c]	n/a	n/a	n/a	(5)
INTERMATE™ (Baxter)[e]	RC	5 mg/mL	D5W, NS	n/a	[a]	24 hr	28 d[d]	30 d	n/a	n/a	n/a	(6)
	RC	5-40 mg/mL	D5W, NS	n/a	[a]	24 hr	21 d[d]	30 d	n/a	n/a	n/a	(6)
	RC	30 mg/mL	SWFI	n/a	[a]	n/a	10 d	n/a	n/a	n/a	n/a	(6)
SMARTeZ® (Progressive Medical)	UN	40 mg/mL	NS	n/a	[a]	24 hr	14 d	n/a	n/a	n/a	n/a	(7)
	UN	10, 50 mg/mL	NS	n/a	[a]	48 hr[c]	14 d[c]	n/a	n/a	n/a	n/a	(7)
COMMERCIAL PREPARATIONS (RTU)												
Duplex® Flexible Dual-Chambered Container (B. Braun)	BRN	20, 40 mg/mL	[h]	iso	[a]	24 hr	7 d	n/a	n/a	n/a	n/a	(8)
GALAXY™ Plastic Container (Baxter)	BA	20, 40 mg/mL	D5W	iso	6-8	n/a	n/a	[g]	48 hr[g]	21 d[g]	n/a	(9)

Flush Compatibility: Sodium chloride 0.9%, heparin.[1]

Special Considerations: Do not use diluents containing calcium to reconstitute or further dilute cefTRIAXone for administration.[1,2]

Notes

[a] pH of 1% reconstituted solution is 6.7.[2,9]

[b] Lidocaine HCl 1% (without EPINEPHrine) was also studied as a diluent.[1,2]

[c] Manufacturer extrapolated data from other sources.

[d] Followed by 24 hr at room temperature.

[e] INTERMATE™/INFUSOR™ Portable Elastomeric Infusion System devices are no longer available in the United States.

[f] Bacteriostatic Water for Injection contained Benzyl Alcohol 0.9% as a preservative.

[g] Frozen expiration date per manufacturer's label. Do not extrapolate commercial premix stability data to extemporaneously compounded solutions. Do not re-freeze.[9]

[h] Diluent in the Duplex® Dual-Chamber system (BRN) is Hydrous Dextrose Injection at a concentration that renders the reconstituted solution iso-osmotic.[8]

REFERENCES

1. ASHP's Interactive Handbook on Injectable Drugs, 2020. Bethesda, MD: American Society of Health-System Pharmacists; Accessed August 2020.
2. Rocephin® (Ceftriaxone Sodium) Injection [package insert]. South San Francisco, CA: Genentech USA, Inc.; June 2015.
3. *Drug Stability Table - Dosi-Fuser® Elastomeric Pump (S-CL-00-001v16)*, 2021. Barcelona, Spain: Leventon SAU; Updated May 2021.
4. *Drug Stability for Easypump® ST/LT*, 2020. Bethlehem, PA: B. Braun USA; Updated June 2020.
5. *Stability Data for Drugs Using Homepump Disposable Ambulatory Infusion Systems (MK-00314 rev 3)*, 2015. Alpharetta, GA: Halyard Health; Updated June 2015.
6. Stabforum - Stability Database: CefTRIAXone, Ontario, Canada: Baxter Healthcare; Accessed December 2020.
7. *SMARTeZ® - Stability Data for Drugs Using Elastomeric Infusion Pumps*, 2020. Fenton, MO: Progressive Medical, Inc.; Updated May 2020.
8. Ceftriaxone and Dextrose Injection [package insert]. Bethlehem, PA: B. Braun Medical Inc.; April 2020.
9. Ceftriaxone Injection in Dextrose in GALAXY™ Container [package insert]. Deerfield, IL: Baxter Healthcare Corporation; May 2018.

Cefuroxime Sodium

Storage Conditions

	Drug Manufacturer	Concentration	Diluents	Osmolality (mOsm/kg)	pH	Temperature Room	Temperature Refrig	Temperature Frozen	Post-thaw Temp Room	Post-thaw Temp Refrig	Body Temp	Refer.
CONTAINER												
Bag, Polyolefin	UN	15 mg/mL	D5W	[f]	[e]	n/a	31 d	14 wk	n/a	21 d	n/a	(1)
Bag, Polyvinyl Chloride (PVC)	GL	5, 10 mg/mL	NS, D5W	[f]	[e]	24 hr	30 d	30 d	n/a	n/a	n/a	(1)(11)
	UN	6 mg/mL	NS, D5W	[f]	[e]	24 hr	24 hr	n/a	n/a	n/a	n/a	(1)
	COV	7.5, 15, 30 mg/mL	NS, D5W	[f]	[e]	n/a	n/a	6 m	24 hr	7 d	n/a	(1)(2)
Syringe, Polypropylene	GL	50 mg/mL	NS	335	6.9-7.3	48 hr	21 d	n/a	n/a	n/a	n/a	(7)
	GL	90 mg/mL	NS	[f]	[e]	48 hr	14 d[g]	n/a	n/a	n/a	n/a	(8)
	PAN	10 mg/mL	NS	331	7.28	16 hr[g]	21 d[g]	365 d[g]	n/a	n/a	n/a	(4)
Unspecified	COV	1-30 mg/mL	NS, D5W, D5NS, R, D10W, LR	[f]	[e]	24 hr	7 d	n/a	n/a	n/a	n/a	(1)(2)
	SAG	225 mg/mL	SWFI	[f]	[e]	24 hr	48 hr	n/a	n/a	n/a	n/a	(2)
Vial, Glass	GL	15 mg/mL	D5W	[f]	[e]	n/a	11 d	n/a	n/a	n/a	n/a	(1)
	GL	5, 10 mg/mL	NS, D5W	[f]	4.5-7.3	24 hr	30 d	30 d	n/a	n/a	n/a	(1)(11)
	GL	30, 60 mg/mL	SWFI	[f]	[e]	n/a	n/a	30 d	n/a	4 d	n/a	(1)
	GL	15 mg/mL	NS, D5W	[f]	[e]	48 hr	n/a	n/a	n/a	n/a	n/a	(1)
OTHER INFUSION CONTAINERS												
CADD® Cassette (Smiths Medical)	GL	22.5, 45 mg/mL	SWFI	[f]	[e]	n/a	7 d	n/a	n/a	n/a	8 hr[c]	(1)
	GL	30, 60 mg/mL	SWFI	[f]	[e]	n/a	n/a	30 d	n/a	4 d	n/a	(1)
Dosi-Fuser® (Leventon)	GL	5-30 mg/mL	NS, D5W	[f]	[e]	n/a	10 d[b]	30 d[b]	n/a	n/a	n/a	(10)
	GL	15-30 mg/mL	D5W	[f]	[e]	15 hr[b]	7 d[b]	n/a	n/a	n/a	n/a	(10)
	UN	60 mg/mL	NS	[f]	[e]	24 hr	14 d	n/a	n/a	n/a	n/a	(10)
Easypump® ST/LT (B. Braun)	UN	1, 30 mg/mL	NS	[f]	[e]	24 hr	72 hr	n/a	n/a	n/a	n/a	(5)
	UN	1, 30 mg/mL	D5W	[f]	[e]	12 hr	72 hr	n/a	n/a	n/a	n/a	(5)
Homepump Eclipse® / Homepump® (Halyard)	UN	1-30 mg/mL	NS, D5W	[f]	[e]	24 hr[b]	7 d[b]	n/a	n/a	n/a	n/a	(6)
	UN	5, 10 mg/mL	NS, D5W	[f]	[e]	n/a	n/a	30 d[b]	n/a	n/a	n/a	(6)
INFUSOR™ (Baxter)[d]	GSK	15-30 mg/mL	D5W	[f]	[e]	15 hr[a]	7 d[a]	n/a	n/a	n/a	n/a	(3)
INTERMATE™ (Baxter)[d]	GSK	5-30 mg/mL	NS	[f]	[e]	5 hr	4 d	n/a	n/a	n/a	n/a	(3)
SMARTeZ® (Progressive Medical)	UN	1, 30 mg/mL	NS	[f]	[e]	24 hr[b]	72 hr[b]	n/a	n/a	n/a	n/a	(9)

DOI 10.37573/9781585286720.039

Flush Compatibility: Sodium chloride 0.9%, heparin.[2]

Special Considerations: n/a

Notes

[a] Followed by 15 hours at room temperature.[3]

[b] Manufacturer(s) extrapolated data from other sources.

[c] Storage temperature: 30°C.[1]

[d] INTERMATE™/INFUSOR™ Portable Elastomeric Infusion System devices are no longer available in the United States.

[e] pH of reconstituted solution is 6-8.5.[1,2]

[f] Osmolality of 30, 50, and 76 mg/mL in D5W is 315, 329, and 568 mOsm/kg; solutions of 30, 50, and 68 mg/mL in NS is 314, 335, and 541 mOsm/kg. At 137 mg/mL in SWFI, osmolality is 489 mOsm/kg.[1]

[g] Protected from light.

REFERENCES

1. ASHP's Interactive Handbook on Injectable Drugs, 2020. Bethesda, MD: American Society of Health-System Pharmacists; Accessed May 2020.
2. Cefuroxime Sodium Injection [package insert]. Schaumburg, IL: Sagent Pharmaceuticals, Inc.; October 2020.
3. Stabforum - Stability Database: Cefuroxime, Ontario, Canada: Baxter Healthcare; Accessed February 2021.
4. Feutry F, Simon N, Genay S, et al. Stability of 10 mg/mL cefuroxime solution for intracameral injection in commonly used polypropylene syringes and new ready-to-use cyclic olefin copolymer sterile vials using the LC-UV stability-indicating method. *Drug Dev Ind Pharm*. 2016; 42(1):166-74.
5. *Drug Stability for Easypump® ST/LT*, 2020. Bethlehem, PA: B. Braun USA; Updated June 2020.
6. *Stability Data for Drugs Using Homepump Disposable Ambulatory Infusion Systems (MK-00314 rev 3)*, 2015. Alpharetta, GA: Halyard Health; Updated June 2015.
7. Gupta VD. Chemical stability of cefuroxime sodium after reconstitution in 0.9% sodium chloride injection and storage in polypropylene syringes for pediatric use. *Int J Pharm Compd*. 2003; 7(4):310-2.
8. Vercheval C, Streel S, Servais AC, et al. Stability of 90 mg/mL cefuroxime sodium solution for administration by continuous infusion. *J Chemother*. 2018; 30(6-8):371-74.
9. *SMARTeZ® - Stability Data for Drugs Using Elastomeric Infusion Pumps*, 2020. Fenton, MO: Progressive Medical, Inc.; Updated May 2020.
10. *Drug Stability Table - Dosi-Fuser® Elastomeric Pump (ES.H.00.73-10)*, 2015. Barcelona, Spain: Leventon SAU; Updated October 2015.
11. Das Gupta V, Stewart KR. Stability of cefuroxime sodium in some aqueous buffered solutions and intravenous admixtures. *J Clin Hosp Pharm*. 1986; 11(1):47-54.

Cetuximab

Storage Conditions

						Temperature			Post-thaw Temp			
	Drug Manufacturer	Concentration	Diluents	Osmolality (mOsm/kg)	pH	Room	Refrig	Frozen	Room	Refrig	Body Temp	Refer.
CONTAINER												
Bag, Polyvinyl Chloride (PVC)	BMS	2 mg/mL	Undiluted	n/a	[b]	n/a	14 d	n/a	n/a	n/a	n/a	(1)
Vial, Glass	BMS	2 mg/mL	Undiluted	n/a	[b]	n/a	14 d	n/a	n/a	n/a	n/a	(1)
OTHER INFUSION CONTAINERS												
INTERMATE™ (Baxter)[a]	BMS	0.83 mg/mL	NS	n/a	n/a	48 hr	5 wk	n/a	n/a	n/a	n/a	(2)
	BMS	5 mg/mL[c]	Undiluted	n/a	[b]	48 hr	5 wk	n/a	n/a	n/a	n/a	(2)

Flush Compatibility: Sodium chloride 0.9%.[2]

Special Considerations: Store unused vials under refrigeration at 2°C to 8°C. Do not freeze or shake. Increased particulate formation may occur at temperatures at or below 0°C.[3] Administer through 0.22 micron in-line filter, with rate not to exceed 10 mg/min, and discard any remaining solution in the infusion container after 8 hours at controlled room temperature or after 12 hours at 2°C to 8°C.[3]

Notes

[a] INTERMATE™/INFUSOR™ Portable Elastomeric Infusion System devices are no longer available in the United States.

[b] pH of undiluted (2 mg/mL) solution is 7-7.4.[3]

[c] Cetuximab 5 mg/mL is available internationally.

REFERENCES

1. Ikesue H, Vermeulen LC, Hoke R, et al. Stability of cetuximab and panitumumab in glass vials and polyvinyl chloride bags. *Am J Health Syst Pharm.* 2010; 67(3):223-6.
2. Stabforum - Stability Database: Cetuximab, Ontario, Canada: Baxter Healthcare; Accessed September 2020.
3. Erbitux® (Cetuximab) Injection [package insert]. Branchburg, NJ: ImClone LLC; November 2020.

DOI 10.37573/9781585286720.040

ChlorproMAZINE Hydrochloride

Storage Conditions

						Temperature			Post-thaw Temp			
	Drug Manufacturer	Concentration	Diluents	Osmolality (mOsm/kg)	pH	Room	Refrig	Frozen	Room	Refrig	Body Temp	Refer.
CONTAINER												
Bag, Polyvinyl Chloride (PVC)	MB	0.009 mg/mL	NS	n/a	[d]	7 d[a]	n/a	[e]	n/a	n/a	n/a	(1)
Syringe, Polypropylene	ES	6.25 mg/mL	[b]	n/a	[d]	12 m[c]	12 m[c]	[e]	n/a	n/a	n/a	(1)

Flush Compatibility: Sodium chloride 0.9%, D5W.[2]

Special Considerations: Parenteral administration should be reserved for non-ambulating patients or acute ambulatory cases due to possible hypotensive effects. Intravenous route is only to be used for severe hiccups, surgery and tetanus. It is recommended that patients lay down for at least 30 minutes after parenteral administration. Avoid injecting undiluted chlorproMAZINE HCl into a vein.[2]

Notes

[a] Evidence of 5% sorption during 7 days of storage in NS PVC bags.[1]

[b] Solution contained hydrOXYzine HCl 12.5 mg/mL (PF) and meperidine HCl 25 mg/mL (WI).

[c] Protected from light.

[d] pH of undiluted solution is 3.4-5.4.[2]

[e] Do not freeze.

REFERENCES

1. ASHP's Interactive Handbook on Injectable Drugs, 2020. Bethesda, MD: American Society of Health-System Pharmacists; Accessed August 2020.
2. Chlorpromazine Hydrochloride Injection [package insert]. E. Windsor, NJ: AuroMedics Pharma LLC; June 2020.

DOI 10.37573/9781585286720.041

Cidofovir

Storage Conditions

						Temperature			Post-thaw Temp			
CONTAINER	Drug Manufacturer	Concentration	Diluents	Osmolality (mOsm/kg)	pH[b]	Room	Refrig	Frozen	Room	Refrig	Body Temp	Refer.
Bag, Polyolefin	GIL	0.085, 3.51 mg/mL	D5½NS	382, 392	6.7–7.0	24 hr[a]	24 hr	n/a	n/a	n/a	n/a	(4)
	GIL	0.21, 8.12 mg/mL	D5W	241, 286	7.2–7.6	24 hr[a]	24 hr	n/a	n/a	n/a	n/a	(4)
	GIL, AB, BA	0.2, 8.1 mg/mL	NS	275, 315	7.1–7.5	n/a	5 d	5 d	n/a	n/a	n/a	(1)(3)
	GIL	0.21, 8.12 mg/mL	NS	275, 315	7.1–7.5	24 hr[a]	24 hr	n/a	n/a	n/a	n/a	(4)
Bag, Polyvinyl Chloride (PVC)	GIL, AB, BA	0.2, 8.1 mg/mL	NS	284, 316	7.1–7.5	n/a	5d	5 d	n/a	n/a	n/a	(3)
	GIL	0.085, 3.51 mg/mL	D5½NS	382, 392	6.7–7.0	24 hr[a]	24 hr	n/a	n/a	n/a	n/a	(4)
	GIL	0.2, 8.1 mg/mL	NS	275, 315	7.1–7.5	n/a	5 d	5 d	n/a	n/a	n/a	(1)
	GIL	0.21, 8.12 mg/mL	NS	275, 315	7.1–7.5	24 hr[a]	24 hr	n/a	n/a	n/a	n/a	(4)
	GIL	0.21, 8.12 mg/mL	D5W	241, 286	7.2–7.6	24 hr[a]	24 hr	n/a	n/a	n/a	n/a	(4)
Syringe, Polypropylene	GIL	6.25 mg/mL	NS	n/a	[b]	150 d	150 d	n/a	n/a	n/a	n/a	(1)

Flush Compatibility: Sodium chloride 0.9%.[2]

Special Considerations: Product labeling recommends dilution in 100 mL NS prior to administration.[2]

Notes

[a] Storage temperature: 30°C.[4]

[b] pH of undiluted solution is 7.4.[2]

REFERENCES

1. ASHP's Interactive Handbook on Injectable Drugs, 2020. Bethesda, MD: American Society of Health-System Pharmacists; Accessed June 2020.
2. Vistide® (Cidofovir) Injection [package insert]. Foster City, CA: Gilead Sciences, Inc.; September 2013.
3. Ennis RD, Dahl TC. Stability of cidofovir in 0.9% sodium chloride injection for five days. *Am J Health Syst Pharm*. 1997; 54(19):2204-6.
4. Yuan LC, Samuels GJ, Visor GC. Stability of cidofovir in 0.9% sodium chloride injection and in 5% dextrose injection. *Am J Health Syst Pharm*. 1996; 53(16):1939-43.

DOI 10.37573/9781585286720.042

Ciprofloxacin

Storage Conditions

						Temperature			Post-thaw Temp			
	Drug Manufacturer	Concentration	Diluents	Osmolality (mOsm/kg)	pH	Room	Refrig	Frozen	Room	Refrig	Body Temp	Refer.
CONTAINER												
Bag, Polyvinyl Chloride (PVC)	MI	2.86 mg/mL	NS, D5W	n/a	[e]	90 d	90 d	n/a	n/a	n/a	n/a	(1)
OTHER INFUSION CONTAINERS												
Dosi-Fuser® (Leventon)	MI	0.5–6 mg/mL	D5W, NS	n/a	[e]	30 d[b]	90 d[b]	n/a	n/a	n/a	n/a	(7)
Easypump® ST/LT (B. Braun)	UN	2 mg/mL	D5W	n/a	[e]	10 d	30 d	n/a	n/a	n/a	n/a	(5)
Homepump Eclipse® / Homepump® (Halyard)	UN	2 mg/mL	n/a	n/a	[e]	24 hr	27 d	n/a	n/a	n/a	n/a	(4)
INTERMATE™ (Baxter)[f]	BAY	0.5–2 mg/mL	D5W, NS	n/a	[e]	30 d[c]	90 d[c]	n/a	n/a	n/a	n/a	(3)
	MI	0.5–6 mg/mL	D5W, NS, SWFI	n/a	[e]	30 d[c]	90 d[c]	n/a	n/a	n/a	n/a	(3)
SMARTeZ® (Progressive Medical)	UN	2 mg/mL	D5W	n/a	[e]	10 d[b]	30 d[b]	n/a	n/a	n/a	n/a	(6)
COMMERCIAL PREPARATIONS (RTU)												
Flexible Container[a] (Hospira)	HOS	2 mg/mL	RTU[g]	n/a	3.5–4.6	[d]	[d]	n/a	n/a	n/a	n/a	(2)

Flush Compatibility: Sodium chloride 0.9%. White precipitate forms immediately with heparin.[1]

Special Considerations: Protect from light. Do not freeze.[1,2]

Notes

[a] Latex-free PVC bag.[2]

[b] Manufacturer extrapolated data from other sources.

[c] Stable for 14 d room temperature following 90 d refrigerated.[3]

[d] Expiration date per manufacturer's label. Do not extrapolate commercial premix stability data to extemporaneously compounded solutions.

[e] pH of undiluted 1% aqueous solution is 3–3.9.[2]

[f] INTERMATE™/INFUSOR™ Portable Elastomeric Infusion System devices are no longer available in the United States.

[g] Premixed solution of 0.2% ciprofloxacin in D5W.[2]

DOI 10.37573/9781585286720.043

REFERENCES

1. ASHP's Interactive Handbook on Injectable Drugs, 2020. Bethesda, MD: American Society of Health-System Pharmacists; Accessed June 2020.
2. Ciprofloxacin Injection [package insert]. Lake Forest, IL: Hospira, Inc.; July 2020.
3. Stabforum - Stability Database: Ciprofloxacin, Ontario, Canada: Baxter Healthcare; Accessed January 2021.
4. *Stability Data for Drugs Using Homepump Disposable Ambulatory Infusion Systems (MK-00314 rev 3)*, 2015. Alpharetta, GA: Halyard Health; Updated June 2015.
5. *Drug Stability for Easypump® ST/LT*, 2020. Bethlehem, PA: B. Braun USA; Updated June 2020.
6. *SMARTeZ® - Stability Data for Drugs Using Elastomeric Infusion Pumps*, 2020. Fenton, MO: Progressive Medical, Inc.; Updated May 2020.
7. *Drug Stability Table - Dosi-Fuser® Elastomeric Pump (S-CL-00-001v16)*, 2021. Barcelona, Spain: Leventon SAU; Updated May 2021.

Cisatracurium Besylate

Storage Conditions

						Temperature			Post-thaw Temp			
	Drug Manufacturer	Concentration	Diluents	Osmolality (mOsm/kg)	pH	Room	Refrig	Frozen	Room	Refrig	Body Temp	Refer.
CONTAINER												
Bag, Polyvinyl Chloride (PVC)	GL	2, 5 mg/mL	D5W	n/a	n/a	7 d[(a)]	30 d[(a)]	n/a	n/a	n/a	n/a	(1)
	GL	0.1, 2, 5 mg/mL	NS	n/a	n/a	7 d[(a)]	30 d[(a)]	n/a	n/a	n/a	n/a	(1)
Syringe, Plastic (Unspecified)	GL	2 mg/mL	Undiluted	n/a	n/a	n/a	30 d[(a)]	n/a	n/a	n/a	n/a	(1)
Vial, Glass	GL	2, 10 mg/mL	Undiluted	n/a	n/a	30 d[(a)]	90 d[(a)]	n/a	n/a	n/a	n/a	(1)

Flush Compatibility: Sodium chloride 0.9%.[(1)]

Special Considerations: n/a

Notes

[a] Protected from light.[(1)]

REFERENCE

1. Xu QA, Zhang YP, Trissel LA, et al. Stability of cisatracurium besylate in vials, syringes, and infusion admixtures. *Am J Health Syst Pharm*. 1998; 55(10):1037-41.

DOI 10.37573/9781585286720.044

CISplatin

Storage Conditions

						Temperature			Post-thaw Temp			
	Drug Manufacturer	Concentration	Diluents	Osmolality (mOsm/kg)	pH	Room	Refrig	Frozen	Room	Refrig	Body Temp	Refer.
CONTAINER												
Bag, Ethylene Vinyl Acetate (EVA)	BEL	0.5, 0.9 mg/mL	NS	n/a	[g]	28 d[b]	n/a	n/a	n/a	n/a	28 d[b][e]	(1)(4)
Bag, Polyethylene	WAS	0.167 mg/mL	NS	n/a	[g]	14 d[b]	n/a	n/a	n/a	n/a	n/a	(4)(7)
Bag, Polypropylene	WAS	0.167 mg/mL	NS	n/a	[g]	14 d[b]	n/a	n/a	n/a	n/a	n/a	(4)(7)
Bag, Polyvinyl Chloride (PVC)	WAS	0.167 mg/mL	NS	n/a	[g]	14 d[b]	n/a	n/a	n/a	n/a	n/a	(4)(7)
	BMS	0.455 mg/mL	NS[c]	n/a	[g]	n/a	24 hr[a][d]	n/a	n/a	n/a	7 d[d]	(2)
	BEL	0.6 mg/mL	NS	n/a	[g]	9 d[b]	n/a	n/a	n/a	n/a	n/a	(4)
	UN	1 mg/mL	NS	n/a	[g]	14 d	n/a	n/a	n/a	n/a	n/a	(3)
Vial, Glass	WAS	0.167 mg/mL	NS	n/a	[g]	14 d[b]	n/a	n/a	n/a	n/a	n/a	(4)(7)
	UN	1 mg/mL	[f]	[h]	[g]	n/a	n/a	n/a	n/a	n/a	10 m[n]	(4)
	FRK	1 mg/mL	Undiluted	n/a	[g]	28 d[b]	n/a	n/a	n/a	n/a	n/a	(11)
	FRK	1 mg/mL	Undiluted	n/a	[g]	7 d[l]	n/a	n/a	n/a	n/a	n/a	(11)
OTHER INFUSION CONTAINERS												
CADD® Cassette (Smiths Medical)	DB	1, 1.6 mg/mL	SWFI[o]	[h]	[g]	14 d[b]	n/a	n/a	n/a	n/a	14 d[b][m]	(8)(13)
Dosi-Fuser® (Leventon)	BEL	1.25 mg/mL	NS	n/a	[g]	4 d[i][j]	n/a	n/a	n/a	n/a	24 hr[i][j]	(12)
	HOS	1 mg/mL	NS	n/a	[g]	14 d	n/a	n/a	n/a	n/a	n/a	(12)
Easypump® ST/LT (B. Braun)	UN	0.1, 0.5 mg/mL	NS	n/a	[g]	14 d	n/a	n/a	n/a	n/a	n/a	(9)
	UN	0.2 mg/mL	NS	n/a	[g]	24 hr	7 d[a]	n/a	n/a	n/a	n/a	(9)
Homepump Eclipse® / Homepump® (Halyard)	UN	0.5 mg/mL	NS	n/a	[g]	28 d[i]	n/a	n/a	n/a	n/a	n/a	(5)
INFUSOR™ (Baxter)[k]	BEL	1.25 mg/mL	NS	n/a	[g]	4 d[b][j]	n/a	n/a	n/a	n/a	24 hr[b][j]	(6)
SMARTeZ® (Progressive Medical)	UN	0.2 mg/mL	NS	n/a	[g]	24 hr[i]	14 d[a][i]	n/a	n/a	n/a	n/a	(10)
	UN	0.1, 0.5 mg/mL	NS	n/a	[g]	14 d	n/a	n/a	n/a	n/a	n/a	(10)

DOI 10.37573/9781585286720.045

Flush Compatibility: Sodium chloride 0.9%, heparin.[(4)]

Special Considerations: Protect from light if solution will not be used within 6 hours.[(4)] Manufacturer states that CISplatin remaining in amber vial following initial entry is stable for 28 days protected from light or 7 days under fluorescent room light.[(4)(11)] Store at room temperature and protect unopened container from light.[(11)]

Notes

[a] Manufacturer recommends not refrigerating because of increased risk of precipitation.[(4)]
[b] Protected from light.
[c] Solution contained: ondansetron (GL) 1.091 mg/mL.
[d] Solution was initially refrigerated for 24 hr prior to storage at 30°C for 7 d. Solutions were protected from light.[(2)]
[e] Storage temperature: 35°C.[(1)(4)]
[f] Solution contained: sodium chloride 9 mg/mL and mannitol 10 mg/mL.[(4)]
[g] pH range is 3.5-4.5.[(4)]
[h] Undiluted product is 285 mOsm/kg.[(4)]
[i] Manufacturer extrapolated data from other sources.
[j] 4 d at 25°C, followed by 24 hr at 33°C.[(6)]
[k] INTERMATE™/INFUSOR™ Portable Elastomeric Infusion System devices are no longer available in the United States.
[l] Exposed to fluorescent light.
[m] Storage temperature: 37°C and 60°C.[(13)]
[n] Storage temperature: 40°C.[(4)]
[o] Solution contained: sodium chloride 9 mg/mL and mannitol 1 mg/mL.[(13)]

REFERENCES

1. Rochard E, Barthes D, Courtois P. Stability of cisplatin in ethylene vinylacetate portable infusion-pump reservoirs. *J Clin Pharm Ther*. 1992; 17(5):315-8.
2. Henry DW, Marshall JL, Nazzaro D, et al. Stability of cisplatin and ondansetron hydrochloride in admixtures for continuous infusion. *Am J Health Syst Pharm*. 1995; 52(22):2570-3.
3. Vyas HM, Baptista RJ, Mitrano FP, et al. Drug stability guidelines for a continuous infusion chemotherapy program. *Hosp Pharm*. 1987; 22(7):685-7.
4. ASHP's Interactive Handbook on Injectable Drugs, 2020. Bethesda, MD: American Society of Health-System Pharmacists; Accessed August 2020.
5. *Stability Data for Drugs Using Homepump Disposable Ambulatory Infusion Systems (MK-00314 rev 3)*, 2015. Alpharetta, GA: Halyard Health; Updated June 2015.
6. Stabforum - Stability Database: Cisplatin, Ontario, Canada: Baxter Healthcare; Accessed February 2021.
7. Cubells MP, Aixela JP, Brumos VG, et al. Stability of cisplatin in sodium chloride 0.9% intravenous solution related to the container's material. *Pharm World Sci*. 1993; 15(1):34-6.
8. *Pharmaceutical report on chemical and physical stability of drugs commonly used with CADD® infusion pumps (IN193109GB-122019)*, 2019. Minneapolis, MN: Smiths Medical ASD, Inc.; Updated December 2019.
9. *Drug Stability for Easypump® ST/LT*, 2020. Bethlehem, PA: B. Braun USA; Updated June 2020.
10. *SMARTeZ® - Stability Data for Drugs Using Elastomeric Infusion Pumps*, 2020. Fenton, MO: Progressive Medical, Inc.; Updated May 2020.
11. Cisplatin Injection [package insert]. Lake Zurich, IL: Fresenius Kabi USA, LLC; December 2019.
12. *Drug Stability Table - Dosi-Fuser® Elastomeric Pump (S-CL-00-001v16)*, 2021. Barcelona, Spain: Leventon SAU; Updated May 2021.
13. Hrubisko M, Mc Gown AT, Prendiville JA, et al. Suitability of cisplatin solutions for 14-day continuous infusion by ambulatory pump. *Cancer Chemother Pharmacol*. 1992; 29(3):252-5.

Cladribine

Storage Conditions

	Drug Manufacturer	Concentration	Diluents	Osmolality (mOsm/kg)	pH	Temperature			Post-thaw Temp			
						Room	Refrig	Frozen	Room	Refrig	Body Temp	Refer.
CONTAINER												
Bag, Polyethylene	JC	0.016 mg/mL	NS	[c]	[b]	30 d[a]	30 d[a]	n/a	n/a	n/a	n/a	(1)(2)
Bag, Polyvinyl Chloride (PVC)	JC	0.016 mg/mL	NS	[c]	[b]	30 d[a]	30 d[a]	n/a	n/a	n/a	n/a	(1)(2)
Vial, Glass	UN	0.024 mg/mL	NS	[c]	[b]	n/a	14 d	n/a	n/a	n/a	n/a	(1)
OTHER INFUSION CONTAINERS												
CADD® Cassette (Smiths Medical)[e]	OB	1 mg/mL	NS, BNS	[c]	[b]	7 d[d]	n/a	n/a	n/a	n/a	n/a	(3)(4)

Flush Compatibility: Sodium chloride 0.9%, heparin.[1]

Special Considerations: Store intact cladribine vials under refrigeration and protected from light.[1] D5W is not recommended as a diluent because of increased cladribine degradation.[1,3]

Notes

[a] Protected from light, and exposed to light.[2]

[b] pH of undiluted solution is 5.5-8.[1]

[c] Undiluted solution is isotonic.[1]

[d] Use BNS (containing 0.9% benzyl alcohol preservative) when preparing a 7 d continuous infusion. Add both drug and diluent to the infusion reservoir through 0.22 micron filters, then aspirate all air bubbles from the reservoir through a dry sterile filter or sterile vent filter assembly. Solutions prepared for patients weighing more than 85 kg may have reduced preservative effectiveness due to dilution of the benzyl alcohol preservative.[3]

[e] Physical and chemical stability noted in the SIMS Deltec Medication Cassette™. CADD® Cassette, now marketed by Smiths Medical, was marketed by SIMS Deltec.[3]

REFERENCES

1. ASHP's Interactive Handbook on Injectable Drugs, 2020. Bethesda, MD: American Society of Health-System Pharmacists; Accessed June 2020.
2. Daouphars M, Vigneron J, Perrin A, et al. Stability of Cladribine in Either Polyethylene Containers or Polyvinyl Chloride Bags. *Eur Hosp Pharm*. 1997; 3(4):154-6.
3. Cladribine Injection [package insert]. Bridgewater, NJ: Hisun Pharmaceuticals USA, Inc.; May 2020.
4. *Pharmaceutical report on chemical and physical stability of drugs commonly used with CADD® infusion pumps (IN193109GB-122019)*, 2019. Minneapolis, MN: Smiths Medical ASD, Inc.; Updated December 2019.

DOI 10.37573/9781585286720.046

Clindamycin Phosphate

Storage Conditions

	Drug Manufacturer	Concentration	Diluents	Osmolality (mOsm/kg)	pH	Temperature Room	Temperature Refrig	Temperature Frozen	Post-thaw Temp Room	Post-thaw Temp Refrig	Body Temp	Refer.
CONTAINER												
Bag, Polyolefin	UP	7.6 mg/mL	D5W	[g]	[d]	n/a	n/a	30 d	n/a	14 d	n/a	(1)
Bag, Polyvinyl Chloride (PVC)	GW	3 mg/mL	NS, D5W	[g]	[d]	24 hr	24 hr	n/a	n/a	n/a	n/a	(1)
	UP	6 mg/mL	D5W	[g]	[d]	n/a	n/a	30 d	24 hr	n/a	n/a	(1)(2)
	UP	6, 9, 12 mg/mL	D5W, LR, NS	[g]	[d]	16 d	32 d	8 wk	n/a	n/a	n/a	(1)
	QU	6, 12 mg/mL	D5W, NS	[g]	[d]	22 d	54 d	68 d	n/a	n/a	n/a	(1)
	PHU, AVG	18 mg/mL	D5W	[g]	[d]	16 d	n/a	n/a	n/a	n/a	n/a	(1)
	UP	18 mg/mL	D5W, NS	[g]	[d]	n/a	n/a	28 d	n/a	n/a	n/a	(1)
Syringe, Plastic (Unspecified)[a]	UN	20, 40, 60, 120 mg/mL	SWFI	n/a	[d]	30 d	n/a	60 d	n/a	n/a	n/a	(1)
Syringe, Polypropylene[a]	UP	150 mg/mL	Undiluted	n/a	[d]	48 hr[e]	n/a	n/a	n/a	n/a	n/a	(1)
	UN	150 mg/mL	Undiluted	n/a	[d]	48 hr	n/a	n/a	n/a	n/a	n/a	(1)
Unspecified	UP	0.25 mg/mL	D5W, D10W, NS, LR, D5NS	[g]	[d]	24 hr	24 hr	n/a	n/a	n/a	n/a	(1)
	UN	0.6 mg/mL	D5NS, NS	n/a	[d]	24 hr	n/a	n/a	n/a	n/a	n/a	(1)
	UN	6 mg/mL	D5W	[g]	[d]	n/a	n/a	79 d	n/a	n/a	n/a	(1)
Vial, Glass[a]	GW	3 mg/mL	NS, D5W	[g]	[d]	24 hr	24 hr	n/a	n/a	n/a	n/a	(1)
	UP	6, 9, 12 mg/mL	D5W, LR, NS	[g]	[d]	16 d	32 d	8 wk	n/a	n/a	n/a	(1)
	AB	15 mg/mL	SWFI	n/a	[d]	13 wk	13 wk	n/a	n/a	n/a	n/a	(1)
	UN	20, 40, 60, 120 mg/mL	SWFI	n/a	[d]	30 d	n/a	60 d	n/a	n/a	n/a	(1)
OTHER INFUSION CONTAINERS												
Accufuser® Elastomeric Pump (Vygon)[h]	SZ	1, 12 mg/mL	NS, D5W	n/a	[d]	7 d	27 d	n/a	n/a	n/a	n/a	(3)
Dosi-Fuser® (Leventon)	UP	2-12 mg/mL	NS	n/a	[d]	24 hr[b]	10 d[b]	30 d[b]	n/a	n/a	n/a	(8)
	UP	12 mg/mL	D5W	n/a	[d]	24 hr[b]	10 d[b]	30 d[b]	n/a	n/a	n/a	(8)

DOI 10.37573/9781585286720.047

Storage Conditions

	Drug Manufacturer	Concentration	Diluents	Osmolality (mOsm/kg)	pH	Temperature Room	Temperature Refrig	Temperature Frozen	Post-thaw Temp Room	Post-thaw Temp Refrig	Body Temp	Refer.
OTHER INFUSION CONTAINERS												
Easypump® ST/LT (B. Braun)	UN	6, 12 mg/mL	NS	[g]	[d]	72 hr	30 d	n/a	n/a	n/a	n/a	(7)
Homepump Eclipse® / Homepump® (Halyard)	UN	10 mg/mL	NS	[g]	[d]	24 hr	10 d	n/a	n/a	n/a	n/a	(5)
INTERMATE™ (Baxter)[f]	UP	2-12 mg/mL	D5W, NS	[g]	[d]	n/a	n/a	30 d	n/a	n/a	n/a	(4)
	UP	12 mg/mL	D5W, NS	[g]	[d]	n/a	10 d	30 d	n/a	n/a	n/a	(4)
	UP	12 mg/mL	D5W	[g]	[d]	24 hr	10 d	30 d	n/a	n/a	n/a	(4)
SMARTeZ® (Progressive Medical)	UN	6-12 mg/mL	NS	[g]	[d]	72 hr	30 d	n/a	n/a	n/a	n/a	(6)
COMMERCIAL PREPARATIONS (RTU)												
GALAXY™ Plastic Container (Baxter)	PF	6, 12, 18 mg/mL	D5W, NS	[g]	[d]	[c]	n/a	n/a	n/a	n/a	n/a	(1)

Flush Compatibility: Sodium chloride 0.9%.

Special Considerations: Clindamycin phosphate infusions should not exceed 18 mg/mL; do not administer undiluted product as an IV bolus.(1) When refrigerated or frozen, solutions form crystals which must be re-dissolved before administration.(1)

Notes

[a] Clindamycin phosphate is incompatible with natural rubber closures because of the risk of crystalline particulate extraction. If clindamycin phosphate is repackaged in vials or disposable syringes, storage at room temperature should be limited to a few days.(1)

[b] Manufacturer(s) extrapolated data from other sources.

[c] Expiration date per manufacturer label. Do not extrapolate commercial premix stability data to extemporaneously compounded solutions.

[d] Clindamycin 150 mg/mL (AVG) injection solution has a pH ranging from 5.5-7. Clindamycin 6,12, and 18 mg/mL (AKN) premixed infusion solutions in dextrose 5% have a pH ranging from 5.9-6.3. Clindamycin 6,12, and 18 mg/mL (BA) premixed infusion solutions in sodium chloride 0.9% have a pH ranging from 5.5-6.5.(1)

[e] Exposed to fluorescent light.(1)

[f] INTERMATE™/INFUSOR™ Portable Elastomeric Infusion System devices are no longer available in the United States.

[g] Osmolality of 12 mg/mL is 293 mOsm/kg in D5W and 309 mOsm/kg in NS; undiluted 150 mg/mL product is reported as 795 mOsm/kg or 835 mOsm/kg as determined by freezing-point depression. However, the manufacturer has stated that the osmolality is usually 825-880 mOsm/kg. Calculated osmolality for 6 mg/mL is 268 mOsm/kg in D5W and 294 mOsm/kg in NS. Calculated osmolality for 12 mg/mL is 279 mOsm/kg in D5W and 306 mOsm/kg in NS.(1)

[h] Accufuser® Elastomeric Pump tested was a 60 mL disposable silicone balloon infuser originally marketed by Woo Young Medical Co Ltd.(3)

REFERENCES

1. ASHP's Interactive Handbook on Injectable Drugs, 2020. Bethesda, MD: American Society of Health-System Pharmacists; Accessed June 2020.
2. Holmes CJ, Ausman RK, Kundsin RB, et al. Effect of freezing and microwave thawing on the stability of six antibiotic admixtures in plastic bags. *Am J Hosp Pharm*. 1982; 39(1):104-8.
3. Walker SE, Iazzetta J, Law S, et al. Stability of commonly used antibiotic solutions in an elastomeric infusion device. *Can J Hosp Pharm*. 2010; 63(3):212-24.
4. Stabforum - Stability Database: Clindamycin, Ontario, Canada: Baxter Healthcare; Accessed January 2021.
5. *Stability Data for Drugs Using Homepump Disposable Ambulatory Infusion Systems (MK-00314 rev 3)*, 2015. Alpharetta, GA: Halyard Health; Updated June 2015.
6. *SMARTeZ® - Stability Data for Drugs Using Elastomeric Infusion Pumps*, 2020. Fenton, MO: Progressive Medical, Inc.; Updated May 2020.
7. *Drug Stability for Easypump® ST/LT*, 2020. Bethlehem, PA: B. Braun USA; Updated June 2020.
8. *Drug Stability Table - Dosi-Fuser® Elastomeric Pump (S-CL-00-001v16)*, 2021. Barcelona, Spain: Leventon SAU; Updated May 2021.

CloNIDine Hydrochloride

Storage Conditions

	Drug Manufacturer	Concentration	Diluents	Osmolality (mOsm/kg)	pH	Temperature Room	Temperature Refrig	Temperature Frozen	Post-thaw Temp Room	Post-thaw Temp Refrig	Body Temp	Refer.
CONTAINER												
Bag, Polypropylene	BI	5 mcg/mL	NS[i][j]	n/a	[p]	30 d[k]	n/a	n/a	n/a	n/a	n/a	(1)(5)
	BI	50 mcg/mL	NS[i]	n/a	[p]	30 d[k]	n/a	n/a	n/a	n/a	n/a	(1)(5)
Bag, Polyvinyl Chloride (PVC)	BI	3 mcg/mL	NS[b]	n/a	[p]	21 d	n/a	n/a	n/a	n/a	n/a	(1)
	BI	9 mcg/mL	NS[g]	n/a	[p]	24 d[c]	28 d[c]	n/a	n/a	n/a	n/a	(1)
Syringe, Polypropylene	ROX	100 mcg/mL	Undiluted	n/a	[p]	7 d	n/a	n/a	n/a	n/a	n/a	(1)
	BI	15 mcg/mL	NS[r]	1030	3.46	n/a	40 d	n/a	n/a	n/a	n/a	(8)
	MDZ	0.5, 5 mcg/mL	D5W, D10W, NS	n/a	n/a	n/a	n/a	n/a	n/a	n/a	24 hr[e]	(1)
	BI	9 mcg/mL	NS[h]	n/a	[a][p]	30 d	30 d	n/a	n/a	n/a	30 d[e]	(1)(4)
Unspecified	UN	200 mcg/mL	NS	n/a	n/a	n/a	n/a	n/a	n/a	n/a	10 wk[c]	(1)
Vial, Glass	SH	200 mcg/mL	NS[d]	n/a	[p]	n/a	n/a	n/a	n/a	n/a	10 wk[c]	(1)(3)
	ROX	100 mcg/mL	Undiluted	n/a	[p]	7 d	n/a	n/a	n/a	n/a	n/a	(1)
	MDZ	0.5, 5 mcg/mL	D5W, D10W, NS	n/a	n/a	n/a	7 d[c]	n/a	n/a	n/a	n/a	(1)
	ASH	150, 500, 1500 mcg/mL	NS	285	6.5	2 yr	2 yr	n/a	n/a	n/a	12 wk	(2)
OTHER INFUSION CONTAINERS												
Pump Reservoir (Bard)	ROX	100 mcg/mL	Undiluted	n/a	[p]	7 d	n/a	n/a	n/a	n/a	n/a	(1)
SynchroMed® EL Implantable Pump (Medtronic)	BI	150 mcg/mL	unspec.[n]	n/a	[p]	n/a	n/a	n/a	n/a	n/a	5 wk	(10)
	BI	50 mcg/mL	unspec.[q]	n/a	n/a	n/a	n/a	n/a	n/a	n/a	12 wk	(1)
	UN	2000 mcg/mL	SWFI[m]	n/a	[p]	n/a	n/a	n/a	n/a	n/a	90 d	(9)
	NVA	250, 500, 1000 mcg/mL	NS[l]	n/a	[p]	n/a	n/a	n/a	n/a	n/a	14 wk	(6)
	BI	1840 mcg/mL	unspec.[s]	n/a	n/a	n/a	n/a	n/a	n/a	n/a	12 wk	(1)
SynchroMed® II Implantable Pump (Medtronic)	BB	2000 mcg/mL	[f][o]	n/a	n/a	n/a	n/a	n/a	n/a	n/a	28 d	(1)
	BI	15 mcg/mL	NS[r]	1030	3.46	n/a	n/a	n/a	n/a	n/a	40 d	(8)

DOI 10.37573/9781585286720.048

Flush Compatibility: Sodium chloride 0.9%, heparin.[1]

Special Considerations: Duraclon® (MYL) is intended for epidural administration only.[1,7] Do not use products or diluents containing preservatives for epidural administration.[1]

Notes

[a] In Terumo® syringes. Solutions in Omnifix® (BRN) syringes demonstrated a pH shift outside the acceptable pH range.[1]

[b] Solution contained: meperidine hydrochloride 8 mg/mL.[1]

[c] Protected from light.[1]

[d] Solutions contained cloNIDine alone, or combined with baclofen 1 mg/mL. Both solutions exhibited same stability.[1,3]

[e] Storage temperature: 35°C.[1,4]

[f] CloNIDine and morphine powder dissolved in ziconotide acetate (ELN) for injection.[1]

[g] Solution contained: bupivacaine hydrochloride 1 mg/mL and fentaNYL citrate 35 mcg/mL.[1]

[h] Solution contained: fentaNYL citrate (JN) 35 mcg/mL and bupivacaine hydrochloride (AST) 1 mg/mL.[4]

[i] Solution contained: ropivacaine hydrochloride (ASZ) 1 mg/mL.[5]

[j] Solution contained: ropivacaine hydrochloride (ASZ) 2 mg/mL.[5]

[k] Storage temperature: 30°C.[1,5]

[l] Solution contained: baclofen (NVA) 0.25, 0.5, and 1 mg/mL, respectively.[6]

[m] Solution contained: bupivacaine hydrochloride 25 mg/mL and morphine sulfate 50 mg/mL.[9]

[n] Solution contained: HYDROmorphone 25 mcg/mL.[10]

[o] Solution contained: ziconotide acetate (ELN) 25 mg/mL.[1]

[p] pH of the undiluted solution is 5-7.[1,7]

[q] Solution contained: morphine sulfate 20 mg/mL (Infumorph).[1]

[r] Combined with ziconotide acetate (EI) 0.1, 0.25, 0.5, or 0.75 mcg/mL, morphine sulfate (LAV) 7.5 mg/mL, and ropivacaine chlorhydrate (ASZ) 7.5 mg/mL. There was a 53.4% residual concentration of ziconotide after 5 wk, with no loss of morphine, ropivacaine, or cloNIDine.[8]

[s] Solution contained: morphine sulfate 2 mg/mL.[1]

REFERENCES

1. ASHP's Interactive Handbook on Injectable Drugs, 2020. Bethesda, MD: American Society of Health-System Pharmacists; Accessed August 2020.
2. Trissel LA, Xu QA, Hassenbusch SJ. Development of clonidine hydrochloride injections for epidural intrathecal administration. *Int J Pharm Compd*. 1997; 1(4):274-7.
3. Godwin D, Kim N, Zuniga R. Stability of a Baclofen and Clonidine Hydrochloride Admixture for Intrathecal Administration. *Hosp Pharm*. 2001; 36: 950-54.
4. Jappinen AMP, Kokki HM, Naaranlahti TP. pH Stability of Injectable Fentanyl, Bupivacaine, or Clonidine Solution or a Ternary Mixture in 0.9% Sodium Chloride in Two Types of Polypropylene Syringes. *Int J Pharm Compd*. 2002; 6(6):471-4.
5. Oster Svedberg K, McKenzie J, Larrivee-Elkins C. Compatibility of ropivacaine with morphine, sufentanil, fentanyl, or clonidine. *J Clin Pharm Ther*. 2002; 27(1):39-45.
6. Alvarez JC, De Mazancourt P, Chartier-Kastler E, et al. Drug stability testing to support clinical feasibility investigations for intrathecal baclofen-clonidine admixture. *J Pain Symptom Manage*. 2004; 28(3):268-72.
7. Duraclon® (Clonidine Hydrochloride) Injection [package insert]. Morgantown, WV: Mylan Institutional LLC; July 2020.
8. Dupoiron D, Richard H, Chabert-Desnot V, et al. In vitro stability of low-concentration ziconotide alone or in admixtures in intrathecal pumps. *Neuromodulation*. 2014; 17(5):472-82; discussion 82.
9. Classen AM, Wimbish GH, Kupiec TC. Stability of admixture containing morphine sulfate, bupivacaine hydrochloride, and clonidine hydrochloride in an implantable infusion system. *J Pain Symptom Manage*. 2004; 28(6):603-11.
10. Rudich Z, Peng P, Dunn E, et al. Stability of clonidine in clonidine-hydromorphone mixture from implanted intrathecal infusion pumps in chronic pain patients. *J Pain Symptom Manage*. 2004; 28(6):599-602.

Coagulation Factor VIIa (F7a) (Recombinant)

Storage Conditions

						Temperature			Post-thaw Temp			
	Drug Manufacturer	Concentration	Diluents	Osmolality (mOsm/kg)	pH	Room	Refrig	Frozen	Room	Refrig	Body Temp	Refer.
CONTAINER												
Bag, Polyvinyl Chloride (PVC)	NVN	[a][e]	SWFI	n/a	[d]	72 hr[h]	n/a	n/a	n/a	n/a	n/a	(1)
Syringe, Plastic (Unspecified)	NVN	[a][e]	SWFI	n/a	[d]	72 hr[h]	n/a	n/a	n/a	n/a	n/a	(1)
Vial, Glass	NVN[c]	[a]	[g]	n/a	[d]	6 hr	24 hr	n/a	n/a	n/a	n/a	(4)
	NVN[c]	0.97-0.99 mg/mL[b]	NS	n/a	6.0	6 hr	24 hr	n/a	n/a	n/a	n/a	(7)
OTHER INFUSION CONTAINERS												
CADD® Cassette (Smiths Medical)	NVN	[a][e]	SWFI	n/a	[d]	72 hr[h]	n/a	n/a	n/a	n/a	n/a	(1)(5)
WalkMed™ Reservoir Bag	NVN	[a][f]	SWFI	n/a	[d]	72 hr	n/a	n/a	n/a	n/a	24 hr	(2)(5)
Continuous-Infusion Pump System (Unspecified)	NVN[c]	unspec.	[g]	n/a	[d]	24 hr	n/a	n/a	n/a	n/a	n/a	(6)

Flush Compatibility: Sodium chloride 0.9%.[3]

Special Considerations: Prior to reconstitution, store product and included histidine diluent between 2-25°C. Store product protected from light. Do not freeze prior to or after reconstitution. If refrigerated, bring product and diluent to room temperature, but not above 37°C, before preparation. Do not inject the diluent directly on the NovoSeven® RT powder. Vials are closed with a chlorobutyl rubber stopper, and not made with natural rubber latex.[3]

Notes

[a] Concentration is at manufacturer's recommended dilution upon reconstitution.

[b] 1 mg reconstituted with 1.15 mL NS.[7]

[c] NovoSeven® RT Coagulation Factor VIIa (Recombinant).

[d] When reconstituted as recommended, the resulting solution is clear and colorless, with a pH of approximately 6.0 and contains no preservatives.[3]

[e] Evaluated alone, with a low molecular weight heparin (LMWH), concentrations unspecified, and with heparin 5-10 units/mL in SWFI. Note that addition of heparin 5-10 units/mL caused a 50% decrease in FVII activity in 4 hours, whereas the LMWH did not affect FVII activity.[1]

[f] Evaluated alone, and with enoxaparin (LMWH) or heparin or NS. LMWH did not affect FVII activity.[2]

[g] Diluent supplied in NovoSeven® RT package is 10 mmol solution of L-histidine in water.[3]

[h] Protected from light.

DOI 10.37573/9781585286720.049

REFERENCES

1. Schulman S, Bech Jensen M, Varon D, et al. Feasibility of using recombinant factor VIIa in continuous infusion. *Thromb Haemost*. 1996; 75(3):432-6.
2. Bonde C, Jensen MB. Continuous infusion of recombinant activated factor VII: stability in infusion pump systems. *Blood Coagul Fibrinolysis*. 1998; 9 Suppl 1:S103-5.
3. Novo Seven® RT (Coagulation Factor VIIa, Recombinant) Injection [package insert]. Plainsboro, NJ: Novo Nordisk; July 2020.
4. Nedergaard H, Vestergaard S, Jensen PT, et al. In vitro stability of lyophilized and reconstituted recombinant activated factor VII formulated for storage at room temperature. *Clin Ther*. 2008; 30(7):1309-15.
5. Stachnik JM, Gabay MP. Continuous infusion of coagulation factor products. *Ann Pharmacother*. 2002; 36(5):882-91.
6. Christensen A, Jensen JT, Nohr AM, et al. Room-temperature-stable recombinant activated coagulation factor VII recombinant: chemical and microbiologic stability over 24 hours during continuous in vitro infusion. *Clin Ther*. 2011; 33(12):1997-2001.
7. Petersson B, Schonwandt AB, Thornstfeldt P, et al. In vitro stability of two formulations of recombinant activated factor VIIa reconstituted in inappropriate solvents or at inappropriate volumes. *Clin Ther*. 2008; 30(5):917-23.

Coagulation Factor VIII (F8)

	Drug Manufacturer	Concentration[a]	Diluents	Osmolality (mOsm/kg)	pH	Storage Conditions: Temperature: Room	Storage Conditions: Temperature: Refrig	Storage Conditions: Temperature: Frozen	Storage Conditions: Post-thaw Temp: Room	Storage Conditions: Post-thaw Temp: Refrig	Body Temp	Refer.
CONTAINER												
Bag, Polyethylene	BAY[d]	83-121 units/mL	SWFI	n/a	n/a	7 d	7 d	n/a	n/a	n/a	n/a	(2)
	BAY[d]	83-121 units/mL	SWFI[j]	n/a	n/a	7 d	n/a	n/a	n/a	n/a	n/a	(2)
Bag, Polyvinyl Chloride (PVC)	BA[g]	22-106 units/mL	SWFI	n/a	n/a	4 d[f]	n/a	n/a	n/a	n/a	n/a	(6)
	BA[g]	22-106 units/mL	SWFI[l]	n/a	n/a	4 d[f]	n/a	n/a	n/a	n/a	n/a	(6)
	BAY[d]	83-121 units/mL	SWFI	n/a	n/a	7 d	7d	n/a	n/a	n/a	n/a	(2)
	BAY[d]	83-121 units/mL	SWFI[j]	n/a	n/a	7 d	n/a	n/a	n/a	n/a	n/a	(2)
Syringe, Plastic	BAY[d]	50, 80, 120 units/mL	SWFI, NS, LR	n/a	n/a	72 hr	n/a	n/a	n/a	n/a	n/a	(1)
	BA[h]	Various	SWFI[k]	n/a	n/a	48 hr	n/a	n/a	n/a	n/a	n/a	(8)
	BA[h]	Various	SWFI	n/a	n/a	48 hr	n/a	n/a	n/a	n/a	n/a	(8)
	AR[e]	100 units/mL	SWFI	n/a	n/a	15 d	n/a	n/a	n/a	n/a	n/a	(3)
	AR[e]	100 units/mL	SWFI[l]	n/a	n/a	15 d	n/a	n/a	n/a	n/a	n/a	(3)
Syringe, Polypropylene	BA[c][g]	unspec.	SWFI	n/a	n/a	28 d[i]	28 d[i]	n/a	n/a	n/a	14 d[i]	(4)
	BAY[b]	Various	SWFI	n/a	n/a	24 hr	n/a	n/a	n/a	n/a	n/a	(5)
Unspecified	GRI[m]	unspec.	SWFI	n/a	n/a	7 d	7 d	n/a	n/a	n/a	n/a	(9)
Vial, Glass	BA[c]	unspec.	SWFI	n/a	n/a	28 d[i]	24 hr[i]	n/a	n/a	n/a	24 hr[i]	(4)
	BA[g]	unspec.	SWFI	n/a	n/a	28 d[i]	28 d[i]	n/a	n/a	n/a	24 hr[i]	(4)
	BA[h]	unspec.	SWFI	n/a	n/a	24 hr	n/a	n/a	n/a	n/a	n/a	(7)
OTHER INFUSION CONTAINERS												
CADD® Cassette (Smiths Medical)	BA[h]	Various	SWFI	n/a	n/a	48 hr	n/a	n/a	n/a	n/a	n/a	(8)
	BA[h]	Various	SWFI[k]	n/a	n/a	48 hr	n/a	n/a	n/a	n/a	n/a	(8)

Flush Compatibility: Sodium chloride 0.9%.[1]

Special Considerations: Avoid exposure to direct sunlight. Do not freeze. Bring refrigerated products and diluents to room temperature before preparation.[7] Stability is defined as retaining > 80% of baseline value indicated by one-state clotting assay. Several continuous factor VIII infusion studies noted variation in the loss of factor VIII activity in PVC or polyethylene tubing upon initial dilution or infusion. This was primarily due to initial adsorption, resolved relatively quickly, was less pronounced with higher flow rates, and the overall impact on a long duration continuous factor infusion was therapeutically negligible.[6]

DOI 10.37573/9781585286720.050

Notes

[a] Concentration is at manufacturer's recommended dilution unless noted.
[b] Kovaltry® (BAY).
[c] Hemofil M® (BA).
[d] Kogenate® FS (BAY).
[e] Monoclate-P® (AR).
[f] Storage temperature: 20-25°C and 30 ± 2°C.
[g] Recombinate® (BA).
[h] Advate® (BA).
[i] Protected from light.
[j] Solution contained: heparin 4 units/mL (LI).[(2)]
[k] Solution contained: heparin 2 units/mL (ES).[(8)]
[l] Solution contained: heparin 1 unit/mL (ES).[(6)]
[m] Koate® DVI (GRI).

REFERENCES

1. Rand M, Schumugge M, Clark D, et al. Stability of dilutions of the recombinant factor VIII Kogenate FS stored in syringes. *J Thromb Haemost*. 2003; 1(Supplement 1): P1625.
2. Hurst D, Zabor S, Malianni D, et al. Evaluation of recombinant factor VIII (Kogenate) stability for continuous infusion using a minipump infusion device. *Haemophilia*. 1998; 4(6): 785-9.
3. Schulman S, Varon D, Keller N, et al. Monoclonal purified F VIII for continuous infusion: stability, microbiological safety and clinical experience. *Thromb Haemost*. 1994; 72(3): 403-7.
4. Schulman S, Gitel S, Martinowitz U. Stability of factor VIII concentrates after reconstitution. *Am J Hematol*. 1994; 45(3): 217-23.
5. Teare JM, Trefethen J, Garger S, et al. Reconstituted Bay 81-8973 Factor VIII Stability Supports Its Suitability for Continuous Infusion for up to 24 Hours. *Blood*. 2018; 132(Supplement 1): 5043.
6. Parti R, Ardosa J, Yang L, et al. In vitro stability of recombinant human factor VIII (Recombinate). *Haemophilia*. 2000; 6(5): 513-22.
7. ASHP's Interactive Handbook on Injectable Drugs, 2020. Bethesda, MD: American Society of Health-System Pharmacists; Accessed August 2020.
8. Fernandez M, Yu T, Bjornson E, et al. Stability of ADVATE, Antihemophilic Factor (Recombinant) Plasma/Albumin-Free Method, during simulated continuous infusion. *Blood Coagul Fibrinolysis*. 2006; 17(3): 165-71.
9. Shields S, Kim A, Elder J. Extended Stability and Sterility of Antihemophilic Factor Human. *J Pediatr Pharmacol Ther*. 2017; 22(3): 203-06.

Coagulation Factor IX (F9)

Storage Conditions

						Temperature			Post-thaw Temp			
	Drug Manufacturer	Concentration	Diluents	Osmolality (mOsm/kg)	pH	Room	Refrig	Frozen	Room	Refrig	Body Temp	Refer.
CONTAINER												
Syringe, Polyethylene	WY[a]	100 units/mL	SWFI[c]	[b]	[b]	4 d	14 d	n/a	n/a	n/a	n/a	(1)
	WY[a]	100 units/mL	SWFI	[b]	[b]	7 d	14 d	n/a	n/a	n/a	n/a	(1)
Syringe, Polypropylene	AR[d]	100 units/mL	SWFI	[b]	[b]	28 d[e]	28 d[e]	n/a	n/a	n/a	7 d[e]	(2)

Flush Compatibility: n/a

Special Considerations: Stability is defined as retaining > 80% of baseline value indicated by one-state clotting assay. Do not freeze.

Notes

[a] BeneFIX® brand.

[b] When reconstituted as recommended, the resulting solution is a clear, colorless, isotonic preparation of neutral pH.

[c] Solution contained: unfractionated heparin 4 units/mL.[1]

[d] Mononine® brand.

[e] Protected from light.

REFERENCES

1. Chowdary P, Dasani H, Jones JA, et al. Recombinant factor IX (BeneFix) by adjusted continuous infusion: a study of stability, sterility and clinical experience. *Haemophilia*. 2001; 7(2):140-5.
2. Schulman S, Gitel S, Zivelin A, et al. The feasibility of using concentrates containing factor IX for continuous infusion. *Haemophilia*. 1995; 1(2):103-10.

DOI 10.37573/9781585286720.051

Colistimethate Sodium

Storage Conditions

	Drug Manufacturer	Concentration	Diluents	Osmolality (mOsm/kg)	pH	Temperature Room	Temperature Refrig	Temperature Frozen	Post-thaw Temp Room	Post-thaw Temp Refrig	Body Temp	Refer.
CONTAINER												
Bag, Polyvinyl Chloride (PVC)	PF	1.5 mg/mL	D5W, NS	n/a	n/a	n/a	48 hr[(a)]	n/a	n/a	n/a	n/a	(1)
Unspecified	PAR	unspec.	NS, D5W, LR, D5¼NS, D5NS, D5½NS	n/a	n/a	24 hr	n/a	n/a	n/a	n/a	n/a	(7)
	APP	75 mg/mL	SWFI	n/a	n/a	24 hr	24 hr[(b)]	24 hr[(c)]	n/a	n/a	n/a	(3)
Vial, Glass	PF	75 mg/mL	SWFI	n/a	n/a	7 d	7 d	n/a	n/a	n/a	n/a	(1)(7)
OTHER INFUSION CONTAINERS												
Dosi-Fuser® (Leventon)	PX	1-3 mg/mL	D5W, NS	n/a	n/a	48 hr[(e)(d)]	30 d[(d)]	n/a	n/a	n/a	n/a	(6)
Easypump® ST/LT (B. Braun)	UN	3 mg/mL	NS	n/a	n/a	2 hr	24 hr	n/a	n/a	n/a	n/a	(4)
INTERMATE™ (Baxter)[(f)]	PX	1-3 mg/mL	NS	n/a	n/a	48 hr[(e)]	30 d	n/a	n/a	n/a	n/a	(2)
SMARTeZ® (Progressive Medical)	UN	3 mg/mL	NS	n/a	n/a	2 hr[(d)]	24 hr[(d)]	n/a	n/a	n/a	n/a	(5)

Flush Compatibility: Sodium chloride 0.9%, heparin.[(1)]

Special Considerations: Dosage and concentration stated as colistin base activity.

Notes

[a] Protected from light.

[b] Storage temperature: 0°C.

[c] Storage temperature: –20°C and –70°C.

[d] Manufacturer extrapolated data from other sources.

[e] After 30 d refrigerated storage.

[f] INTERMATE™/INFUSOR™ Portable Elastomeric Infusion System devices are no longer available in the United States.

DOI 10.37573/9781585286720.052

REFERENCES

1. Wallace SJ, Li J, Rayner CR, et al. Stability of colistin methanesulfonate in pharmaceutical products and solutions for administration to patients. *Antimicrob Agents Chemother*. 2008; 52(9):3047-51.
2. Stabforum - Stability Database: Colistimethate, Ontario, Canada: Baxter Healthcare; Accessed November 2020.
3. Healan AM, Gray W, Fuchs EJ, et al. Stability of Colistimethate Sodium in Aqueous Solution. *Antimicrob Agents Chemother*. 2012; 56(12):6432-33.
4. *Drug Stability for Easypump® ST/LT*, 2020. Bethlehem, PA: B. Braun USA; Updated June 2020.
5. *SMARTeZ® - Stability Data for Drugs Using Elastomeric Infusion Pumps,* 2020. Fenton, MO: Progressive Medical, Inc.; Updated May 2020.
6. *Drug Stability Table - Dosi-Fuser® Elastomeric Pump (S-CL-00-001v16),* 2021. Barcelona, Spain: Leventon SAU; Updated May 2021.
7. Coly-Mycin® M Parenteral (Colistimethate) Injection [package insert]. Chestnut Ridge, NY: Par Pharmaceutical; April 2017.

Cyclophosphamide

Storage Conditions

	Drug Manufacturer	Concentration	Diluents	Osmolality (mOsm/kg)	pH	Temperature Room	Temperature Refrig	Temperature Frozen	Post-thaw Temp Room	Post-thaw Temp Refrig	Body Temp	Refer.
CONTAINER												
Bag, Polyethylene	AM	1.8 mg/mL[f]	D5W	n/a	[d]	6 hr	48 hr	n/a	n/a	n/a	n/a	(6)
	AM	10.8 mg/mL[e]	D5W	n/a	[d]	24 hr	48 hr	n/a	n/a	n/a	n/a	(5)(6)
Bag, Polyvinyl Chloride (PVC)	MJ	0.3, 2 mg/mL[b]	D5W, NS	n/a	[d]	4 d	8 d	n/a	n/a	n/a	n/a	(1)(5)
	CE	4 mg/mL	NS	n/a	[d]	n/a	19 wk	19 wk	n/a	n/a	n/a	(2)(5)
	UN	8 mg/mL	NS	n/a	[d]	6 d	n/a	n/a	n/a	n/a	n/a	(7)
Syringe, Polypropylene	CE	20 mg/mL	SWFI	[a]	[d]	n/a	28 d	n/a	n/a	n/a	n/a	(2)(5)
Unspecified	MJ	0.1, 3.1 mg/mL	D5NS, D5W	n/a	[d]	8 hr	6 d	n/a	n/a	n/a	n/a	(5)
	UN	21 mg/mL	SWFI	[a]	[d]	8 hr	6 d	n/a	n/a	n/a	n/a	(5)
OTHER INFUSION CONTAINERS												
CADD® Cassette (Smiths Medical)	UN	20 mg/mL	SWFI	n/a	[d]	n/a	14 d	n/a	n/a	n/a	24 hr	(3)
Dosi-Fuser® (Leventon)	BA	2-20 mg/mL	NS	n/a	[d]	48 hr[c]	48 d[c]	n/a	n/a	n/a	n/a	(9)
Easypump® ST/LT (B. Braun)	UN	2 mg/mL	NS	n/a	[d]	48 hr	14 d	n/a	n/a	n/a	n/a	(11)
	UN	20 mg/mL	NS	n/a	[d]	48 hr	7 d	n/a	n/a	n/a	n/a	(11)
Homepump Eclipse® / Homepump® (Halyard)	UN	4.5 mg/mL	NS	n/a	[d]	7 d	7 d	n/a	n/a	n/a	n/a	(4)
SMARTeZ® (Progressive Medical)	UN	2 mg/mL	NS	n/a	[d]	48 hr	14 d	n/a	n/a	n/a	n/a	(8)
	UN	20 mg/mL	NS	n/a	[d]	48 hr	7 d	n/a	n/a	n/a	n/a	(8)

Flush Compatibility: Sodium chloride 0.9%, heparin.[5]

Special Considerations: Cyclophosphamide solutions should not be stored at temperatures above 25°C.[5] Do not use benzyl alcohol-preserved diluents.[5] Reconstitute cyclophosphamide with NS only.[5]

DOI 10.37573/9781585286720.053

Notes

[a] Reconstitution with SWFI results in a hypotonic solution, which must be further diluted with an appropriate infusion solution prior to administration.[5][10]

[b] Solution contained ondansetron (GL) 0.05 mg/mL and ondansetron (GL) 0.4 mg/mL, respectively.

[c] Manufacturer extrapolated data from other sources.

[d] pH of reconstituted solution is 3-9; 22 mg/mL is pH 6.87.[5]

[e] Solution contained mesna (AM) 3.2 mg/mL.

[f] Solution contained mesna (AM) 0.54 mg/mL.

REFERENCES

1. Fleming RA, Olsen DJ, Savage PD, et al. Stability of ondansetron hydrochloride and cyclophosphamide in injectable solutions. *Am J Health Syst Pharm*. 1995; 52(5): 514-6.
2. Kirk B, Melia CD, Wilson JV. Chemical stability of cyclophosphamide injection. The effect of low temperature storage and microwave thawing. *Br J Parenter Ther*. 1984; 5(3): 90-97.
3. *Pharmaceutical report on chemical and physical stability of drugs commonly used with CADD® infusion pumps (IN193109GB-122019)*, 2019. Minneapolis, MN: Smiths Medical ASD, Inc.; Updated December 2019.
4. *Stability Data for Drugs Using Homepump Disposable Ambulatory Infusion Systems (MK-00314 rev 3)*, 2015. Alpharetta, GA: Halyard Health; Updated June 2015.
5. ASHP's Interactive Handbook on Injectable Drugs, 2020. Bethesda, MD: American Society of Health-System Pharmacists; Accessed August 2020.
6. Menard C, Bourguignon C, Schlatter J, et al. Stability of cyclophosphamide and mesna admixtures in polyethylene infusion bags. *Ann Pharmacother*. 2003; 37(12): 1789-92.
7. Vyas HM, Baptista RJ, Mitrano FP, et al. Drug stability guidelines for a continuous infusion chemotherapy program. *Hosp Pharm*. 1987; 22(7): 685-7.
8. *SMARTeZ® - Stability Data for Drugs Using Elastomeric Infusion Pumps*, 2020. Fenton, MO: Progressive Medical, Inc.; Updated May 2020.
9. *Drug Stability Table - Dosi-Fuser® Elastomeric Pump (S-CL-00-001v16)*, 2021. Barcelona, Spain: Leventon SAU; Updated May 2021.
10. Cyclophosphamide Injection [package insert]. Deerfield, IL: Baxter Healthcare Corporation; March 2017.
11. *Drug Stability for Easypump® ST/LT*, 2020. Bethlehem, PA: B. Braun USA; Updated June 2020.

CycloSPORINE

Storage Conditions

	Drug Manufacturer	Concentration	Diluents	Osmolality (mOsm/kg)	pH	Temperature: Room	Temperature: Refrig	Temperature: Frozen	Post-thaw Temp: Room	Post-thaw Temp: Refrig	Body Temp	Refer.
CONTAINER												
Bag, Ethylene Vinyl Acetate (EVA)	NVA	0.2 mg/mL	D5W, NS	n/a	n/a	7 d	n/a	n/a	n/a	n/a	n/a	(3)
Bag, Polyolefin[c]	NVA	0.2, 2.5 mg/mL	D5W, NS	n/a	n/a	14 d	n/a	n/a	n/a	n/a	n/a	(1)(2)
Bag, Polyvinyl Chloride (PVC)[b]	SZ	2 mg/mL	D5W, NS	n/a	n/a	24 hr[b]	n/a	n/a	n/a	n/a	n/a	(1)
Unspecified	SZ	1 mg/mL	D5W	n/a	n/a	72 hr	n/a	n/a	n/a	n/a	n/a	(1)
	UN	2 mg/mL	NS	n/a	n/a	24 hr	24 hr	n/a	n/a	n/a	n/a	(1)
Vial, Glass	SZ	2 mg/mL	D5W	n/a	n/a	48 hr[a]	48 hr[a]	n/a	n/a	n/a	n/a	(1)
	SZ	2 mg/mL	NS	n/a	n/a	24 hr	n/a	n/a	n/a	n/a	n/a	(1)

Flush Compatibility: Sodium chloride 0.9%.[1]

Special Considerations: Due to leaching of syringe plunger components, polypropylene syringes cannot be recommended for storage of cycloSPORINE solutions. Short term (less than 10 min) syringe use for preparation and transfer is considered safe.[1][2] Do not use DEHP-containing containers or tubing to administer cycloSPORINE. Use non-PVC administration sets and containers for administration.

Notes

[a] Exposed to fluorescent light.

[b] Cremophor® EL can cause phthalate stripping from PVC.[1]

[c] AVIVA™ polypropylene-polyolefin bag (BA).

REFERENCES

1. ASHP's Interactive Handbook on Injectable Drugs, 2020. Bethesda, MD: American Society of Health-System Pharmacists; Accessed September 2020.
2. Li M, Forest JM, Coursol C, et al. Stability of cyclosporine solutions stored in polypropylene-polyolefin bags and polypropylene syringes. *Am J Health Syst Pharm*. 2011; 68(17):1646-50.
3. Li M, Coursol C, Leclair G. Stability of cyclosporine diluted with 0.9% sodium chloride injection or 5% dextrose injection and stored in ethylene-vinyl acetate containers. *Am J Health Syst Pharm*. 2013; 70(22):1970-2.

DOI 10.37573/9781585286720.054

Cytarabine (Conventional)

Storage Conditions

	Drug Manufacturer	Concentration	Diluents	Osmolality (mOsm/kg)	pH	Temperature Room	Temperature Refrig	Temperature Frozen	Post-thaw Temp Room	Post-thaw Temp Refrig	Body Temp	Refer.
CONTAINER												
Bag, Ethylene Vinyl Acetate (EVA)	UP	1.25, 25 mg/mL	D5W, NS	n/a	[e]	28 d[a]	28 d[a]	n/a	n/a	n/a	7 d[a][c]	(1)(6)
Bag, Plastic (Unspecified)	HOS	unspec.	D5W, NS, SWFI	n/a	[e]	8 d	n/a	n/a	n/a	n/a	n/a	(7)
Bag, Polyvinyl Chloride (PVC)	UP	8, 24, 32 mg/mL	D5W, D5¼NS, NS	n/a	[e]	7 d	7 d	7 d	n/a	n/a	n/a	(6)
	UN	20 mg/mL	BWFI, NS[d]	n/a	[e]	8 d	n/a	n/a	n/a	n/a	n/a	(2)
Syringe, Polypropylene	DB	20, 50 mg/mL	SWFI	n/a	[e]	29 d[a]	29 d[a]	n/a	n/a	n/a	n/a	(3)
	UN	40, 80 mg/mL	BWFI	n/a	n/a	15 d	15 d	n/a	n/a	n/a	7 d[i]	(6)
	UP	20 mg/mL	unspec.	n/a	[e]	7 d	7 d	n/a	n/a	n/a	n/a	(6)
Unspecified	UP	0.5 mg/mL	D5W, NS	n/a	[e]	7 d	n/a	n/a	n/a	n/a	n/a	(6)
	UN	0.5-5 mg/mL	D5W, NS, LR	n/a	[e]	14 d	n/a	n/a	n/a	n/a	n/a	(6)
	UN	20, 250 mg/mL[g]	BWFI	n/a	[e]	5 d	n/a	n/a	n/a	n/a	n/a	(6)
Vial, Glass	UP	8, 24, 32 mg/mL	D5W, D5¼NS, NS	n/a	[e]	7 d	7 d	7 d	n/a	n/a	n/a	(6)
	HOS	unspec.	D5W, NS, SWFI	n/a	[e]	8 d	n/a	n/a	n/a	n/a	n/a	(6)(7)
	UP	20 mg/mL	unspec.	n/a	n/a	7 d	7 d	n/a	n/a	n/a	n/a	(6)
OTHER INFUSION CONTAINERS												
CADD® Cassette (Smiths Medical)	UN	20 mg/mL	NS	n/a	n/a	n/a	12 d	n/a	n/a	n/a	8 d	(8)
Dosi-Fuser® (Leventon)	HOS	4 mg/mL	NS	n/a	n/a	7 d	n/a	n/a	n/a	n/a	n/a	(9)
Infusaid® Model 400 Implantable Pump (Infusaid)	UP	1 mg/mL	[b]	n/a	[e]	n/a	n/a	n/a	n/a	n/a	15 d	(4)(6)
INFUSOR™ (Baxter)[h]	UP	5 mg/mL	D5W	n/a	[e]	7 d[a][f]	n/a	n/a	n/a	n/a	24 hr[a][f]	(5)

Flush Compatibility: Sodium chloride 0.9%.[6]

Special Considerations: Some preparations contain preservatives and should not be used for intrathecal administration. Preservative-free bulk vials should only be used for preparation of intravenous infusions.[6]

DOI 10.37573/9781585286720.055

Notes

[a] Protected from light.

[b] Elliott's B artificial spinal fluid.

[c] Storage temperature: 35°C.

[d] NS with and without bacteriostat.

[e] pH of preservative-free commercial injection 20 mg/mL is 7.4 and 100 mg/mL is 7.7. pH of 20 mg/mL multi-dose vial containing benzyl alcohol is 7.6.[(6)]

[f] Storage temperature: 25°C for 7 d, followed by 24 hr at 33°C.[(5)]

[g] Cytarabine has an aqueous solubility of 100 mg/mL. Precipitation from more concentrated solutions has been observed.[(6)]

[h] INTERMATE™/INFUSOR™ Portable Elastomeric Infusion System devices are no longer available in the United States.

[i] Storage temperature: 37°C.

REFERENCES

1. Rochard EB, Barthes DM, Courtois PY. Stability of fluorouracil, cytarabine, or doxorubicin hydrochloride in ethylene vinylacetate portable infusion-pump reservoirs. *Am J Hosp Pharm*. 1992; 49(3): 619-23.
2. Vyas HM, Baptista RJ, Mitrano FP, et al. Drug stability guidelines for a continuous infusion chemotherapy program. *Hosp Pharm*. 1987; 22(7): 685-7.
3. Weir PJ, Ireland DS. Chemical stability of cytarabine and vinblastine injections. *Br J Pharm Pract*. 1990; 12: 53-55.
4. Keller JH, Ensminger WD. Stability of cancer chemotherapeutic agents in a totally implanted drug delivery system. *Am J Hosp Pharm*. 1982; 39(8): 1321-3.
5. Cytarabine Stability Information Letter (Ref#: N/A) [personal communication]. Mississauga, ON: Baxter Corporation; 2020:1.
6. ASHP's Interactive Handbook on Injectable Drugs, 2020. Bethesda, MD: American Society of Health-System Pharmacists; Accessed June 2020.
7. Cytarabine Injection [package insert]. Lake Forest, IL: Hospira, Inc.; March 2021.
8. *Pharmaceutical report on chemical and physical stability of drugs commonly used with CADD® infusion pumps (IN193109GB-122019)*, 2019. Minneapolis, MN: Smiths Medical ASD, Inc.; Updated December 2019.
9. *Drug Stability Table - Dosi-Fuser® Elastomeric Pump (S-CL-00-001v16)*, 2021. Barcelona, Spain: Leventon SAU; Updated May 2021.

Dacarbazine

Storage Conditions

						Temperature			Post-thaw Temp			
	Drug Manufacturer	Concentration	Diluents	Osmolality (mOsm/kg)	pH	Room	Refrig	Frozen	Room	Refrig	Body Temp	Refer.
CONTAINER												
Bag, Polyolefin	UN	1.7 mg/mL	D5W	n/a	[b]	24 hr[e]	n/a	n/a	n/a	n/a	n/a	(1)
Bag, Polyvinyl Chloride (PVC)	AVE	1.4 mg/mL	D5W	n/a	[b]	48 hr[c]	7 d[c]	n/a	n/a	n/a	n/a	(1)(2)
	UN	1.7 mg/mL	D5W	n/a	[b]	24 hr[e]	n/a	n/a	n/a	n/a	n/a	(1)
Glass Vial	AVE	11 mg/mL	SWFI	n/a	[b]	24 hr[e]	4 d[c]	n/a	n/a	n/a	n/a	(2)
	UN	1.7 mg/mL	D5W	n/a	[b]	24 hr[e]	n/a	n/a	n/a	n/a	n/a	(1)
	TE	10 mg/mL[d]	SWFI	n/a	[b]	8 hr	72 hr	n/a	n/a	n/a	n/a	(3)
OTHER INFUSION CONTAINERS												
Dosi-Fuser® (Leventon)	UN	7.3 mg/mL	D5W[a]	n/a	[b]	n/a	5 d[c]	5 d[c]	n/a	n/a	n/a	(4)

Flush Compatibility: Sodium chloride 0.9%.[1]

Special Considerations: Manufacturer recommends protection from light.[3]

Notes

[a] Solution contained: DOXOrubicin.[4]

[b] pH of reconstituted preparation 10 mg/mL in SWFI is 3-4.[3]

[c] Protected from light.

[d] Manufacturer original vial.[3]

[e] Exposed to fluorescent light.

REFERENCES

1. ASHP's Interactive Handbook on Injectable Drugs, 2020. Bethesda, MD: American Society of Health-System Pharmacists; Accessed December 2020.
2. El Aatmani M, Poujol S, Astre C, et al. Stability of dacarbazine in amber glass vials and polyvinyl chloride bags. *Am J Health Syst Pharm*. 2002; 59(14):1351-6.
3. Dacarbazine Injection [package insert]. Parsippany, NJ: Teva Pharmaceuticals USA, Inc.; June 2020.
4. *Drug Stability Table - Dosi-Fuser® Elastomeric Pump (ES.H.00.73-10)*, 2015. Barcelona, Spain: Leventon SAU; Updated October 2015.

DOI 10.37573/9781585286720.056

Dalbavancin

Storage Conditions

						Temperature			Post-thaw Temp			
	Drug Manufacturer	Concentration	Diluents	Osmolality (mOsm/kg)	pH	Room	Refrig	Frozen	Room	Refrig	Body Temp	Refer.
CONTAINER												
Bag, Plastic (Unspecified)	DRT	1-5 mg/mL	D5W	n/a	n/a	48 hr[(a)]	48 hr	n/a	n/a	n/a	n/a	(1)(2)
Vial, Glass	DRT	20 mg/mL	D5W, SWFI	n/a	n/a	48 hr[(a)]	48 hr	n/a	n/a	n/a	n/a	(2)

Flush Compatibility: D5W.[(2)]

Special Considerations: Do not shake. Avoid mixture or co-infusion with saline-based infusion solutions due to precipitation. Do not freeze.[(2)]

Notes

[a] Storage temperature: 20-25°C.[(2)]

REFERENCES

1. ASHP's Interactive Handbook on Injectable Drugs, 2020. Bethesda, MD: American Society of Health-System Pharmacists; Accessed May 2020.
2. Dalvance® (dalbavancin) Injection [package insert]. Madison, NJ: Allergan USA, Inc.; October 2018.

DOI 10.37573/9781585286720.057

DAPTOmycin

Storage Conditions

	Drug Manufacturer	Concentration	Diluents	Osmolality (mOsm/kg)	pH	Temperature			Post-thaw Temp			
						Room	Refrig	Frozen	Room	Refrig	Body Temp	Refer.
CONTAINER												
Bag, Polypropylene	NVA	5.6, 14 mg/mL	NS	n/a	4.5-4.6	48 hr	7 d	n/a	n/a	n/a	n/a	(1)
Bag, Polyvinyl Chloride (PVC)	ME	2.5, 10, 20 mg/mL	NS	n/a	n/a	12 hr	10 d	n/a	n/a	n/a	n/a	(2)
	ME[(a)]	1, 14 mg/mL	NS[(b)]	n/a	n/a	48 hr	10 d	n/a	n/a	n/a	n/a	(3)(4)
Syringe, Polypropylene	CUB	5 mg/mL	LR[(e)]	n/a	n/a	n/a	14 d	14 d	n/a	n/a	n/a	(9)
	ME	50 mg/mL	NS	n/a	n/a	12 hr	10 d	n/a	n/a	n/a	n/a	(5)
	ME[(a)]	50 mg/mL	BWFI	n/a	n/a	48 hr	10 d	n/a	n/a	n/a	n/a	(3)(4)
Syringe, Polyvinyl Chloride (PVC)	ME	20 mg/mL	NS	n/a	n/a	12 hr	10 d	n/a	n/a	n/a	n/a	(5)
Vial, Glass	NVA	50 mg/mL	NS	n/a	4.5-4.6	48 hr	7 d	n/a	n/a	n/a	n/a	(1)
	ME[(a)]	50 mg/mL	BWFI	n/a	6.8	48 hr	72 hr	n/a	n/a	n/a	n/a	(3)
OTHER INFUSION CONTAINERS												
Easypump® ST/LT (B. Braun)	UN	1, 5, 20 mg/mL	NS	n/a	n/a	24 hr	10 d	n/a	n/a	n/a	n/a	(8)
Homepump Eclipse® / Homepump® (Halyard)	ME	20 mg/mL	NS	n/a	n/a	12 hr	10 d	n/a	n/a	n/a	n/a	(5)
	ME[(a)]	20 mg/mL	SWFI, BWFI	n/a	n/a	48 hr	14 d	n/a	n/a	n/a	n/a	(6)(10)
INTERMATE™ (Baxter)[(c)]	ME	20 mg/mL	NS	n/a	n/a	12 hr	10 d	n/a	n/a	n/a	n/a	(5)
	ME[(a)]	20 mg/mL	SWFI, BWFI	n/a	n/a	48 hr	14 d	n/a	n/a	n/a	n/a	(6)(10)
SMARTeZ® (Progressive Medical)	UN	20 mg/mL	NS	n/a	4.5	24 hr[(d)]	10 d[(d)]	n/a	n/a	n/a	n/a	(7)

Flush Compatibility: Sodium chloride 0.9%.[(3)]

Special Considerations: Cubicin®/daptomycin and Cubicin® RF differ in reconstitution and storage requirements.

Notes

[a] Cubicin® RF data.

[b] Cubicin® RF vials reconstituted with BWFI, and diluted in sodium chloride 0.9%.[(3)]

[c] INTERMATE™/INFUSOR™ Portable Elastomeric Infusion System devices are no longer available in the United States.

[d] Manufacturer extrapolated data from other sources.

[e] Solution contained: Heparin sodium 100 units/mL.[(9)]

DOI 10.37573/9781585286720.058

REFERENCES

1. Sanchez-Rubio Ferrandez J, Vazquez Sanchez R, Cordoba Diaz D, et al. Stability of daptomycin reconstituted vials and infusion solutions. *Eur J Hosp Pharm*. 2018; 25(2):107-10.
2. Cubicin® Stability in PVC Information Letter (Ref#: US20-10294) [personal communication]. North Wales, PA: Merck & Co., Inc.; 2020:2.
3. Cubicin® RF (Daptomycin) Injection, Lyophilized [package insert]. Whitehouse Station, NJ: Merck Sharp & Dohme, Corp.; August 2020.
4. Cubicin® RF Stability in Mini-Bags & Syringes Information Letter (Ref#: US20-11584) [personal communication]. North Wales, PA: Merck & Co., Inc.; 2020:2.
5. Cubicin® Stability in Elastomeric Pumps, Syringes & Minibag Systems Information Letter (Ref#: US20-10295) [personal communication]. North Wales, PA: Merck & Co., Inc.; 2020:6.
6. Cubicin® RF Stability in Elastomeric Pumps, Syringes & Minibag Systems Information Letter (Ref#: US20-10296) [personal communication]. North Wales, PA: Merck & Co., Inc.; 2020:5.
7. *SMARTeZ® - Stability Data for Drugs Using Elastomeric Infusion Pumps*, 2020. Fenton, MO: Progressive Medical, Inc.; Updated May 2020.
8. *Drug Stability for Easypump® ST/LT*, 2020. Bethlehem, PA: B. Braun USA; Updated June 2020.
9. Ortega R, Salmeron-Garcia A, Cabeza J, et al. Stability of daptomycin 5 mg/mL and heparin sodium 100 units/mL combined in lactated Ringer's injection and stored in polypropylene syringes at 4 and -20 degrees C. *Am J Health Syst Pharm*. 2014; 71(11):956-9.
10. Cubicin® RF Stability in Elastomeric Pumps Information Letter (Ref#: US20-17708) [personal communication]. North Wales, PA: Merck & Co., Inc.; 2020:2.

DAUNOrubicin Hydrochloride (Conventional)

Storage Conditions

						Temperature			Post-thaw Temp			
	Drug Manufacturer	Concentration	Diluents	Osmolality (mOsm/kg)	pH	Room	Refrig	Frozen	Room	Refrig	Body Temp	Refer.
CONTAINER												
Bag, Polyvinyl Chloride (PVC)	RP	0.1 mg/mL	NS, D5W	n/a	[c]	43 d[a]	43 d[a]	43 d[a][b]	n/a	n/a	n/a	(1)(2)
	BEL	0.016 mg/mL	D5W, NS	n/a	[c]	n/a	7 d[a]	n/a	n/a	n/a	n/a	(1)
Syringe, Polypropylene	RP	2 mg/mL	SWFI	n/a	[c]	n/a	43 d[a]	n/a	n/a	n/a	n/a	(1)(2)
Test Tube, Polypropylene[e]	RP	0.1 mg/mL	D5W, LR, NS, D3.3$^1/_3$NS	n/a	[c]	28 d[a]	n/a	n/a	n/a	n/a	n/a	(3)
Unspecified	RP	0.1 mg/mL	D5W, LR, NS	n/a	[c]	4 wk[a]	n/a	n/a	n/a	n/a	n/a	(1)
	BEL	0.0157 mg/mL	D5W	n/a	[c]	48 hr[d]	48 hr	n/a	n/a	n/a	n/a	(1)
	NCI	0.020 mg/mL	D5W, LR, NS	n/a	[c]	24 hr	n/a	n/a	n/a	n/a	n/a	(1)

Flush Compatibility: Sodium chloride 0.9%.[1]

Special Considerations: n/a

Notes

[a] Protected from light.

[b] Frozen samples were subjected to 11 freeze/thaw cycles with no apparent loss in potency between cycles.

[c] pH of a 5 mg/mL aqueous solution is 4-5 (HIK)[4]; pH of a 5 mg/mL aqueous solution is 3-4 (HP, TE)[5,6]; maximum stability is at pH 4.5-5.5.[1]

[d] Exposed to light.

[e] Test tubes sealed with stoppers.[3]

REFERENCES

1. ASHP's Interactive Handbook on Injectable Drugs, 2020. Bethesda, MD: American Society of Health-System Pharmacists; Accessed August 2020.
2. Wood MJ, Irwin WJ, Scott DK. Stability of doxorubicin, daunorubicin and epirubicin in plastic syringes and minibags. *J Clin Pharm Ther*. 1990; 15(4):279-89.
3. Beijnen JH, Rosing H, de Vries PA, et al. Stability of anthracycline antitumour agents in infusion fluids. *J Parenter Sci Technol*. 1985; 39(6):220-2.
4. Daunorubicin Hydrochloride Injection [package insert]. Eatontown, NJ: Hikma Pharmaceuticals USA, Inc.; December 2019.
5. Daunorubicin Hydrochloride Injection [package insert]. Bridgewater, NJ: Hisun Pharmaceuticals USA, Inc.; February 2020.
6. Daunorubicin Hydrochloride Injection [package insert]. Irvine, CA: Teva Parenteral Medicines, Inc.; December 2012.

DOI 10.37573/9781585286720.059

Deferoxamine Mesylate

Storage Conditions

	Drug Manufacturer	Concentration	Diluents	Osmolality (mOsm/kg)	pH	Temperature Room	Temperature Refrig	Temperature Frozen	Post-thaw Temp Room	Post-thaw Temp Refrig	Body Temp	Refer.
CONTAINER												
Syringe, Polypropylene	CG	250 mg/mL	SWFI	[f]	n/a	14 d[a]	n/a	n/a	n/a	n/a	n/a	(1)
OTHER INFUSION CONTAINERS												
CADD® Cassette (Smiths Medical)	CG	210, 370 mg/mL	SWFI	[f]	n/a	8 d	n/a	n/a	n/a	n/a	n/a	(3)
Dosi-Fuser® (Leventon)	NVA	10-100 mg/mL	SWFI	[f]	n/a	21 d	n/a	n/a	n/a	n/a	n/a	(7)
Easypump® ST/LT (B. Braun)	UN	5, 100 mg/mL	NS	[f]	n/a	48 hr	14 d	n/a	n/a	n/a	n/a	(6)
	UN	0.022 mg/mL	NS	[f]	n/a	48 hr	14 d	n/a	n/a	n/a	n/a	(6)
Homepump Eclipse® / Homepump® (Halyard)	UN	5 mg/mL	NS	[f]	n/a	12 d	n/a	n/a	n/a	n/a	n/a	(2)
	UN	5-160 mg/mL	SWFI	[f]	n/a	n/a	28 d	n/a	n/a	n/a	n/a	(2)
	UN	73 mg/mL	NS	[f]	n/a	7 d	28 d	n/a	n/a	n/a	n/a	(2)
INFUSOR™ (Baxter)[b]	CG	25 mg/mL	NS	[f]	n/a	72 hr	15 d[c]	n/a	n/a	n/a	7 d[d]	(4)
	CG	83.3 mg/mL	SWFI	[f]	n/a	4 d	31 d[g]	n/a	n/a	n/a	72 hr[d]	(4)
	CG	83.3 mg/mL	SWFI	[f]	n/a	72 hr	5 wk[e]	n/a	n/a	n/a	72 hr[d]	(4)
	CG	83.3 mg/mL	SWFI	[f]	n/a	20 d	n/a	n/a	n/a	n/a	n/a	(4)
	CG	90 mg/mL	SWFI	[f]	n/a	72 hr	15 d[c]	n/a	n/a	n/a	7 d[d]	(4)
	CG	100-200 mg/mL	SWFI	[f]	n/a	10 d	n/a	n/a	n/a	n/a	n/a	(4)
SMARTeZ® (Progressive Medical)	UN	95 mg/mL	NS	n/a	n/a	24 hr	14 d	n/a	n/a	n/a	n/a	(5)

Flush Compatibility: Sodium chloride 0.9%.[1]

Special Considerations: Precipitate may form at higher concentrations and over longer time periods.[1]

DOI 10.37573/9781585286720.060

Notes

[a] Storage temperature: 30°C.[1]

[b] INTERMATE™/INFUSOR™ Portable Elastomeric Infusion System devices are no longer available in the United States.

[c] Followed by 72 hr at 25°C, followed by 7 d at 33°C.[4]

[d] Storage temperature: 33°C.[4]

[e] Followed by 72 hr at 25°C, followed by 72 hr at 33°C.[4]

[f] Reconstituted deferoxamine 95 mg/mL is isotonic.[1]

[g] Followed by 4 d at 25°C, followed by 72 hr at 33°C.[4]

REFERENCES

1. ASHP's Interactive Handbook on Injectable Drugs, 2020. Bethesda, MD: American Society of Health-System Pharmacists; Accessed November 2020.
2. *Stability Data for Drugs Using Homepump Disposable Ambulatory Infusion Systems (MK-00314 rev 3)*, 2015. Alpharetta, GA: Halyard Health; Updated June 2015.
3. Hayes D, Reilly RM, Lee M. The Pharmaceutical Stability of Deferoxamine Mesylate. *Can J Hosp Pharm*. 1994; 47(1):9-14.
4. Stabforum - Stability Database: Deferoxamine, Ontario, Canada: Baxter Healthcare; Accessed November 2020.
5. *SMARTeZ® - Stability Data for Drugs Using Elastomeric Infusion Pumps*, 2020. Fenton, MO: Progressive Medical, Inc.; Updated May 2020.
6. *Drug Stability for Easypump® ST/LT*, 2020. Bethlehem, PA: B. Braun USA; Updated June 2020.
7. *Drug Stability Table - Dosi-Fuser® Elastomeric Pump (S-CL-00-001v16)*, 2021. Barcelona, Spain: Leventon SAU; Updated May 2021.

DexAMETHasone Sodium Phosphate

Storage Conditions

	Drug Manufacturer	Concentration	Diluents	Osmolality (mOsm/kg)	pH	Temperature: Room	Temperature: Refrig	Temperature: Frozen	Post-thaw Temp: Room	Post-thaw Temp: Refrig	Body Temp	Refer.
CONTAINER												
Bag, Polyolefin	OR	0.1 mg/mL	D5W[k]	[n]	[g]	n/a	n/a	12 wk	n/a	30 d	n/a	(1)
Bag, Polyvinyl Chloride (PVC)	AMR	0.092, 0.66 mg/mL	NS	[n]	[g]	14 d[b]	n/a	n/a	n/a	n/a	n/a	(1)
	AMR	0.092, 0.66 mg/mL	D5W, NS[d]	[n]	[g]	14 d[b]	14 d[b]	n/a	n/a	n/a	n/a	(1)
	AMR	0.094, 0.658 mg/mL	D5W	[n]	[g]	14 d[b]	n/a	n/a	n/a	n/a	n/a	(1)
	ES	0.2, 0.4 mg/mL	NS[s]	[n]	[g]	n/a	30 d[c][f]	n/a	n/a	n/a	n/a	(1)
	AMR	0.2, 0.4 mg/mL	D5W, NS[r]	[n]	[g]	48 hr	14 d	n/a	n/a	n/a	n/a	(1)
	MSD	0.4 mg/mL	NS[q]	[n]	[g]	28 d	28 d	n/a	n/a	n/a	n/a	(3)
	MSD	0.43 mg/mL	NS, D5W[a]	[n]	[g]	28 d	28 d	n/a	n/a	n/a	n/a	(3)
	FRK	0.08 to 0.4 mg/mL	D5W, NS	n/a	[e]	14 d	14d	n/a	n/a	n/a	n/a	(7)
Syringe, Glass	OT	10 mg/mL	Undiluted	[n]	[g]	13 wk	13 wk	n/a	n/a	n/a	n/a	(1)
Syringe, Polypropylene	OT	10 mg/mL	Undiluted	[n]	[g]	55 d	n/a	n/a	n/a	n/a	n/a	(1)
	OR	0.07 mg/mL	NS[l]	[n]	[l]	8 d	8 d	n/a	n/a	n/a	8 d	(1)(4)
	APP	0.1, 1 mg/mL	NS	[n]	[m]	22 d	n/a	n/a	n/a	n/a	n/a	(1)(8)
	ME	0.33, 1.33, 1.67, 3.33 mg/mL	NS[o]	[n]	n/a	5 d[b]	n/a	n/a	n/a	n/a	n/a	(1)(5)
	ME	0.33-3.33 mg/mL	NS[p]	[n]	n/a	5 d	5 d	n/a	n/a	n/a	n/a	(1)(6)
Vials, Glass	LY	1 mg/mL	BNS	[n]	[g]	28 d	28 d	n/a	n/a	n/a	n/a	(1)
OTHER INFUSION CONTAINERS												
CADD® Cassette (Smiths Medical)	AMR	0.4 mg/mL	NS[h]	[n]	[g]	14 d[j]	14 d	n/a	n/a	n/a	n/a	(1)
	UN	0.02 mg/mL	unspec.[i]	[n]	[g]	7 d	n/a	n/a	n/a	n/a	n/a	(2)
Dosi-Fuser® (Leventon)	HOS	0.8 mg/mL	NS	n/a	n/a	24 hr	48 hr	n/a	n/a	n/a	n/a	(9)
	HOS	0.8 mg/mL	D5W	n/a	n/a	24 hr	n/a	n/a	n/a	n/a	n/a	(9)

DOI 10.37573/9781585286720.061

Flush Compatibility: Sodium chloride 0.9%, heparin.[1]

Special Considerations: n/a

Notes

[a] Solution contained: ondansetron hydrochloride (GL) 0.15 mg/mL.[3]

[b] Protected from light.[1,5]

[c] 30 d refrigerated followed by 48 hr at room temperature.[1]

[d] Solution contained: granisetron hydrochloride (SKB) 0.01 and 0.04 mg/mL.[1]

[e] The initial pH values were 6.4-6.8 and 7.0-7.8 for samples in NS and D5W, respectively. The pH of all samples remained within one pH unit from the initial values.[7]

[f] Stored for 30 days at 4°C followed by 2 days at 23°C.[1]

[g] pH of undiluted solutions is 7-8.5. Dilutions of 0.5, 1, and 2 mg/mL in NS are 7.3, 7.3, and 7.5.[1]

[h] Solution contained: 200 mg diphenhydrAMINE (ES), 4 mg LORazepam (WY), and 400 mg metoclopramide hydrochloride (DU) in 100 mL NS. Above stability pertains to dexAMETHasone, diphenhydrAMINE, and metoclopramide only.[1]

[i] Solution contained: morphine sulfate 15 mg/mL.[2]

[j] Storage temperatures: 23°C and 30°C.[1]

[k] Solution contained: ondansetron 0.08 mg/mL (GSK).[1]

[l] Solution contained: ketamine hydrochloride (PF) 3.6 mg/mL (pH 5.29-5.40) or 42.9 mg/mL (pH 4.26-4.37), exposed to normal fluorescent light.[1,4]

[m] The pH of 1 mg/mL decreased from 7.3 to 7.2 in 22 days, while the pH of 0.1 mg/mL decreased from 6.5 to 6.3.[1,8]

[n] Osmolality of a dexAMETHasone injection (UN) reported to be 255 mOsm/kg. Osmolality of 4 mg/mL (ES) is 356 mOsm/kg. Dilutions of 0.5, 1, and 2 mg/mL (DB) in NS were 269, 260, and 238 mOsm/kg.[1]

[o] Solution contained: traMADol (GRU) 8.3, 16.66, 33.33 mg/mL.[1,5]

[p] Solution contained: furosemide (HO) 3.33-10 mg/mL.[1,6]

[q] Solution contained: ondansetron 0.14 mg/mL (GL).[3]

[r] Solution contained: palonosetron hydrochloride (MGI) 0.005 mg/mL.[1]

[s] Solution contained: ondansetron hydrochloride (CER) 0.1, 0.2, 0.4, and 0.64 mg/mL.[1]

REFERENCES

1. ASHP's Interactive Handbook on Injectable Drugs, 2020. Bethesda, MD: American Society of Health-System Pharmacists; Accessed June 2020.
2. Swanson G, Smith J, Bulich R, et al. Patient-controlled analgesia for chronic cancer pain in the ambulatory setting: a report of 117 patients. *J Clin Oncol*. 1989; 7(12):1903-8.
3. Evrard B, Ceccato A, Gaspard O, et al. Stability of ondansetron hydrochloride and dexamethasone sodium phosphate in 0.9% sodium chloride injection and in 5% dextrose injection. *Am J Health Syst Pharm*. 1997; 54(9):1065-8.
4. Watson DG, Lin M, Morton A, et al. Compatibility and stability of dexamethasone sodium phosphate and ketamine hydrochloride subcutaneous infusions in polypropylene syringes. *J Pain Symptom Manage*. 2005; 30(1):80-6.
5. Negro S, Salama A, Sanchez Y, et al. Compatibility and stability of tramadol and dexamethasone in solution and its use in terminally ill patients. *J Clin Pharm Ther*. 2007; 32(5):441-4.
6. Negro S, Rendon AL, Azuara ML, et al. Compatibility and stability of furosemide and dexamethasone combined in infusion solutions. *Arzneimittelforschung*. 2006; 56(10):714-20.
7. Buga I, Uzoma JI, Reindel K, et al. Physical and Chemical Stability of Dexamethasone Sodium Phosphate in Intravenous Admixtures Used to Prevent Chemotherapy-Induced Nausea and Vomiting. *Hosp Pharm*. 2019; 83(5):964-5.
8. Gupta VD. Chemical stability of dexamethasone sodium phosphate after reconstitution in 0.9% sodium chloride injection and storage in polypropylene syringes. *Int J Pharm Compd*. 2002; 6(5):395-7.
9. *Drug Stability Table - Dosi-Fuser® Elastomeric Pump (S-CL-00-001v16)*, 2021. Barcelona, Spain: Leventon SAU; Updated May 2021.

DexMEDEtomidine

Storage Conditions

						Temperature			Post-thaw Temp			
	Drug Manufacturer	Concentration	Diluents	Osmolality (mOsm/kg)	pH	Room	Refrig	Frozen	Room	Refrig	Body Temp	Refer.
CONTAINER												
Bag, Polyolefin	HOS	4 mcg/mL	NS	n/a	n/a	14 d	14 d	n/a	n/a	n/a	n/a	(2)
Bag, Polyvinyl Chloride (PVC)	UN	4 mcg/mL	NS	n/a	4.7-5.8	48 hr	14 d	n/a	n/a	n/a	n/a	(1)
	HOS	4 mcg/mL	NS	n/a	n/a	14 d	14 d	n/a	n/a	n/a	n/a	(2)
	HOS	4, 8, 12, 20 mcg/mL	NS	n/a	5.8-6.4	48 hr	n/a	n/a	n/a	n/a	n/a	(4)
Syringe, Polypropylene	HOS	4 mcg/mL	NS	n/a	n/a	48 hr[a]	14 d	n/a	n/a	n/a	n/a	(5)

Flush Compatibility: D5W, Sodium chloride 0.9%.[(3)]

Special Considerations: n/a

Notes

[a] Exposed to light.[(5)]

REFERENCES

1. Marquis K, Hohlfelder B, Szumita PM. Stability of Dexmedetomidine in 0.9% Sodium Chloride in Two Types of Intravenous Infusion Bags. *Int J Pharm Compd*. 2017; 21(5): 436-39.
2. ASHP's Interactive Handbook on Injectable Drugs, 2020. Bethesda, MD: American Society of Health-System Pharmacists; Accessed September 2020.
3. Precedex™ (Dexmedetomidine Hydrochloride) Injection [package insert]. Lake Forest, IL: Hospira, Inc.; September 2020.
4. Preslaski CR, Mueller SW, Wempe MF, et al. Stability of dexmedetomidine in polyvinyl chloride bags containing 0.9% sodium chloride injection. *Am J Health Syst Pharm*. 2013; 70(15):1336-41.
5. Anderson CR, MacKay MW, Holley M, et al. Stability of dexmedetomidine 4 mug/mL in polypropylene syringes. *Am J Health Syst Pharm*. 2012; 69(7):595-7.

DOI 10.37573/9781585286720.062

DiazePAM

Storage Conditions

CONTAINER	Drug Manufacturer	Concentration	Diluents	Osmolality (mOsm/kg)	pH	Temperature: Room	Temperature: Refrig	Temperature: Frozen	Post-thaw Temp: Room	Post-thaw Temp: Refrig	Body Temp	Refer.
Bag, Polyethylene	RC, BRN, ON	0.01-0.2 mg/mL	D5W, NS	n/a	n/a	24 hr	24 hr	n/a	n/a	n/a	n/a	(1)
	UN	0.05 mg/mL	NS	n/a	n/a	7 d	n/a	n/a	n/a	n/a	n/a	(1)
Bag, Polyethylene, multilayer[f]	RC	0.04 mg/mL	D5W, NS	n/a	n/a	48 hr	n/a	n/a	n/a	n/a	n/a	(3)
Bag, Polypropylene, multilayer[e]	ON, SJN	0.04-1.2 mg/mL	NS	n/a	n/a	24 hr[a]	n/a	n/a	n/a	n/a	n/a	(1)(2)
Syringe, Glass	UN	5 mg/mL	n/a	n/a	n/a	90 d[a]	90 d[a]	n/a	n/a	n/a	n/a	(1)
Syringe, Plastic	UN	5 mg/mL	n/a	n/a	n/a	24 hr[a]	7 d[a]	30 d[a][d]	n/a	n/a	n/a	(1)
Vial, Glass	UN	unspec.	n/a	[b]	6.2-6.9	28 d[c]	n/a	n/a	n/a	n/a	n/a	(1)
	RC, ON	0.04-0.2 mg/mL	D5W, R, LR, NS	n/a	n/a	24 hr	n/a	n/a	n/a	n/a	n/a	(1)
	BRN	0.04 mg/mL	D5W, NS	n/a	n/a	24 hr	24 hr	n/a	n/a	n/a	n/a	(1)

Flush Compatibility: Sodium chloride 0.9%.

Special Considerations: The drug is most stable at pH 4 to 8 and is subject to acid-catalyzed hydrolysis below pH 3. Sorption of diazePAM occurs in PVC containers. A 24% loss of drug was observed at 30 minutes, and 80-90% of the drug was lost at 24 hours. Significant loss occurs with multiple types of infusion tubing.(1)

Notes

a Protected from light.

b The osmolality of diazePAM (RC) was determined to be 7775 mOsm/kg. Diazemuls® (KA) has an osmolality of 349 mOsm/kg.(1)

c Storage temperature: 26-38°C (simulated summer conditions in paramedic vehicles).(1)

d 5-13% loss.(1)

e Polypropylene multilayer bag, TechFlex®, consists of three layers, polypropylene, styrene-based rubber, and polypropylene. Manufactured by Choongwae Pharma (Seoul, Korea).(2)

f Macopharma Laboratories (Tourcoing, France) Multilayer M312 Bag is made of five layers; the inner layer in direct contact with the solution is made of a co-polymer of polyethylene and polypropylene; from inner to outer surface: polyethylene, polypropylene and polyester.(3)

DOI 10.37573/9781585286720.063

REFERENCES

1. ASHP's Interactive Handbook on Injectable Drugs, 2020. Bethesda, MD: American Society of Health-System Pharmacists; Accessed August 2020.
2. Noh DI, Park KN, Chun HJ, et al. Compatibility of Diazepam with Polypropylene Multilayer Infusion Container. *Macromol Res*. 2009; 17(7):516-21.
3. Kambia NK, Dine T, Dupin-Spriet T, et al. Compatibility of nitroglycerin, diazepam and chlorpromazine with a new multilayer material for infusion containers. *J Pharm Biomed Anal*. 2005; 37(2):259-64.

DilTIAZem Hydrochloride

Storage Conditions

						Temperature			Post-thaw Temp			
	Drug Manufacturer	Concentration	Diluents	Osmolality (mOsm/kg)	pH	Room	Refrig	Frozen	Room	Refrig	Body Temp	Refer.
CONTAINER												
Bag, Polyethylene	BRN, GO	0.05 mg/mL	D5W, NS	n/a	n/a	24 hr	24 hr	n/a	n/a	n/a	n/a	(1)
Bag, Polyolefin	BA	1 mg/mL	D5W	n/a	3.83-4.17	30 d[(a)]	30 d	30 d	n/a	n/a	n/a	(1)(2)
Bag, Polyvinyl Chloride (PVC)	GRI	1 mg/mL	D5W, NS	n/a	n/a	90 d	90 d	n/a	n/a	n/a	n/a	(1)
Unspecified	SYO	1 mg/mL	D5W	n/a	n/a	48 hr	n/a	n/a	n/a	n/a	n/a	(1)
Vial, Glass	BRN, GO	0.05 mg/mL	D5W, NS	n/a	n/a	24 hr	24 hr	n/a	n/a	n/a	n/a	(1)
OTHER INFUSION CONTAINERS												
ADD-Vantage® Flexible Container System (Pfizer)	HOS	1 mg/mL	D5W, NS	n/a	n/a	24 hr	24 hr	n/a	n/a	n/a	n/a	(1)

Flush Compatibility: D5W, Sodium chloride 0.9%.[(2)]

Special Considerations: n/a

Notes

[a] Exposed to fluorescent light.[(2)]

REFERENCES

1. ASHP's Interactive Handbook on Injectable Drugs, 2020. Bethesda, MD: American Society of Health-System Pharmacists; Accessed September 2020.
2. Kaushal G, Sayre BE, Prettyman T. Stability of extemporaneously compounded diltiazem hydrochloride infusions stored in polyolefin bags. *Am J Health Syst Pharm*. 2013; 70(10):894-9.

DOI 10.37573/9781585286720.064

DimenhyDRINATE

Storage Conditions

						Temperature			Post-thaw Temp			
	Drug Manufacturer	Concentration	Diluents	Osmolality (mOsm/kg)	pH	Room	Refrig	Frozen	Room	Refrig	Body Temp	Refer.
CONTAINER												
Bag, Polyvinyl Chloride (PVC)	SAB	0.5, 1, 2 mg/mL	D5W, NS	n/a	[a]	7 d[b]	13 wk[c]	n/a	n/a	n/a	n/a	(2)
Syringe, Polypropylene	SAB	2.5, 5, 10 mg/mL	NS	n/a	[a]	60 d[b]	60 d[c]	n/a	n/a	n/a	n/a	(2)
Unspecified	UN	unspec.	D5W, NS	n/a	[a]	10 d	n/a	n/a	n/a	n/a	n/a	(1)

Flush Compatibility: Sodium chloride 0.9%, heparin.[(1)]

Special Considerations: Do not freeze.[(2)]

Notes

[a] The pH of undiluted solution is 6.4-7.2.[(1)]

[b] Exposed to light.

[c] Protected from light.

REFERENCES

1. ASHP's Interactive Handbook on Injectable Drugs, 2020. Bethesda, MD: American Society of Health-System Pharmacists; Accessed August 2020.
2. Donnelly RF. Chemical Stability of Dimenhydrinate in Minibags and Polypropylene Syringes. *Can J Hosp Pharm*. 2002; 55(5):307-12.

DOI 10.37573/9781585286720.065

DiphenhydrAMINE Hydrochloride

Storage Conditions

						Temperature			Post-thaw Temp			
	Drug Manufacturer	Concentration	Diluents	Osmolality (mOsm/kg)	pH	Room	Refrig	Frozen	Room	Refrig	Body Temp	Refer.
CONTAINER												
Bag, Polyvinyl Chloride (PVC)	PD	0.25, 0.5, 1 mg/mL	D5W, NS	n/a	n/a	91 d[b]	91 d[b]	n/a	n/a	n/a	n/a	(2)
	FRK	0.2, 1 mg/mL	D5W, NS	n/a	[c]	n/a	14 d	n/a	n/a	n/a	n/a	(3)
Syringe, Polypropylene[d]	PD	1.25, 2.5, 5 mg/mL	NS	n/a	n/a	28 d[b]	28 d[b]	n/a	n/a	n/a	n/a	(2)
OTHER INFUSION CONTAINERS												
CADD® Cassette (Smiths Medical)	ES	2 mg/mL	NS[a]	n/a	n/a	14 d[c]	14 d	n/a	n/a	n/a	n/a	(1)

Flush Compatibility: Sodium chloride 0.9%, heparin.[1]

Special Considerations: Protect from light; avoid freezing.[1]

Notes

[a] Solution contained: 40 mg dexAMETHasone (AMR), 4 mg LORazepam (WY), and 400 mg metoclopramide (DU) in 100 mL NS. Stability pertains to dexAMETHasone, diphenhydrAMINE, and metoclopramide only.

[b] Protected from light.[2]

[c] Initial pH readings ranged from 4.44 to 4.60.[1]

[d] Sealed with friction caps.[2]

REFERENCES

1. ASHP's Interactive Handbook on Injectable Drugs, 2020. Bethesda, MD: American Society of Health-System Pharmacists; Accessed August 2020.
2. Donnelly RF. Chemical stability of diphenhydramine hydrochloride in minibags and polypropylene. *Can J Hosp Pharm*. 1999; 52:150-5.
3. Sabins D, Diep T, McCartan P, et al. Stability and Compatibility of Diphenhydramine Hydrochloride in Intravenous Admixtures: A New Look at an Old Drug. *Hosp Pharm*. 2019; 54(5):330-34.

DOI 10.37573/9781585286720.066

DOBUTamine Hydrochloride

Storage Conditions

						Temperature			Post-thaw Temp			
	Drug Manufacturer	Concentration	Diluents	Osmolality (mOsm/kg)	pH	Room	Refrig	Frozen	Room	Refrig	Body Temp	Refer.
CONTAINER												
Bag, Polyvinyl Chloride (PVC)	LI	0.25 mg/mL	NS, D5W	n/a	[c]	48 hr	7 d	n/a	n/a	n/a	n/a	(1)
	LI	1 mg/mL	D5W	n/a	[c]	48 hr	234 d[a]	n/a	n/a	n/a	n/a	(1)
	LI	1 mg/mL	NS	n/a	[c]	48 hr	n/a	n/a	n/a	n/a	n/a	(1)
	AB	4 mg/mL	D5W	n/a	[c]	30 d[a]	30 d[a]	n/a	n/a	n/a	n/a	(1)
	LI	5 mg/mL	D5W	361[g]	[c]	n/a	100 d[a]	n/a	n/a	n/a	n/a	(1)
Syringe, Polypropylene	LI	5 mg/mL	D5W	361[g]	[c]	48 hr	48 hr	n/a	n/a	n/a	n/a	(1)
Syringe, Unspecified	PHX	10 mg/mL	D5W	n/a	n/a	5 wk[a]	6 wk[a]	n/a	n/a	n/a	n/a	(3)
OTHER INFUSION CONTAINERS												
CADD® Cassette (Smiths Medical)	HOS	10 mg/mL	D5W, NS	n/a	n/a	n/a	7 d[e]	n/a	n/a	n/a	n/a	(4)
COMMERCIAL PREPARATIONS (RTU)												
ViaFlex™ Container (Baxter)	BA	1, 2, 4 mg/mL	D5W	259, 266, 280[f]	[c]	7 d[b][d]	n/a	n/a	n/a	n/a	n/a	(2)(5)

Flush Compatibility: Sodium chloride 0.9%, heparin.[1]

Special Considerations: n/a

Notes

[a] Protected from light.[1,3]

[b] Expiration date per manufacturer's label when stored in the protective overwrap under labeled storage conditions.

[c] pH of premixed solution and undiluted solutions is 2.5-5.5.[1]

[d] Do not use beyond this date after removal of manufacturer's protective overwrap.[5]

[e] Chemically stable at 4°C for 7 days, followed by 12 hours at 35°C, followed by 12 hours at 25°C.[4]

[f] Calculated (mOsmol/L).[2]

[g] Osmolality at 5 mg/mL, unspecified manufacturer and diluent.[1]

DOI 10.37573/9781585286720.067

REFERENCES

1. ASHP's Interactive Handbook on Injectable Drugs, 2020. Bethesda, MD: American Society of Health-System Pharmacists; Accessed June 2020.
2. Dobutamine Hydrochloride in Dextrose Injection [package insert]. Deerfield, IL: Baxter Healthcare Corporation; March 2019.
3. Patel N, Taki M, Tunstell P, et al. Stability of dobutamine 500 mg in 50 ml syringes prepared using a Central Intravenous Additive Service. *Eur J Hosp Pharm*. 2012; 19(1):52-56.
4. Al Madfai F, Valah B, Zaidi STR, et al. Stability of dobutamine in continuous ambulatory delivery devices. *J Clin Pharm Ther*. 2018; 43(4):530-35.
5. Dobutamine Premixed Injection Medication Information Letter (Ref#: USM15-24707) [personal communication]. Deerfield, IL: Baxter Healthcare Corp; 2015:2.

DOCEtaxel

Storage Conditions

						Temperature			Post-thaw Temp			
	Drug Manufacturer	Concentration	Diluents	Osmolality (mOsm/kg)	pH	Room	Refrig	Frozen	Room	Refrig	Body Temp	Refer.
CONTAINER												
Bag, Polyethylene	RPR	0.3, 0.9 mg/mL	NS	n/a	n/a	28 d[a]	n/a	n/a	n/a	n/a	n/a	(1)(3)
	UN	0.3 mg/mL	D5W, NS	n/a	n/a	28 d	n/a	n/a	n/a	n/a	n/a	(5)
	SAA[e]	1.8 mg/mL	NS	n/a	n/a	n/a	7 d	n/a	n/a	n/a	n/a	(6)
Bag, Polyolefin[b]	AVE	0.4, 0.8 mg/mL	NS	n/a	[d]	5 wk	n/a	n/a	n/a	n/a	n/a	(1)(2)
Bag, Polypropylene	RPR	0.3, 0.9 mg/mL	D5W	n/a	n/a	28 d[a]	n/a	n/a	n/a	n/a	n/a	(1)(3)
Vial, Glass	RPR	0.3, 0.9 mg/mL	D5W, NS	n/a	n/a	28 d[a]	n/a	n/a	n/a	n/a	n/a	(1)(3)
	AVE	10 mg/mL	[c]	n/a	n/a	21 d	21 d	n/a	n/a	n/a	n/a	(2)
	RPR	10 mg/mL	[c]	n/a	n/a	28 d[a]	28 d[a]	n/a	n/a	n/a	n/a	(1)(3)

Flush Compatibility: Sodium chloride 0.9%, heparin.[1]

Special Considerations: Manufacturer recommends use of glass or polyolefin (polyethylene or polypropylene) containers and polyethylene-lined administration sets to minimize patient exposure to plasticizer (DEHP) from PVC.[1] A one-vial (liquid) formulation (SAA), available as 20 mg/mL in a 50/50 (v/v) ratio polysorbate 80/dehydrated alcohol, is ready for addition to infusion solutions.[4]

Notes

[a] Protected from light.[1,3]

[b] PAB® (Partial Additive Bag) is a polypropylene-polyethylene copolymer container (BRN).

[c] Two-vial formulation, Ethanol-Polysorbate 80 provided by the manufacturer with the undiluted product.

[d] Initial pH values for 0.4 mg/mL solution were 5.13-5.16 and 4.80 for 0.8 mg/mL. Within 5 week test period, pH changed by less than 0.06 pH unit for all tested solutions.[2]

[e] Taxotere® (SAA) is a one-vial formulation.[4,6]

DOI 10.37573/9781585286720.068

REFERENCES

1. ASHP's Interactive Handbook on Injectable Drugs, 2020. Bethesda, MD: American Society of Health-System Pharmacists; Accessed June 2020.
2. Walker S, Charbonneau F, Law S. Stability of Docetaxel Solution after Dilution in Ethanol and Storage in Vials and after Dilution in Normal Saline and Storage in Bags. *Can J Hosp Pharm*. 2007; 60(4):231-7.
3. Thiesen J, Kramer I. Physico-chemical stability of docetaxel premix solution and docetaxel infusion solutions in PVC bags and polyolefine containers. *Pharm World Sci*. 1999; 21(3):137-41.
4. Taxotere® (Docetaxel) Injection [package insert]. Bridgewater, NJ: Sanofi-Aventis U.S., LLC; December 2019.
5. Lazzarini R, Salvadori S, Trapella C, et al. Physicochemical stability of cabazitaxel and docetaxel solutions. *Eur J Hosp Pharm*. 2015; 22(3):150-55.
6. Hart M, Acott S. Physical and chemical stability of Taxotere (docetaxel) one-vial (20 mg/ml) infusion solution following refrigerated storage. *Ecancermedicalscience*. 2010; 4:202.

DOPamine Hydrochloride

Storage Conditions

	Drug Manufacturer	Concentration	Diluents	Osmolality (mOsm/kg)	pH	Temperature Room	Temperature Refrig	Temperature Frozen	Post-thaw Temp Room	Post-thaw Temp Refrig	Body Temp	Refer.
CONTAINER												
Bag, Polyvinyl Chloride (PVC)	ES	0.4, 3.2 mg/mL	D5W, NS	[c]	[e]	48 hr	n/a	n/a	n/a	n/a	n/a	(1)
	UN	0.3 mg/mL	D10W	[c]	[e]	4 d[b]	n/a	n/a	n/a	n/a	n/a	(1)
	DB	3.2 mg/mL	D5W	[c]	[e]	n/a	14 d[a]	n/a	n/a	n/a	n/a	(1)
	SO	6.1 mg/mL	D5W	[c]	[e]	24 hr	n/a	n/a	n/a	n/a	n/a	(1)
Syringe, Plastic (Unspecified)	AB	4 mg/mL	D5W	[c]	[e]	24 hr	n/a	n/a	n/a	n/a	n/a	(1)
Syringe, Polypropylene	TLP	4 mg/mL	D5W	[c]	[e]	48 hr	48 hr	n/a	n/a	n/a	n/a	(1)
	NY	0.5 mg/mL	D5W	[c]	3.9-3.98	7 d[a]	12 wk[a]	6 m[a][d]	n/a	n/a	n/a	(3)
Vial, Glass	AS	0.8 mg/mL	D5W	[c]	4.0-4.1	48 hr	7 d	n/a	n/a	n/a	n/a	(5)
	AS	0.8 mg/mL	NS, D5NS, D5½NS, LR	[c]	4.0-6.05	48 hr	n/a	n/a	n/a	n/a	n/a	(5)
COMMERCIAL PREPARATIONS (RTU)												
ViaFlex™ Plus Container (Baxter)	BA	0.8, 1.6, 3.2 mg/mL	D5W	[c]	[e]	7 d[f]	n/a	n/a	n/a	n/a	n/a	(2)(4)

Flush Compatibility: Sodium chloride 0.9%, heparin.[1]

Special Considerations: DOPamine decomposes in alkaline solutions forming a pink to violet or yellow to brown color. Discolored solutions should not be used.[1]

Notes

[a] Protected from light.

[b] Exposed to fluorescent light.

[c] Osmolality of 40 mg/mL solution determined by freezing point depression was 619 mOsm/kg and 581 mOsm/kg determined by vapor pressure. A 10 mg/mL solution with unspecified diluent was 277 mOsm/kg.[4]

[d] Frozen stability data was consistent only in Codan™ syringes. The authors recommend to not use B. Braun syringes if preparation will be frozen.[3]

[e] pH of premixed solution range is 2.5-4.5 and undiluted solution is 2.5-5.[1]

[f] Do not use beyond this date after removal of manufacturer's protective overwrap.

DOI 10.37573/9781585286720.069

REFERENCES

1. ASHP's Interactive Handbook on Injectable Drugs, 2020. Bethesda, MD: American Society of Health-System Pharmacists; Accessed July 2020.
2. Dopamine Premixed Injection Medication Information Letter (Ref#: USM15-24707) [personal communication]. Deerfield, IL: Baxter Healthcare Corp; 2015:2.
3. Braenden JU, Stendal TL, Fagernaes CB. Stability of dopamine hydrochloride 0.5 mg/mL in polypropylene syringes. *J Clin Pharm Ther*. 2003; 28(6):471-4.
4. Dopamine Hydrochloride and Dextrose Injection [package insert]. Deerfield, IL: Baxter Healthcare Corporation; July 2017.
5. Gardella LA, Zaroslinski JF, Possley LH. Intropin (dopamine hydrochloride) intravenous admixture compatibility. Part 1: stability with common intravenous fluids. *Am J Hosp Pharm*. 1975; 32(6):575-8.

DOXOrubicin Hydrochloride (Conventional)

Storage Conditions

CONTAINER	Drug Manufacturer	Concentration	Diluents	Osmolality (mOsm/kg)	pH	Temperature: Room	Temperature: Refrig	Temperature: Frozen	Post-thaw Temp: Room	Post-thaw Temp: Refrig	Body Temp	Refer.
Bag, Ethylene Vinyl Acetate (EVA)	BEL	0.5 mg/mL	D5W	n/a	[j]	14 d[a]	28 d[a]	n/a	n/a	n/a	14 d[a](s)	(1)(2)
	BEL	0.5 mg/mL	NS	n/a	[j]	14 d[a]	14 d[a]	n/a	n/a	n/a	7 d[a](s)	(1)(2)
	BEL	1.25 mg/mL	NS, D5W	n/a	[j]	28 d[a]	28 d[a]	n/a	n/a	n/a	7 d[a](s)	(1)(2)
Bag, Polyolefin	PHU	0.12 mg/mL	NS[l]	n/a	[j]	n/a	124 hr	n/a	n/a	n/a	124 hr[r]	(8)
	PHU	0.24 mg/mL	NS[m]	n/a	[j]	n/a	124 hr	n/a	n/a	n/a	124 hr[r]	(8)
	PHU	0.4 mg/mL	NS[n]	n/a	[j]	n/a	124 hr	n/a	n/a	n/a	124 hr[q]	(8)
Bag, Polyvinyl Chloride (PVC)	UN	0.04 mg/mL	NS, D5W	n/a	[j]	n/a	7 d[a]	n/a	n/a	n/a	n/a	(2)
	FA	0.1 mg/mL	NS, D5W	n/a	[j]	43 d[a]	43 d[a]	43 d[a](b)	n/a	n/a	n/a	(2)(14)
	UN	1 mg/mL	NS	n/a	[j]	14 d	n/a	n/a	n/a	n/a	n/a	(10)
	FA	1.4 mg/mL	NS	n/a	[j]	n/a	n/a	30 d	n/a	n/a	n/a	(2)
Syringe, Polypropylene	AD	1, 2 mg/mL	NS	n/a	[j]	124 d[c]	124 d[c]	n/a	n/a	n/a	n/a	(2)
	FA	2 mg/mL	Undiluted	n/a	[j]	n/a	43 d	n/a	n/a	n/a	n/a	(14)
Vial, Glass	AD	0.01, 0.02 mg/mL	D5W, LR, NS	n/a	[j]	24 hr[c]	n/a	n/a	n/a	n/a	n/a	(2)
	UN	0.18 mg/mL	D5W	n/a	[j]	48 hr	n/a	n/a	n/a	n/a	n/a	(2)
	AD	2 mg/mL	NS	n/a	[j]	124 d[c]	124 d[c]	n/a	n/a	n/a	n/a	(2)
Unspecified	FA	1.4 mg/mL	D5½NS, NS[o]	n/a	[j]	14 d	n/a	n/a	n/a	n/a	14 d	(2)
	UN	0.1 mg/mL	D3.3⅓NS, D5W	n/a	[j]	28 d[a]	n/a	n/a	n/a	n/a	n/a	(2)
	UN	0.1 mg/mL	LR	n/a	[j]	40 hr[a]	n/a	n/a	n/a	n/a	n/a	(2)
	UN	0.1 mg/mL	NS	n/a	[j]	6 d[a]	n/a	n/a	n/a	n/a	n/a	(2)

DOI 10.37573/9781585286720.070

Storage Conditions

						Temperature			Post-thaw Temp			
	Drug Manufacturer	Concentration	Diluents	Osmolality (mOsm/kg)	pH	Room	Refrig	Frozen	Room	Refrig	Body Temp	Refer.
OTHER INFUSION CONTAINERS												
CADD® Cassette (Smiths Medical)	NYC	1.67 mg/mL	NS[d]	n/a	[j]	n/a	7 d[k]	n/a	n/a	n/a	4 d[s]	(2)(3)
	CET	2 mg/mL	NS	n/a	[j]	14 d	14 d	n/a	n/a	n/a	28 d[h][p]	(2)(4)
Dosi-Fuser® (Leventon)	PF	0.2-5 mg/mL	NS	n/a	[j]	14 d	60 d	n/a	n/a	n/a	n/a	(13)
	UN	0.2-5 mg/mL	NS	n/a	[j]	9 d[f]	34 d[f]	n/a	n/a	n/a	n/a	(13)
	UN	3 mg/mL	D5W	n/a	[j]	30 d[f]	30 d[f]	30 d[f]	n/a	n/a	n/a	(13)
Easypump® ST/LT (B. Braun)	UN	2 mg/mL	NS	n/a	[j]	14 d[f]	22 d[f]	n/a	n/a	n/a	n/a	(12)
Graseby™ 9000 Cassette (Graseby Medical)	PHU	2 mg/mL	SWFI[g]	n/a	[j]	n/a	14 d[a]	n/a	n/a	n/a	7 d[a]	(2)(7)
Homepump Eclipse® / Homepump® (Halyard)	UN	2 mg/mL	NS	n/a	[j]	n/a	48 hr[f]	n/a	n/a	n/a	n/a	(6)
INFUSOR™ (Baxter)[i]	AD	0.2-2 mg/mL	NS	n/a	[j]	5 d	6 wk	n/a	n/a	n/a	n/a	(5)
	AD	0.2-5 mg/mL	NS	n/a	[j]	9 d	34 d	n/a	n/a	n/a	n/a	(5)
	AD	1 mg/mL	NS	n/a	[j]	9 d	96 d	n/a	n/a	n/a	n/a	(5)
	NYC	1.67 mg/mL	NS[d]	n/a	[j]	n/a	7 d[k]	n/a	n/a	n/a	4 d[s]	(2)(3)
	ARR	0.12, 0.24, 0.4 mg/mL	NS[t][u][v]	n/a	[j]	10 hr	14 d[e]	n/a	n/a	n/a	7 d[s][a]	(9)
SMARTeZ® (Progressive Medical)	UN	2 mg/mL	NS	n/a	[j]	14 d[f]	22 d[f]	n/a	n/a	n/a	n/a	(11)

Flush Compatibility: Sodium chloride 0.9%.[2]

Special Considerations: n/a

Notes

[a] Protected from light.

[b] Frozen samples were subjected to 11 freeze/thaw cycles with no apparent loss in potency between cycles.[14]

[c] Exposed to fluorescent light.

[d] Solution contained: vinCRIStine sulfate (LI) 0.036 mg/mL.[2,3]

[e] Followed by 7 d at 35°C.[9]

[f] Manufacturer extrapolated data from other sources.

[g] Solution contained: vinCRIStine sulfate (FAU) 0.2 mg/mL.[2,7]

[h] Storage temperature: 30°C.[2,4]

[i] INTERMATE™/INFUSOR™ Portable Elastomeric Infusion System devices are no longer available in the United States.

[j] The pH of lyophilized product reconstituted in NS is 3.8-6.5. The pH of undiluted solution product is 3.0.[2]

[k] Followed by 4 d at 35°C.[2,3]

[l] Solution contained: etoposide phosphate (BMS) 0.6 mg/mL and vinCRIStine sulfate (LI) 5 mcg/mL.[2,8]

[m] Solution contained: etoposide phosphate (BMS) 1.2 mg/mL and vinCRIStine sulfate (LI) 10 mcg/mL.[2,8]

[n] Solution contained: etoposide phosphate (BMS) 2 mg/mL and vinCRIStine sulfate (LI) 16 mcg/mL.[2,8]

[o] Solution contained: vinCRIStine sulfate (LI) 33 mcg/mL; stored at 25°C, 30°C, and 37°C.[2]

[p] Following 14 d at 3°C or 23°C.[2,4]

[q] Storage temperature: 35-40°C.[2,8]

[r] Storage temperature: 40°C.[2,8]

[s] Storage temperature: 35°C.[2,3]

[t] Solution contained: DOXOrubicin hydrochloride (conventional) (AAR) 0.24 mg/mL, etoposide phosphate (BMS) 1.2 mg/mL and vinCRIStine sulfate (HOS) 10 mcg/mL.[9]

[u] Solution contained: DOXOrubicin hydrochloride (conventional) (AAR) 0.4 mg/mL, etoposide phosphate (BMS) 2 mg/mL and vinCRIStine sulfate (HOS) 16 mcg/mL.[9]

[v] Solution contained: DOXOrubicin hydrochloride (conventional) (AAR) 0.12 mg/mL, etoposide phosphate (BMS) 0.6 mg/mL and vinCRIStine sulfate (HOS) 5 mcg/mL.[9]

REFERENCES

1. Rochard EB, Barthes DM, Courtois PY. Stability of fluorouracil, cytarabine, or doxorubicin hydrochloride in ethylene vinylacetate portable infusion-pump reservoirs. *Am J Hosp Pharm*. 1992; 49(3):619-23.
2. ASHP's Interactive Handbook on Injectable Drugs, 2020. Bethesda, MD: American Society of Health-System Pharmacists; Accessed September 2020.
3. Nyhammar EK, Johansson SG, Seiving BE. Stability of doxorubicin hydrochloride and vincristine sulfate in two portable infusion-pump reservoirs. *Am J Health Syst Pharm*. 1996; 53(10):1171-3.
4. Stiles ML, Allen LV, Jr. Stability of doxorubicin hydrochloride in portable pump reservoirs. *Am J Hosp Pharm*. 1991; 48(9):1976-7.
5. Stabforum - Stability Database: Doxorubicin, Ontario, Canada: Baxter Healthcare; Accessed November 2020.
6. *Stability Data for Drugs Using Homepump Disposable Ambulatory Infusion Systems (MK-00314 rev 3)*, 2015. Alpharetta, GA: Halyard Health; Updated June 2015.
7. Priston MJ, Sewell GJ. Stability of three cytotoxic drug infusions in the Graseby 9000 ambulatory infusion pump. *J Oncol Pharm Pract*. 1998; 4(3):143-49.
8. Yuan P, Grimes GJ, Shankman SE, et al. Compatibility and stability of vincristine sulfate, doxorubicin hydrochloride, and etoposide phosphate in 0.9% sodium chloride injection. *Am J Health Syst Pharm*. 2001; 58(7):594-8.
9. Svirskis D, Behera S, Naidoo N, et al. Stability of vincristine sulfate, doxorubicin hydrochloride and etoposide phosphate admixtures in polyisoprene elastomeric pump supporting transition of the EPOCH regimen to outpatient care. *J Oncol Pharm Pract*. 2019; 25(4):831-40.
10. Vyas HM, Baptista RJ, Mitrano FP, et al. Drug stability guidelines for a continuous infusion chemotherapy program. *Hosp Pharm*. 1987; 22(7):685-7.
11. *SMARTeZ® - Stability Data for Drugs Using Elastomeric Infusion Pumps*, 2020. Fenton, MO: Progressive Medical, Inc.; Updated May 2020.
12. *Drug Stability for Easypump® ST/LT*, 2020. Bethlehem, PA: B. Braun USA; Updated June 2020.
13. *Drug Stability Table - Dosi-Fuser® Elastomeric Pump (S-CL-00-001v16)*, 2021. Barcelona, Spain: Leventon SAU; Updated May 2021.
14. Wood MJ, Irwin WJ, Scott DK. Stability of doxorubicin, daunorubicin and epirubicin in plastic syringes and minibags. *J Clin Pharm Ther*. 1990; 15(4):279-89.

Doxycycline Hyclate

Storage Conditions

	Drug Manufacturer	Concentration	Diluents	Osmolality (mOsm/kg)	pH	Temperature Room	Temperature Refrig	Temperature Frozen	Post-thaw Temp Room	Post-thaw Temp Refrig	Body Temp	Refer.
CONTAINER												
Bag, Polyvinyl Chloride (PVC)	PF	0.1-1 mg/mL	D5W, NS	[f]	[e]	48 hr[a]	72 hr[b]	n/a	n/a	n/a	n/a	(1)
	PF	0.8, 1 mg/mL	D5W, NS	[f]	[e]	4 d	7 d	n/a	n/a	n/a	n/a	(1)
	PF	1 mg/mL	D5W	292	[e]	n/a	n/a	8 wk	n/a	n/a	n/a	(1)
Vial, Glass	PF	10 mg/mL	SWFI	507	[e]	n/a	n/a	8 wk	n/a	n/a	n/a	(1)(2)
OTHER INFUSION CONTAINERS												
CADD® Cassette (Smiths Medical)	ES	2 mg/mL	NS	[f]	[e]	n/a	24 hr[d]	n/a	n/a	n/a	24 hr[d]	(1)
Dosi-Fuser® (Leventon)	PF	1 mg/mL	D5W	[f]	[e]	12 hr[c]	72 hr[c]	8 wk[c]	n/a	n/a	n/a	(4)
	PF	1 mg/mL	NS	[f]	[e]	12 hr[c]	72 hr[c]	n/a	n/a	n/a	n/a	(4)
	PF	1.5 mg/mL	D5W, NS	[f]	[e]	48 hr[c]	72 hr[c]	8 wk[c]	n/a	n/a	n/a	(4)
Easypump® ST/LT (B. Braun)	UN	1, 1.5 mg/mL	D5W, NS	[f]	[e]	12 hr[c]	72 hr	n/a[c]	n/a	n/a	n/a	(5)
Homepump Eclipse® / Homepump® (Halyard)	UN	0.1-1 mg/mL	D5W, NS	[f]	[e]	48 hr[c]	72 hr[c]	n/a	n/a	n/a	n/a	(3)
	UN	1 mg/mL	D5W	292	[e]	n/a	n/a	8 wk[c]	n/a	n/a	n/a	(1)(3)
SMARTeZ® (Progressive Medical)	UN	1-1.5 mg/mL	D5W, NS	[f]	[e]	12 hr[c]	72 hr[c]	n/a	n/a	n/a	n/a	(6)

Flush Compatibility: Sodium chloride 0.9%. Incompatible with heparin.[1]

Special Considerations: Administer by slow intravenous infusion over 1-4 hr. Avoid extravasation. Protect from direct sunlight.[1]

DOI 10.37573/9781585286720.071

Notes

[a] Protected from sunlight.[1]

[b] When protected from artificial light and sunlight, 0.1-1 mg/mL infusions can be stored under refrigeration for 72 hr prior to start of infusion. Infusion must then be completed within 12 hr.[2]

[c] Manufacturer extrapolated data from other sources.

[d] Simulated administration at 30°C. 5% loss in freshly prepared solution after 24 hr; > 5% loss in 6 hr after storage at 5°C for 24 hr.[1]

[e] pH of reconstituted solutions of 10 mg/mL is 1.8-3.3.[1]

[f] Osmolality of 1 mg/mL (ES) is 292 mOsm/kg in dextrose 5% and 310 mOsm/kg in sodium chloride 0.9%.[1]

REFERENCES

1. ASHP's Interactive Handbook on Injectable Drugs, 2020. Bethesda, MD: American Society of Health-System Pharmacists; Accessed September 2020.
2. Doxy 100™ (Doxycycline Hyclate) Injection, lyophilized [package insert]. Lake Zurich, IL: Fresenius Kabi USA, LLC; June 2020.
3. *Stability Data for Drugs Using Homepump Disposable Ambulatory Infusion Systems (MK-00314 rev 3)*, 2015. Alpharetta, GA: Halyard Health; Updated June 2015.
4. *Drug Stability Table - Dosi-Fuser® Elastomeric Pump (ES.H.00.73-10)*, 2015. Barcelona, Spain: Leventon SAU; Updated October 2015.
5. *Drug Stability for Easypump® ST/LT*, 2020. Bethlehem, PA: B. Braun USA; Updated June 2020.
6. *SMARTeZ® - Stability Data for Drugs Using Elastomeric Infusion Pumps*, 2020. Fenton, MO: Progressive Medical, Inc.; Updated May 2020.

Droperidol

Storage Conditions

CONTAINER	Drug Manufacturer	Concentration	Diluents	Osmolality (mOsm/kg)	pH	Temperature Room	Temperature Refrig	Temperature Frozen	Post-thaw Temp Room	Post-thaw Temp Refrig	Body Temp	Refer.
Bag, Polyolefin	PS	0.025 mg/mL	D5W[b]	[a]	5	n/a	32 d	n/a	n/a	n/a	n/a	(1)
	XU	0.033 mg/mL	NS[d]	[a]	4.7-4.8	14 d[c]	14 d[c]	n/a	n/a	n/a	n/a	(2)
Bag, Polyvinyl Chloride (PVC)	JN	0.02 mg/mL	D5W, NS	[a]	[e]	7 d	n/a	n/a	n/a	n/a	n/a	(3)
	JN	0.02 mg/mL	LR	[a]	[e]	24 hr	n/a	n/a	n/a	n/a	n/a	(3)
	JN	0.05 mg/mL	NS[f]	[a]	[e]	30 d	30 d	n/a	n/a	n/a	n/a	(3)
	JN	0.05 mg/mL	NS[g]	[a]	3.8-4.1	30 d	30 d	n/a	n/a	n/a	n/a	(4)
	XU	0.05 mg/mL	NS[h]	[a]	4.6-4.8	15 d[c]	15 d[c]	n/a	n/a	n/a	n/a	(3)(5)
Syringe, Polypropylene	JN	0.2 mg/mL	NS[i]	388	5.6	14 d[c]	14 d[c]	n/a	n/a	n/a	n/a	(6)
	JN	0.2 mg/mL	NS[j]	255	6.1	14 d[c]	14 d[c]	n/a	n/a	n/a	n/a	(6)
	UN	0.625 mg/mL	NS	[a]	2.9-3.3	180 d[c]	n/a	n/a	n/a	n/a	n/a	(7)
	AMR	1.25 mg/mL	NS	[a]	[e]	24 hr	[k]	n/a	n/a	n/a	n/a	(3)
	UN	2.5 mg/mL	Undiluted	[a]	[e]	28 d[c]	n/a	n/a	n/a	n/a	n/a	(3)
Vial, Glass	JN	0.02 mg/mL	D5W, NS, LR	[a]	[e]	7 d	n/a	n/a	n/a	n/a	n/a	(3)
	XU	0.05 mg/mL	NS[h]	[a]	[e]	15 d[c]	15 d[c]	n/a	n/a	n/a	n/a	(3)
	JN	0.05 mg/mL	NS[f]	[a]	[e]	30 d	n/a	n/a	n/a	n/a	n/a	(3)
	JN	0.05 mg/mL	NS[g]	[a]	3.8-4.1	30 d	n/a	n/a	n/a	n/a	n/a	(4)

Flush Compatibility: Sodium chloride 0.9%. Incompatible with heparin.[3]

Special Considerations: Protect from light.[8]

DOI 10.37573/9781585286720.072

Notes

[a] The osmolality of 2.5 mg/mL solution is 16 mOsm/kg.[3]

[b] Solution contained: traMADol hydrochloride (GRU) 1 mg/mL.[1]

[c] Protected from light.

[d] Solution contained: butorphanol tartrate (JIN) 0.067 mg/mL and ketamine hydrochloride (SHN) 1.33 mg/mL.[2]

[e] pH of undiluted solution is 3-3.8.[3]

[f] Solution contained: fentaNYL citrate (DB) 0.1 mg/mL and ketamine hydrochloride (JN) 1 mg/mL.[3]

[g] Solution contained: fentaNYL citrate (DVL) 0.01 mg/mL and ketamine hydrochloride (PD) 1 mg/mL.[4]

[h] Solution contained: butorphanol tartrate (HE) 0.08 mg/mL.[3,5]

[i] Solution contained: morphine tartrate (DB) 40 mg/mL, dexAMETHasone sodium phosphate (DB) 0.8 mg/mL, hycosine butylbromide (BI) 2 mg/mL, and midazolam (RC) 0.8 mg/mL. Midazolam concentration maintained within 10% for 12 d RT.[6]

[j] Solution contained: morphine tartrate (DB) 4 mg/mL, dexAMETHasone sodium phosphate (DB) 0.8 mg/mL, hycosine butylbromide (BI) 2 mg/mL, and midazolam (RC) 0.5 mg/mL. Midazolam concentration maintained within 10% for 5 d RT.[6]

[k] Droperidol precipitated during refrigeration.[3]

REFERENCES

1. Lebitasy M, Hecq JD, Vanbeckbergen D, et al. Long-term stability of tramadol hydrochloride and droperidol mixture in 5% dextrose infusion polyolefin bags at 5+/-3 degrees C. *Ann Pharm Fr*. 2009; 67(4):272-7.
2. Fang B, Wang L, Gu J, et al. Physicochemical stability of ternary admixtures of butorphanol, ketamine, and droperidol in polyolefin bags for patient-controlled analgesia use. *Drug Des Devel Ther*. 2016; 10:3873-78.
3. ASHP's Interactive Handbook on Injectable Drugs, 2020. Bethesda, MD: American Society of Health-System Pharmacists; Accessed August 2020.
4. Lee DK, Wang DP, Harsono R, et al. Compatibility of fentanyl citrate, ketamine hydrochloride, and droperidol in 0.9% sodium chloride injection stored in polyvinyl chloride bags. *Am J Health Syst Pharm*. 2005; 62(11):1190-2.
5. Chen FC, Fang BX, Li P, et al. Compatibility of butorphanol and droperidol in 0.9% sodium chloride injection. *Am J Health Syst Pharm*. 2013; 70(6):515-9.
6. Targett PL, Keefe PA, Merridew CG. Compatibility and Stability of Drug Adjuvants and Morphine Tartrate in 10 mL Polypropylene Syringes. *Aust J Hosp Pharm*. 1997; 27(3):207-12.
7. McClusky SV, Lovely JK. Stability of Droperidol 0.625 mg/mL Diluted with 0.9% Sodium Chloride Injection and Stored in Polypropylene Syringes. *Int J Pharm Compd*. 2011; 15(2):170-5.
8. Droperidol Injection [package insert]. Shirley, NY: American Regent, Inc.; October 2019.

Enoxaparin Sodium

Storage Conditions

						Temperature			Post-thaw Temp			
	Drug Manufacturer	Concentration	Diluents	Osmolality (mOsm/kg)	pH	Room	Refrig	Frozen	Room	Refrig	Body Temp	Refer.
CONTAINER												
Bag, Polyvinyl Chloride (PVC)	RPR	1.2 mg/mL	NS	n/a	n/a	48 hr[g]	n/a	n/a	n/a	n/a	n/a	(1)
Syringe, Plastic (Unspecified)	RPR	100 mg/mL	Undiluted	n/a	[d]	n/a	10 d	n/a	n/a	n/a	n/a	(1)
	SAN	100 mg/mL	Undiluted	n/a	[d]	5 d[e]	n/a	n/a	n/a	n/a	n/a	(1)
	AVE	20 mg/mL	SWFI	n/a	n/a	14 d	14 d	7 d[a]	n/a	n/a	n/a	(1)
	AVE	20 mg/mL	D4W	n/a	n/a	n/a	31 d	31 d	n/a	n/a	n/a	(1)
	AVE	100 mg/mL	Undiluted	n/a	[d]	n/a	31 d	7 d[a]	n/a	n/a	n/a	(1)
Syringe, Polypropylene	UN	100 mg/mL	Undiluted	n/a	[d]	10 d	10 d	n/a	n/a	n/a	n/a	(1)
	UN	20 mg/mL	SWFI	n/a	n/a	14 d	14 d	n/a	n/a	n/a	n/a	(1)
	SAA	20 mg/mL	NS	n/a	n/a	43 d[b]	43 d[c]	n/a	n/a	n/a	n/a	(2)
	AVE	8 mg/mL	SWFI	n/a	n/a	n/a	14 d[f]	n/a	n/a	n/a	n/a	(1)
Vial, Glass	AVE	20 mg/mL	SWFI	n/a	n/a	29 d	n/a	n/a	n/a	n/a	n/a	(1)
	AVE	20 mg/mL	D4W	n/a	n/a	n/a	31 d	31 d	n/a	n/a	n/a	(1)

Flush Compatibility: Sodium chloride 0.9%.[1]

Special Considerations: Multidose vial contains benzyl alcohol as preservative; should not be stored for more than 28 days after first use. Benzyl alcohol has not been found to influence stability compared to preservative-free solutions.[1]

Notes

[a] Stability listed is for frozen solutions at -12°C. More than 10% loss for solutions diluted (20 mg/mL) with SWFI or undiluted (100 mg/mL) when stored at -80°C.[1]

[b] Protected from and exposed to light.[2]

[c] Protected from light.[2]

[d] pH of undiluted product is 5.5 – 7.5.[1]

[e] 100 mg/mL undiluted solution containing benzyl alcohol 15 mg/mL.[1]

[f] Substantial amount of variability in anti-factor Xa activity due to an unknown mechanism.

[g] Exposed to fluorescent light.[1]

DOI10.37573/9781585286720.073

REFERENCES

1. ASHP's Interactive Handbook on Injectable Drugs, 2020. Bethesda, MD: American Society of Health-System Pharmacists; Accessed August 2020.
2. Summerhayes R, Chan M, Ignjatovic V, et al. Stability and sterility of diluted enoxaparin under three different storage conditions. *J Paediatr Child Health*. 2011; 47(5):299-301.

EPHEDrine

Storage Conditions

CONTAINER	Drug Manufacturer	Concentration	Diluents	Osmolality (mOsm/kg)	pH	Temperature: Room	Temperature: Refrig	Temperature: Frozen	Post-thaw Temp: Room	Post-thaw Temp: Refrig	Body Temp	Refer.
Syringe, Polypropylene	UN[b]	10 mg/mL	Undiluted	n/a	4.5-7	28 d[a]	n/a	n/a	n/a	n/a	n/a	(1)
	BV[c]	5 mg/mL	NS	n/a	4.5-7	60 d	60 d	n/a	n/a	n/a	n/a	(1)
	HAG[d]	10 mg/mL	[e]	n/a	6	12 m	n/a	n/a	n/a	n/a	12 m[f]	(2)

Flush Compatibility: Sodium chloride 0.9%, heparin.[1]

Special Considerations: n/a

Notes

[a] Protected from light.

[b] Salt form not specified.

[c] Sulfate salt form.

[d] Hydrochloride salt form.

[e] Sodium chloride 0.6%.

[f] Storage temperature: 40°C.

REFERENCES

1. ASHP's Interactive Handbook on Injectable Drugs, 2020. Bethesda, MD: American Society of Health-System Pharmacists; Accessed August 2020.
2. Griffiths W, Ing H, Kern C, et al. The stability of ready-to-use (RTU) ephedrine hydrochloride in polypropylene syringes for use in maternal hypotension. *Eur J Hosp Pharm Science.* 2005; 11(5):107-10.

DOI 10.37573/9781585286720.074

EPINEPHrine

Storage Conditions

	Drug Manufacturer	Concentration	Diluents	Osmolality (mOsm/kg)	pH	Temperature Room	Temperature Refrig	Temperature Frozen	Post-thaw Temp Room	Post-thaw Temp Refrig	Body Temp	Refer.
CONTAINER												
Bag, Polyolefin	HOS	0.025, 0.05, 0.1 mg/mL	D5W	n/a	3.5	30 d[(a)]	30 d[(a)]	n/a	n/a	n/a	n/a	(6)
Bag, Polyvinyl Chloride (PVC)	PD	0.001 mg/mL	D5LR, D5NS, D5W, LR, NS	n/a	[(h)]	n/a	24 hr	n/a	n/a	n/a	n/a	(1)
	ANT	0.016 mg/mL	D5W	n/a	[(h)]	n/a	20 d[(a)]	n/a	n/a	n/a	n/a	(1)
	IMS	0.016, 0.064 mg/mL	NS	n/a	4-4.4	60 d	60 d	n/a	n/a	n/a	n/a	(3)
	AMR	0.087 mg/mL	D5W	n/a	[(h)]	24 hr[(a)]	n/a	n/a	n/a	n/a	n/a	(1)
Syringe, Glass	UN	0.1 mg/mL	unspec.	n/a	n/a	n/a	12 wk[(a)(g)]	n/a	n/a	n/a	n/a	(9)
	UN	0.1 mg/mL	NS	n/a	3.3	48 hr[(k)]	n/a	48 hr[(k)]	n/a	n/a	48 hr[(k)]	(11)
Syringe, Plastic (Unspecified)	UN	0.1 mg/mL	SWFI	273	[(h)]	7 d[(a)]	n/a	n/a	n/a	n/a	n/a	(1)
	UN	0.7 mg/mL	SWFI	n/a	[(h)]	8 wk[(a)]	n/a	n/a	n/a	n/a	n/a	(1)
	SAA	0.02 mg/mL	D5W	[(d)]	4.5-5.8	72 hr[(e)]	1 yr	n/a	n/a	n/a	n/a	(5)
	UN, AB	1 mg/mL	unspec.	n/a	3.2	12 wk[(a)]	n/a	n/a	n/a	n/a	8 wk[(f)]	(7)(8)
Syringe, Polycarbonate	MCO	1 mg/mL	SWFI	n/a	n/a	6 m[(a)]	6 m[(a)]	n/a	n/a	n/a	n/a	(17)
Syringe, Polypropylene	AMR	0.02, 0.3, 0.9 mg/mL	D5W, D10W, NS	n/a	4-5	84 hr[(c)]	n/a	n/a	n/a	n/a	n/a	(4)
	ASZ	0.0091 mg/mL	unspec.[(l)]	n/a	7.5-7.8	n/a	7 d[(a)]	n/a	n/a	n/a	n/a	(13)
Unspecified, Glass	PD	0.001 mg/mL	D5LR, D5NS, D5W, LR, NS	n/a	[(h)]	n/a	24 hr	n/a	n/a	n/a	n/a	(1)
	AMR	0.087 mg/mL	D5W	n/a	[(h)]	24 hr[(a)]	n/a	n/a	n/a	n/a	n/a	(1)
	UN	0.1 mg/mL	SWFI	273	[(h)]	7 d[(a)]	n/a	n/a	n/a	n/a	n/a	(1)
	UN	0.7 mg/mL	SWFI	n/a	[(h)]	8 wk[(a)]	n/a	n/a	n/a	n/a	n/a	(1)
	UN	0.1 mg/mL	unspec.	n/a	n/a	n/a	n/a	n/a	n/a	n/a	7 d[(s)]	(12)
OTHER INFUSION CONTAINERS												
CADD® Cassette (Smiths Medical)	UN	0.002 mg/mL	NS[(b)]	n/a	[(h)]	184 d	184 d	n/a	n/a	n/a	n/a	(2)

DOI 10.37573/9781585286720.075

Storage Conditions

	Drug Manufacturer	Concentration	Diluents	Osmolality (mOsm/kg)	pH	Temperature			Post-thaw Temp		Body Temp	Refer.
						Room	Refrig	Frozen	Room	Refrig		
COMMERCIAL PREPARATIONS (RTU)												
Ampules, Glass	UN	1 mg/mL	unspec.	n/a	n/a	n/a	12 wk[a][g]	n/a	n/a	n/a	12 wk[a][i]	(9)
	UN	1 mg/mL	unspec.	n/a	n/a	1 yr[q]	n/a	n/a	n/a	n/a	1 yr[p]	(19) (20)
	STP	0.8 mg/mL	unspec.	n/a	n/a	1 yr	1 yr	n/a	n/a	n/a	1 yr[r]	(14)
Cartridge, Unspecified	UN	0.1 mg/mL	unspec.	n/a	n/a	n/a	n/a	n/a	n/a	n/a	72 hr[m]	(16)
	AST, NVC, IDX, SCN	0.001 mg/mL	unspec.[j]	n/a	n/a	n/a	n/a	n/a	n/a	n/a	30 d	(10) (11)
Syringe, Autoinjector	AB	0.1 mg/mL	unspec.	n/a	n/a	n/a	n/a	n/a	n/a	n/a	45 d[n]	(18)
	MYL	1 mg/mL	unspec.	n/a	2.2-5.0	n/a	10 d[a]	10 d[a][o]	n/a	n/a	n/a	(15)

Flush Compatibility: Sodium chloride 0.9%, heparin.[1]

Special Considerations: Sensitive to light and air. Protection from light is recommended. Withdrawal of doses from multiple-dose vials introduces air, which results in oxidation. As EPINEPHrine oxidizes, it changes from colorless to pink, as adrenochrome forms, to brown, as melanin forms. Discolored solutions or solutions containing a precipitate should not be used.

EPINEPHrine hydrochloride is rapidly destroyed by alkalies or oxidizing agents and is unstable in dextrose 5% at a pH above 5.5.[1]

Notes

[a] Protected from light

[b] Solution contained: bupivacaine 1 mg/mL and fentaNYL citrate 0.002 mg/mL.[2]

[c] Protected from light and exposed to light.[4]

[d] Osmolality ranged from 258 to 307 mOsmol/kg.[5]

[e] Storage temperature: 27°C protected from light and exposed to light. Stability was 14 days when stored at 21°C and protected from light.[5]

[f] Solution contained: sodium metabisulfite 0.9 mg/mL. Protected from light and exposed to light. Stability was 8 weeks at 15% humidity, and 12 weeks at 85% humidity.[7,8]

[g] Samples were cooled in a freezer from room temperature to 2.5°C over a 2 hour period, then allowed to return to room temperature over a 6 hour period. This cycle was repeated once every 24 hours over the 12 week period.[9]

[h] pH ranges from 2.2 to 5.0.

[i] Samples were warmed in an oven for 6 hours until they reached 70°C then allowed to cool to room temperature for 2 hours. This cycle was repeated once every 24 hours over the 12 week period.[9]

[j] Solution contained: lidocaine. The AST and IDX brands were stable for 8 weeks.[10,11]

[k] Storage temperature: −20°C for 4 hours twice every 24 hours with 2 hours in between; this was repeated for 48 hours. Another sample was tested alternating between −20°C and 70°C for 4 hours each every 24 hours for 48 hours. This alternating solution was stable after 48 hours.[11]

[l] Solution contained: sodium bicarbonate and lidocaine.[13]

[m] Storage temperature: 65°C for 8 hours every 24 hours, followed by room temperature storage.[16]

[n] Storage temperature: up to 28.9°C for up to 45 days, and temperature increased up to 51.7°C for a cumulative time of 795 minutes (13.25 hours) without undergoing degradation.[18]

[o] Storage temperature: -25°C constant temperature, and when cycled from -25°C to room temperature for 4 hours out of every 24 hour storage period.[15]

[p] Storage temperature: 40°C.[19,20]

[q] Storage temperature: ranged from -10.4°C to 50.8°C in emergency vehicles and clinics. The mean dose remaining when compared to control was 98.4%.[19,20]

[r] Storage temperature: varied in emergency vehicles from 8°C to 35.8°C; mean, 10.3°C.[14]

[s] Storage temperature: cycled from -6°C to 54°C for 12 hours each.[12]

REFERENCES

1. ASHP's Interactive Handbook on Injectable Drugs, 2020. Bethesda, MD: American Society of Health-System Pharmacists; Accessed September 2020.
2. *Pharmaceutical report on chemical and physical stability of drugs commonly used with CADD® infusion pumps (IN193109GB-122019)*, 2019. Minneapolis, MN: Smiths Medical ASD, Inc.; Updated December 2019.
3. Van Matre ET, Ho KC, Lyda C, et al. Extended Stability of Epinephrine Hydrochloride Injection in Polyvinyl Chloride Bags Stored in Amber Ultraviolet Light-Blocking Bags. *Hosp Pharm*. 2017; 52(8):570-73.
4. Ghanayem NS, Yee L, Nelson T, et al. Stability of dopamine and epinephrine solutions up to 84 hours. *Pediatr Crit Care Med*. 2001; 2(4):315-7.
5. Heeb RM, Stollhof B, Reichhold J, et al. Stability of Ready-to-Administer and Ready-to-Use Epinephrine and Norepinephrine Injection Solutions. *Pharm Technol Hosp Pharm*. 2017; 2(4):159-71.
6. Carr RR, Decarie D, Ensom MH. Stability of epinephrine at standard concentrations. *Can J Hosp Pharm*. 2014; 67(3):197-202.
7. Kerddonfak S, Manuyakorn W, Kamchaisatian W, et al. The stability and sterility of epinephrine prefilled syringe. *Asian Pac J Allergy Immunol*. 2010; 28(1):53-7.
8. Rawas-Qalaji M, Simons FE, Collins D, et al. Long-term stability of epinephrine dispensed in unsealed syringes for the first-aid treatment of anaphylaxis. *Ann Allergy Asthma Immunol*. 2009; 102(6):500-3.
9. Grant TA, Carroll RG, Church WH, et al. Environmental temperature variations cause degradations in epinephrine concentration and biological activity. *Am J Emerg Med*. 1994; 12(3):319-22.
10. Fry BW, Ciarlone AE. Storage at body temperature alters concentration of vasoconstrictors in local anesthetics. *J Dent Res*. 1980; 59(6):1069.
11. Johansen RB, Schafer NC, Brown PI. Effect of extreme temperatures on drugs for prehospital ACLS. *Am J Emerg Med*. 1993; 11(5):450-2.
12. Gammon DL, Su S, Jordan J, et al. Alteration in prehospital drug concentration after thermal exposure. *Am J Emerg Med*. 2008; 26(5):566-73.
13. Pascuet E, Donnelly RF, Garceau D, et al. Buffered lidocaine hydrochloride solution with and without epinephrine: stability in polypropylene syringes. *Can J Hosp Pharm*. 2009; 62(5):375-80.
14. De Winter S, Vanbrabant P, Vi NT, et al. Impact of temperature exposure on stability of drugs in a real-world out-of-hospital setting. *Ann Emerg Med*. 2013; 62(4):380-87 e1.
15. Rachid O, Simons FE, Rawas-Qalaji M, et al. Epinephrine autoinjectors: does freezing or refrigeration affect epinephrine dose delivery and enantiomeric purity? *J Allergy Clin Immunol Pract*. 2015; 3(2):294-6.
16. Church WH, Hu SS, Henry AJ. Thermal degradation of injectable epinephrine. *Am J Emerg Med*. 1994; 12(3):306-9.
17. Zenoni D, Priori G, Bellan C, et al. Stability of diluted epinephrine in prefilled syringes for use in neonatology. *Eur J Hosp Pharm*. 2012; 19(4):378-80.
18. Gill MA, Kislik AZ, Gore L, et al. Stability of advanced life support drugs in the field. *Am J Health Syst Pharm*. 2004; 61(6):597-602.
19. Zeisel U, Bauer M, Tas P, et al. Temperature stability of epinephrine under various storage conditions. *Anasthesiologie und Intensivmedizin*. 1998; 39:139-45.
20. Parish HG, Bowser CS, Morton JR, et al. A systematic review of epinephrine degradation with exposure to excessive heat or cold. *Ann Allergy Asthma Immunol*. 2016; 117(1):79-87.

EpiRUBicin Hydrochloride

Storage Conditions

						Temperature			Post-thaw Temp			
	Drug Manufacturer	Concentration	Diluents	Osmolality (mOsm/kg)	pH	Room	Refrig	Frozen	Room	Refrig	Body Temp	Refer.
CONTAINER												
Bag, Polyethylene	FA	0.05 mg/mL	D5W	n/a	[c]	n/a	30 d[a]	n/a	n/a	n/a	n/a	(1)
	FA	0.05 mg/mL	NS	n/a	[c]	n/a	25 d[a]	n/a	n/a	n/a	n/a	(1)
Bag, Polyvinyl Chloride (PVC)	FA	0.04 mg/mL	D5W, NS	n/a	[c]	n/a	7 d[a]	n/a	n/a	n/a	n/a	(1)
	FA	0.05 mg/mL	D5W	n/a	[c]	n/a	30 d[a]	n/a	n/a	n/a	n/a	(1)
	FA	0.05 mg/mL	NS	n/a	[c]	n/a	25 d[a]	n/a	n/a	n/a	n/a	(1)
	FA	0.1 mg/mL	D5W, NS	n/a	[c]	43 d[a]	43 d[a]	43 d[a]	n/a	n/a	n/a	(5)
	UN	1 mg/mL	NS	n/a	[c]	n/a	n/a	4 wk	n/a	n/a	n/a	(1)
Syringe, Plastic (Unspecified)	UN	0.5 mg/mL	NS	n/a	[c]	28 d	28 d	n/a	n/a	n/a	n/a	(1)
Syringe, Polypropylene	PH	1 mg/mL	NS	n/a	3.39-5.04	2 hr[b]	12 wk[b]	n/a	n/a	n/a	1 hr[b]	(1)(3)
	FA	2 mg/mL	NS	n/a	[c]	14 d	180 d[a]	n/a	n/a	n/a	n/a	(1)(2)
	FA	2 mg/mL	SWFI	n/a	[c]	n/a	43 d[a]	n/a	n/a	n/a	n/a	(5)
	PF	8.33 mg/mL	NS	n/a	4.49-4.61	4 hr[a][d]	72 hr[a]	n/a	n/a	n/a	n/a	(1)(4)
Vial, Glass	FA	0.05 mg/mL	D5W	n/a	[c]	n/a	30 d[a]	n/a	n/a	n/a	n/a	(1)
	FA	0.05 mg/mL	NS	n/a	[c]	n/a	25 d[a]	n/a	n/a	n/a	n/a	(1)

Flush Compatibility: Sodium chloride 0.9%.[1]

Special Considerations: Store intact vials at 2°C to 8°C. Do not freeze. Protect from light. Refrigerated storage of 2 mg/mL commercial solution can result in formation of gelled product, which will return to slightly viscous to mobile solution after 2-4 hr at controlled room temperature.

Notes

[a] Protected from light.

[b] Storage temperature: 8°C followed by 2 hr at 25°C, then 1 hr at 37°C.

[c] pH of undiluted preparation is 3.0.[1]

[d] Followed by 4 hr at 22°C.

DOI 10.37573/9781585286720.076

REFERENCES

1. ASHP's Interactive Handbook on Injectable Drugs, 2020. Bethesda, MD: American Society of Health-System Pharmacists; Accessed August 2020.
2. Pujol M, Munoz M, Prat J, et al. Stability study of epirubicin in NaCl 0.9% injection. *Ann Pharmacother*. 1997; 31(9):992-5.
3. Sewell GJ, Rigby-Jones AE, Priston MJ. Stability of intravesical epirubicin infusion: a sequential temperature study. *J Clin Pharm Ther*. 2003; 28(5):349-53.
4. Bennis Y, Savry A, Correard F, et al. Stability of a highly concentrated solution of epirubicin for conventional transcatheter arterial chemoembolization. *Int J Pharm*. 2015; 495(2):956-62.
5. Wood MJ, Irwin WJ, Scott DK. Stability of doxorubicin, daunorubicin and epirubicin in plastic syringes and minibags. *J Clin Pharm Ther*. 1990; 15(4):279-89.

Epoetin Alfa

Storage Conditions

CONTAINER	Drug Manufacturer	Concentration	Diluents	Osmolality (mOsm/kg)	pH	Temperature: Room	Temperature: Refrig	Temperature: Frozen	Post-thaw Temp: Room	Post-thaw Temp: Refrig	Body Temp	Refer.
Syringe, Plastic (Unspecified)	ORT	0.1 units/mL[a]	D10W	n/a	n/a	24 hr	n/a	n/a	n/a	n/a	n/a	(1)
	UN	2,000, 10,000 units/mL	Undiluted	iso	[b][c]	14 d	14 d	n/a	n/a	n/a	n/a	(1)
	AMG	20,000 units/mL	Undiluted	iso	[b][c]	n/a	6 wk	n/a	n/a	n/a	n/a	(3)
Syringe, Polypropylene	JC	40,000 units/mL	Undiluted	n/a	n/a	n/a	120 d[e]	n/a	n/a	n/a	n/a	(5)
Vial, Glass	ORT	4,000, 5,000 units/mL	NS[d]	n/a	n/a	12 wk	12 wk	n/a	n/a	n/a	n/a	(4)

Flush Compatibility: Sodium chloride 0.9%[1]

Special Considerations: Intact vials should be stored at refrigerated temperature with excursion data allowing single dose vials to be stored for 14 days at room temperature, and multidose vials for 7 days at room temperature. Do not freeze. Do not shake (inappropriate for pneumatic transport systems).[2]

Notes

[a] Solutions contained a final concentration of albumin 0.05% or 0.1%.[1]

[b] pH of undiluted epoetin alfa from single use vials is 6.6-7.2.[1]

[c] pH of undiluted epoetin alfa from multidose vials is 5.8-6.4.[1]

[d] NS preserved with 0.9% benzyl alcohol was added to single-use epoetin vials at a dilution of 1:1 (5,000 units/mL) and 1.5:1 (4,000 units/mL).[4]

[e] Eprex® commercially available product (JC), 1 mL, stored in polypropylene syringes (BD) at 4°C.[5]

REFERENCES

1. ASHP's Interactive Handbook on Injectable Drugs, 2020. Bethesda, MD: American Society of Health-System Pharmacists; Accessed September 2020.
2. Epogen® (Epoetin Alfa) Injection [package insert]. Thousand Oaks, CA: Amgen, Inc.; July 2018.
3. Naughton CA, Duppong LM, Forbes KD, et al. Stability of multidose, preserved formulation epoetin alfa in syringes for three and six weeks. *Am J Health Syst Pharm*. 2003; 60(5):464-8.
4. Corbo DC, Suddith RL, Sharma B, et al. Stability, potency, and preservative effectiveness of epoetin alfa after addition of a bacteriostatic diluent. *Am J Hosp Pharm*. 1992; 49(6):1455-8.
5. Marsili A, Puorro G, Pane C, et al. Stability of erythropoietin repackaging in polypropylene syringes for clinical use. *Saudi Pharm J*. 2017; 25(2):290-93.

DOI 10.37573/9781585286720.077

Epoprostenol Sodium

Storage Conditions

	Drug Manufacturer	Concentration	Diluents	Osmolality (mOsm/kg)	pH	Temperature			Post-thaw Temp		Body Temp	Refer.
						Room	Refrig	Frozen	Room	Refrig		
OTHER INFUSION CONTAINERS												
Bag/Vial, (Polyvinyl Chloride, Polypropylene, or Glass)	ACN[f]	3,000 to < 15,000 ng/mL	SWFI, NS	n/a	11-13	48 hr[h]	8 d[j]	n/a	n/a	n/a	n/a	(1)(4)
	ACN[f]	15,000 to < 60,000 ng/mL	SWFI, NS	n/a	11-13	48 hr[h]	8 d[j]	n/a	n/a	n/a	n/a	(1)(4)
	ACN[f]	≥ 60,000 ng/mL	SWFI, NS	n/a	11-13	72 hr[h]	8 d[j]	n/a	n/a	n/a	n/a	(1)(4)
	GSK[d]	up to 15,000 ng/mL	[e]	n/a	11.7-12.3	72 hr[g]	8 d[g]	n/a	n/a	n/a	n/a	(2)
	GSK[d]	3,000-15,000 ng/mL	[a]	n/a	10.2-10.8	8 hr[b]	40 hr[c]	n/a	n/a	n/a	n/a	(1)(2)
	TE[i]	3,000-15,000 ng/mL	[a]	n/a	11.0-11.8	8 hr[b]	40 hr[c]	n/a	n/a	n/a	n/a	(3)

Flush Compatibility: Sodium chloride 0.9%.[1]

Special Considerations: Protect product and reconstituted solutions from light. Do not freeze. Product labeling states preparation and administration concentrations in nanograms per mL (ng/mL). Administer with non-diethylhexyl phthalate (non-DEHP) infusion set with an inline 0.22 micron filter.[2,4,5] Stability is formulation dependent; do not extrapolate stability data across brands.[1]

Notes

[a] Sterile diluent provided by manufacturer contains 94 mg glycine, 73.3 mg sodium chloride, and sodium hydroxide (to adjust pH) in 50 mL of sterile water for injection.[1–3]

[b] Solutions prepared with sterile diluent for Flolan® or sterile diluent for epoprostenol sodium must be used with a cold pouch if not administered within 8 hr of reconstitution or removal from refrigeration. When used with a cold pouch and frozen gel packs, reconstituted solutions may be used for up to 24 hr. Change gel packs every 12 hr. May be stored refrigerated prior to use provided that total time of refrigerated storage plus administration using a cold pouch does not exceed 48 hr.

[c] Inclusive of administration time. Protect reconstituted product from temperatures < 0°C and > 20°C.

[d] Flolan® (GSK).[1,2]

[e] Prepared with pH-12 Sterile Diluent provided by the manufacturer.[2]

[f] Veletri® (ACN).[4]

[g] Solutions prepared with pH-12 Sterile Diluent may be stored for up to 8 d at 2-8°C prior to administration. Ambient temperature affects the stability for administration: 72 hr at up to 25°C, 48 hr at up to 30°C, 24 hr at up to 35°C, and 12 hr at up to 40°C.[2]

[h] Used after reconstitution and immediate dilution to final concentration and immediate administration.[1,4]

[i] Epoprostenol sodium for injection (TE).[3]

[j] If stored for up to 8 d at 2-8°C, administration time at 25°C is 24 hr for concentrations ≥ 3,000 up to 15,000 ng/mL and 48 hr for ≥ 15,000 ng/mL at 25°C. See package insert for concentration- and temperature-dependent stability data when administered above controlled room temperature.[4]

DOI 10.37573/9781585286720.078

REFERENCES

1. ASHP's Interactive Handbook on Injectable Drugs, 2020. Bethesda, MD: American Society of Health-System Pharmacists; Accessed August 2020.
2. Flolan® (Epoprostenol Sodium) Injection [package insert]. Research Triangle Park, NC: GlaxoSmithKline LLC; November 2019.
3. Epoprostenol Sodium Injection [package insert]. North Wales, PA: Teva Pharmaceuticals USA, Inc.; March 2019.
4. Veletri® (Epoprostenol) Injection [package insert]. South San Francisco, CA: Actelion Pharmaceuticals US, Inc.; January 2021.

Eravacycline Dihydrochloride

Storage Conditions

	Drug Manufacturer	Concentration	Diluents	Osmolality (mOsm/kg)	pH	Temperature			Post-thaw Temp			
						Room	Refrig	Frozen	Room	Refrig	Body Temp	Refer.
CONTAINER												
Bag, Polyolefin	TPI	0.2-0.6 mg/mL	NS	n/a	5.5-7	24 hr	10 d	n/a	n/a	n/a	n/a	(1)(3)
Bag, Polyvinyl Chloride (PVC)	TPI	0.2-0.6 mg/mL	NS	n/a	5.5-7	24 hr	10 d	n/a	n/a	n/a	n/a	(1)(3)
OTHER INFUSION CONTAINERS												
Easypump® ST/LT (B. Braun)	TPI	0.2, 0.6 mg/mL	NS	n/a	n/a	24 hr	8 d	n/a	n/a	n/a	n/a	(1)
Homepump Eclipse® / Homepump® (Halyard)	TPI	0.2, 0.6 mg/mL	NS	n/a	n/a	24 hr	8 d	n/a	n/a	n/a	n/a	(1)
SMARTeZ® (Progressive Medical)	TPI	0.2, 0.6 mg/mL	NS	n/a	n/a	24 hr[a]	8 d[a]	n/a	n/a	n/a	n/a	(2)

Flush Compatibility: Sodium chloride 0.9%.[3]

Special Considerations: Reconstituted eravacycline solutions and diluted eravacycline infusion solutions should not be frozen.[3]

Notes

[a] Manufacturer extrapolated data from other sources.[2]

REFERENCES

1. Xerava™ Medication Information Letter (Ref#: 3070 (XERAVA-025 V5 5 SEPT2019) [personal communication]. Watertown, MA: Tetraphase Pharmaceuticals; 2020:4.
2. *SMARTeZ® - Stability Data for Drugs Using Elastomeric Infusion Pumps*, 2020. Fenton, MO: Progressive Medical, Inc.; Updated May 2020.
3. Xerava™ (Eravacycline) Injection [package insert]. Watertown, MA: Tetraphase Pharmaceuticals, Inc.; June 2020.

DOI 10.37573/9781585286720.079

Ertapenem Sodium

Storage Conditions

	Drug Manufacturer	Concentration	Diluents	Osmolality (mOsm/kg)	pH	Temperature			Post-thaw Temp			
						Room	Refrig	Frozen	Room	Refrig	Body Temp	Refer.
CONTAINER												
Bag, Polyvinyl Chloride (PVC)	ME	10, 20 mg/mL	NS, ¼NS, R	n/a	[a]	6 hr	4 d	n/a	n/a	n/a	n/a	(7)
Syringe, Polypropylene	ME	20 mg/mL	NS	n/a	[a]	17 hr[c]	110 hr[c]	n/a	n/a	n/a	n/a	(4)
	ME	20 mg/mL	SWFI	n/a	[a]	19 hr[c]	110 hr[c]	n/a	n/a	n/a	n/a	(4)
	ME	100 mg/mL	NS	n/a	[a]	30 min[b]	24 hr[b]	28 d	1 hr	n/a	n/a	(3)
OTHER INFUSION CONTAINERS												
Easypump® ST/LT (B. Braun)	UN	5 mg/mL	NS	n/a	[a]	6 hr	7 d	n/a	n/a	n/a	n/a	(5)
	UN	10 mg/mL	NS	n/a	[a]	24 hr	7 d	n/a	n/a	n/a	n/a	(5)
	UN	20 mg/mL	NS	n/a	[a]	24 hr	5 d	n/a	n/a	n/a	n/a	(5)
Homepump Eclipse® / Homepump® (Halyard)	ME	10 mg/mL	NS	n/a	[a]	24 hr	7 d	n/a	n/a	n/a	n/a	(2)
	ME	20 mg/mL	NS	n/a	[a]	18 hr	5 d	n/a	n/a	n/a	n/a	(2)
SMARTeZ® (Progressive Medical)	UN	10 mg/mL	NS	n/a	[a]	24 hr[d]	7 d[d]	n/a	n/a	n/a	n/a	(6)
	UN	20 mg/mL	NS	n/a	[a]	24 hr[d]	5 d[d]	n/a	n/a	n/a	n/a	(6)

Flush Compatibility: Sodium chloride 0.9%, heparin.[3]

Special Considerations: Do not reconstitute or dilute with dextrose-containing solutions.[1,3]

Notes

[a] pH of reconstituted solution is 7.5.[3]

[b] Stable for 4 hr at room temperature after 24 hr under refrigeration.[3]

[c] Storage in 60 mL luer-lock tip plastic syringes (BD) with tubing (RMS) attached and capped.[4]

[d] Manufacturer extrapolated data from other sources.

DOI 10.37573/9781585286720.080

REFERENCES

1. INVANZ® (Ertapenem) Injection [package insert]. Whitehouse Station, NJ: Merck & Co., Inc.; February 2020.
2. *Stability Data for Drugs Using Homepump Disposable Ambulatory Infusion Systems (MK-00314 rev 3)*, 2015. Alpharetta, GA: Halyard Health; Updated June 2015.
3. ASHP's Interactive Handbook on Injectable Drugs, 2020. Bethesda, MD: American Society of Health-System Pharmacists; Accessed August 2020.
4. Fugit KD, Anderson BD. Antibiotic Stability in Freedom 60 Syringe Report by HealthTek™ and the University of Kentucky, Lexington. Chester, NY: RMS Medical Products; 2015.
5. *Drug Stability for Easypump® ST/LT*, 2020. Bethlehem, PA: B. Braun USA; Updated June 2020.
6. *SMARTeZ® - Stability Data for Drugs Using Elastomeric Infusion Pumps*, 2020. Fenton, MO: Progressive Medical, Inc.; Updated May 2020.
7. McQuade MS, Van Nostrand V, Schariter J, et al. Stability and compatibility of reconstituted ertapenem with commonly used i.v. infusion and coinfusion solutions. *Am J Health Syst Pharm*. 2004; 61(1):38-45. Erratum in: *Am J Health Syst Pharm*. 2004; 61(5):437.

Erythromycin Lactobionate

Storage Conditions

	Drug Manufacturer	Concentration	Diluents	Osmolality (mOsm/kg)	pH	Temperature			Post-thaw Temp			
						Room	Refrig	Frozen	Room	Refrig	Body Temp	Refer.
CONTAINER												
Bag, Polyvinyl Chloride (PVC)	AB	1 mg/mL	NS, D5W, D5NS	[a]	n/a	n/a	24 hr	n/a	n/a	n/a	n/a	(1)
	AB	4, 5 mg/mL	NS	[a]	n/a	n/a	20 d	n/a	n/a	n/a	n/a	(1)(5)
	AB	4, 5 mg/mL	NS[b]	[a]	7.5-8.0	n/a	60 d	n/a	n/a	n/a	n/a	(5)
	AB	4 mg/mL	NS	[a]	n/a	24 hr	n/a	n/a	n/a	n/a	n/a	(1)
	AB	4.55 mg/mL	NS	[a]	n/a	n/a	n/a	12 m	n/a	n/a	n/a	(1)
	AB	8.3 mg/mL	NS	[a]	6.75-6.9	n/a	60 d	n/a	n/a	n/a	n/a	(6)
Unspecified	UN	50 mg/mL	SWFI	[a]	[d]	24 hr	14 d	n/a	n/a	n/a	n/a	(1)
Vial, Glass	AB	1 mg/mL	NS, D5W, D5NS	[a]	n/a	n/a	24 hr	n/a	n/a	n/a	n/a	(1)
OTHER INFUSION CONTAINERS												
ADD-Vantage® Flexible Container System (Pfizer)	PF	5 mg/mL	NS	[a]	n/a	8 hr[e]	n/a	n/a	n/a	n/a	n/a	(2)
	PF	5 mg/mL	D5W	[a]	n/a	2 hr[e]	n/a	n/a	n/a	n/a	n/a	(2)
CADD® Cassette (Smiths Medical)	ES	20 mg/mL	NS, SWFI	[a]	[d]	24 hr	24 hr	n/a	n/a	n/a	n/a	(4)
INTERMATE™ (Baxter)[f]	AB	2.5-10 mg/mL	NS	[a]	n/a	24 hr	10 d	n/a	n/a	n/a	n/a	(3)
	AB	2.5-10 mg/mL	D5W	[a]	n/a	n/a	10 d[c]	n/a	n/a	n/a	n/a	(3)
	AB	10 mg/mL	D5W	[a]	n/a	24 hr[c]	10 d[c]	n/a	n/a	n/a	n/a	(3)

Flush Compatibility: Sodium chloride 0.9%. Incompatible with heparin; forms precipitate.[1]

Special Considerations: Do not use sodium chloride 0.9% or other solutions containing inorganic ions to reconstitute vials; precipitate will result. Maximum stability occurs at pH 6-8; degradation accelerates rapidly outside of these values.[1] The manufacturer recommends adding 1 mL sodium bicarbonate 4% for every 100 mL of diluent when using the following diluents: D5W, D5LR, D5NS. Per the manufacturer, preferred diluents are NS, LR and Normosol™-R.[7]

Notes

[a] Osmolality for erythromycin 50 mg/mL in SWFI is 223 mOsm/kg. At concentrations of 5, 10 and 20 mg/mL osmolality of erythromycin in D5W was 265, 273 and 287 mOsm/kg respectively, and 291, 299 and 313 mOsm/kg when diluted in NS.[1]

[b] Solution buffered with 0.2 mL sodium bicarbonate 8.4% per 100 mL NS.[5]

[c] Solution did not contain sodium bicarbonate.[3]

[d] pH of reconstituted product is 6.5-7.5 in SWFI.[1]

[e] After vial activation.[2]

[f] INTERMATE™/INFUSOR™ Portable Elastomeric Infusion System devices are no longer available in the United States.

DOI 10.37573/9781585286720.081

REFERENCES

1. ASHP's Interactive Handbook on Injectable Drugs, 2020. Bethesda, MD: American Society of Health-System Pharmacists; Accessed August 2020.
2. Erythrocin™ Lactobionate - IV (Erythromycin Lactobinate) Injection, Lyophilized ADD-Vantage™ Vials [package insert]. Lake Forest, IL: Hospira, Inc.; March 2020.
3. Stabforum - Stability Database: Erythromycin, Ontario, Canada: Baxter Healthcare; Accessed December 2020.
4. *Pharmaceutical report on chemical and physical stability of drugs commonly used with CADD® infusion pumps (IN193109GB-122019)*, 2019. Minneapolis, MN: Smiths Medical ASD, Inc.; Updated December 2019.
5. Allwood MC. The influence of buffering on the stability of erythromycin injection in small-volume infusions. *Int J Pharm*. 1992; 80(1):R7-R9.
6. Allwood MC. The stability of erythromycin injection in small-volume infusions. *Int J Pharm*. 1990; 62(1):R1-R3.
7. Erythrocin™ Lactobionate - IV (Erythromycin Lactobinate) Injection, Lyophilized [package insert]. Lake Forest, IL: Hospira, Inc.; December 2019.

Ethanol (Catheter/Line Lock)

Storage Conditions

						Temperature			Post-thaw Temp			
	Drug Manufacturer	Concentration	Diluents	Osmolality (mOsm/kg)	pH	Room	Refrig	Frozen	Room	Refrig	Body Temp	Refer.
CONTAINER												
Syringe, Polypropylene	AMR	70%	SWFI	n/a	n/a	14 d	n/a	n/a	n/a	n/a	n/a	(2)
	AMR	70%	BWFI[a]	n/a	n/a	14 d	n/a	n/a	n/a	n/a	n/a	(2)
	AAP	50%[b]	SWFI	n/a	n/a	28 d	n/a	n/a	n/a	n/a	n/a	(4)
	TYS	23.3%[c]	SWFI	n/a	n/a	10 d	10 d	n/a	n/a	n/a	n/a	(1)

Flush Compatibility: Sodium chloride 0.9%.[3,5] Incompatible with heparin.[2,5]

Special Considerations: Ethanol concentrations above 40% are required to inhibit bacterial growth in established biofilms.[3] Ethanol may cause deterioration of certain plastic materials, including polyurethane catheters; check with the device manufacturer to verify compatibility or potential for degradation due to extended exposure to ethanol catheter lock.[5]

Notes

[a] BWFI containing benzyl alcohol as a preservative.

[b] Diluted solution was filtered through two 0.22-micron filters.

[c] Solution contained: 1 mL of each: ethanol 70%, ispropanol 70%, heparin 10 units/mL. Ethanol activity remained above 90% for 10 days. Heparin activity fell by > 10% after 24 hours.[6]

REFERENCES

1. Cullis PS, Keene DJ, Zaman A, et al. Chemical stability of heparin, isopropanol, and ethanol line lock solutions. *J Pediatr Surg*. 2015; 50(2):315-9.
2. Cober MP, Johnson CE. Stability of 70% alcohol solutions in polypropylene syringes for use in ethanol-lock therapy. *Am J Health Syst Pharm*. 2007; 64(23):2480-2.
3. Cober MP, Kovacevich DS, Teitelbaum DH. Ethanol-lock therapy for the prevention of central venous access device infections in pediatric patients with intestinal failure. *J Parenter Enteral Nutr*. 2011; 35(1):67-73.
4. Pomplun M, Johnson JJ, Johnston S, et al. Stability of a heparin-free 50% ethanol lock solution for central venous catheters. *J Oncol Pharm Pract*. 2007; 13(1):33-7.
5. Bing CM, Ross KL. Antibiotic and ethanol lock therapy. *Home Infusion Continuum*. 2008; 2(1):10-1.

DOI 10.37573/9781585286720.082

Etoposide

Storage Conditions

						Temperature			Post-thaw Temp			
	Drug Manufacturer	Concentration	Diluents	Osmolality (mOsm/kg)	pH	Room	Refrig	Frozen	Room	Refrig	Body Temp	Refer.
CONTAINER												
Bag, Polyolefin	BMS	0.125, 0.175 mg/mL[g]	NS[e]	n/a	[i]	4 d	n/a	n/a	n/a	n/a	n/a	(4)
	BMS	0.2 mg/mL[g]	NS[d]	n/a	[i]	72 hr[b][c]	n/a	n/a	n/a	n/a	n/a	(4)
	MYL	0.38, 0.74 mg/mL	D5W	n/a	3.4-3.9	61 d	28 d[m]	n/a	n/a	n/a	n/a	(7)
	MYL	1.26 mg/mL	D5W	n/a	3.4-3.9	61 d	61 d	n/a	n/a	n/a	n/a	(7)
	MYL	1.75 mg/mL	D5W	n/a	3.4-3.9	28 d[m]	9 d[m]	n/a	n/a	n/a	n/a	(7)
	MYL	0.38 mg/mL	NS	n/a	3.3-4	61 d	61 d	n/a	n/a	n/a	n/a	(7)
	MYL	0.74 mg/mL	NS	n/a	3.3-4	28 d[m]	28 d[m]	n/a	n/a	n/a	n/a	(7)
	MYL	1.26 mg/mL	NS	n/a	3.3-4	61 d	21 d[m]	n/a	n/a	n/a	n/a	(7)
	MYL	1.75 mg/mL	NS	n/a	3.3-4	28 d[m]	n/a	n/a	n/a	n/a	n/a	(7)
Bag, Polyvinyl Chloride (PVC)[k]	SZ	0.157 mg/mL	D5W[a]	n/a	[i]	48 hr	48 hr	n/a	n/a	n/a	n/a	(6)
	BR	0.4 mg/mL	NS	n/a	[i]	4 d	n/a	n/a	n/a	n/a	n/a	(1)(6)
Syringe, Plastic (Unspecified)	UN	1 mg/mL	NS	n/a	[i]	28 d	28 d	n/a	n/a	n/a	n/a	(2)
	UN	0.4 mg/mL	NS	n/a	[i]	24 hr	24 hr	n/a	n/a	n/a	n/a	(6)
Unspecified	UN	0.2 mg/mL	NS	n/a	[i]	22 d	22 d	n/a	n/a	n/a	n/a	(6)
	UN	11 mg/mL	NS	n/a	[i]	7 d	22 d	n/a	n/a	n/a	n/a	(6)
	UN	12 mg/mL	NS	n/a	[i]	7 d	14 d	n/a	n/a	n/a	n/a	(6)
Vial, Glass	BR	0.05-0.4 mg/mL	NS	n/a	[i]	4 d	n/a	n/a	n/a	n/a	n/a	(1)(6)
	NOP	0.2 mg/mL	NS	n/a	[i]	22 d	14 d	n/a	n/a	n/a	n/a	(5)
	NOP	0.3 mg/mL	NS	n/a	[i]	48 hr	7 d	n/a	n/a	n/a	n/a	(5)
	BR	0.4 mg/mL	D5W, LR, NS	n/a	[i]	4 d	n/a	n/a	n/a	n/a	n/a	(1)(6)
	BR	0.5 mg/mL	NS	n/a	[i]	48 hr	n/a	n/a	n/a	n/a	n/a	(6)
	NOP	10 mg/mL	NS	n/a	[i]	5 d	7 d	n/a	n/a	n/a	n/a	(5)
	NOP	10.5 mg/mL	NS	n/a	[i]	14 d	22 d	n/a	n/a	n/a	n/a	(5)
	NOP	11 mg/mL	NS	n/a	[i]	7 d	22 d	n/a	n/a	n/a	n/a	(5)
	NOP	12 mg/mL	NS	n/a	[i]	7 d	14 d	n/a	n/a	n/a	n/a	(5)

DOI 10.37573/9781585286720.083

Storage Conditions

	Drug Manufacturer	Concentration	Diluents	Osmolality (mOsm/kg)	pH	Temperature Room	Temperature Refrig	Temperature Frozen	Post-thaw Temp Room	Post-thaw Temp Refrig	Body Temp	Refer.
OTHER INFUSION CONTAINERS												
Dosi-Fuser® (Leventon)	TE	0.24 mg/mL	NS	n/a	[i]	9 d[f]	n/a	n/a	n/a	n/a	n/a	(8)
Easypump® ST/LT (B. Braun)	UN	0.2 mg/mL	NS	n/a	[i]	4 d	n/a	n/a	n/a	n/a	n/a	(11)
	UN	0.4 mg/mL	NS	n/a	[i]	24 hr	n/a	n/a	n/a	n/a	n/a	(11)
Homepump Eclipse® / Homepump® (Halyard)	UN	0.1-0.4 mg/mL	NS	n/a	[i]	9 d[f]	n/a	n/a	n/a	n/a	n/a	(3)
INTERMATE™ (Baxter)[l]	TE	0.1 mg/mL	D5W	n/a	n/a	12 hr	n/a	n/a	n/a	n/a	12 hr[j]	(10)
	TE	0.1 mg/mL	NS	n/a	n/a	24 hr	n/a	n/a	n/a	n/a	24 hr[j]	(10)
	TE	0.4 mg/mL	NS, D5W	n/a	n/a	24 hr	n/a	n/a	n/a	n/a	24 hr[j]	(10)
	TE	0.6 mg/mL	NS, D5W	n/a	n/a	8 hr	n/a	n/a	n/a	n/a	6 hr[j]	(10)
SMARTeZ® (Progressive Medical)	UN	0.2 mg/mL	NS	n/a	[i]	4 d[f]	n/a	n/a	n/a	n/a	n/a	(9)
	UN	0.4 mg/mL	NS	n/a	[i]	24 hr	n/a	n/a	n/a	n/a	n/a	(9)

Flush Compatibility: Sodium chloride 0.9%.[6]

Special Considerations: Etoposide crystallization is unpredictable and occurs more frequently at concentrations above 0.4 mg/mL. Risk of precipitation of etoposide increases with the use of peristaltic pumps, especially at concentrations of 0.4 mg/mL or above.[6]

Notes

[a] Solution contained: cytarabine (UP) 0.157 mg/mL and DAUNOrubicin HCl (BEL) 15.7 mcg/mL.[6]

[b] Protected from light.[4]

[c] Storage temperature: 31-33°C.[4]

[d] Solution contained: vinCRIStine 1.6 mcg/mL and DOXOrubicin 40 mcg/mL.[4]

[e] 0.125 mg/mL etoposide solution contained vinCRIStine 1 mcg/mL and DOXOrubicin 25 mcg/mL. 0.175 mg/mL etoposide solution contained vinCRIStine 1.4 mcg/mL and DOXOrubicin 35 mcg/mL.[4]

[f] Manufacturer extrapolated data from other sources.[3,8,9]

[g] Container: Excel® polyolefin-lined bag (McGaw).[4]

[i] pH of undiluted solution is 3-4.[6]

[j] Storage temperature: 33°C.[10]

[k] The polysorbate-80 surfactant in the etoposide formulation leaches DEHP plasticizer from PVC containers and tubing. Use non-PVC containers and tubing to reduce patient exposure to DEHP.[6]

[l] INTERMATE™/INFUSOR™ Portable Elastomeric Infusion System devices are no longer available in the United States.

[m] Precipitation observed at sample testing intervals (e.g., 9, 16, 21, 28 & 61 days) beyond the length of time noted.[7]

REFERENCES

1. Beijnen JH, Beijnen-Bandhoe AU, Dubbelman AC, et al. Chemical and physical stability of etoposide and teniposide in commonly used infusion fluids. *J Parenter Sci Technol*. 1991; 45(2):108-12.
2. Adams P, Haines-Nutt R, Bradford E, et al. Pharmaceutical aspects of home infusion therapy for cancer patients. *Pharm J*. 1987; 238:476-78.
3. *Stability Data for Drugs Using Homepump Disposable Ambulatory Infusion Systems (MK-00314 rev 3)*, 2015. Alpharetta, GA: Halyard Health; Updated June 2015.
4. Wolfe JL, Thoma LA, Du C, et al. Compatibility and stability of vincristine sulfate, doxorubicin hydrochloride, and etoposide in 0.9% sodium chloride injection. *Am J Health Syst Pharm*. 1999; 56(10):985-9.
5. Lepage R, Walker S, Godin J. Stability and Compatibility of Etoposide in Normal Saline. *Can J Hosp Pharm*. 2000; 53(5):338-45.
6. ASHP's Interactive Handbook on Injectable Drugs, 2020. Bethesda, MD: American Society of Health-System Pharmacists; Accessed September 2020.
7. D'Huart E, Vigneron J, Lider P, et al. Physicochemical stability of etoposide diluted at range concentrations between 0.38 and 1.75 mg/mL in polyolefin bags. *Eur J Hosp Pharm*. 2020; 27(1):43-48.
8. *Drug Stability Table - Dosi-Fuser® Elastomeric Pump (S-CL-00-001v16)*, 2021. Barcelona, Spain: Leventon SAU; Updated May 2021.
9. *SMARTeZ® - Stability Data for Drugs Using Elastomeric Infusion Pumps*, 2020. Fenton, MO: Progressive Medical, Inc.; Updated May 2020.
10. Klasen A, Kessari R, Mercier L, et al. Stability of etoposide solutions in disposable infusion devices for day hospital cancer practices. *Drugs R D*. 2014; 14(1):13-23.
11. *Drug Stability for Easypump® ST/LT*, 2020. Bethlehem, PA: B. Braun USA; Updated June 2020.

Etoposide Phosphate

Storage Conditions

	Drug Manufacturer	Concentration	Diluents	Osmolality (mOsm/kg)	pH	Temperature			Post-thaw Temp			
						Room	Refrig	Frozen	Room	Refrig	Body Temp	Refer.
CONTAINER												
Bag, Polyolefin	BMS	0.6 mg/mL	NS[e]	n/a	4.25-4.5	n/a	5 d[c]	n/a	n/a	n/a	5 d[h][c]	(1)(2)
	BMS	1.2 mg/mL	NS[f]	n/a	4.25-4.5	n/a	5 d[c]	n/a	n/a	n/a	5 d[h][c]	(1)(2)
	BMS	2 mg/mL	NS[g]	n/a	4.25-4.5	n/a	5 d[d]	n/a	n/a	n/a	5 d[h][d]	(1)(2)
Bag, Polyvinyl Chloride (PVC)	BR	0.1, 10 mg/mL	D5W, NS	n/a	n/a	31 d	31 d	n/a	n/a	n/a	7 d[a]	(1)
Syringe, Polypropylene	BR	10, 20 mg/mL	BWFI[b]	n/a	n/a	31 d	31 d	n/a	n/a	n/a	7 d[a]	(1)
Vial, Glass	BMS	10, 20 mg/mL[k]	SWFI, D5W, NS	n/a	n/a	24 hr	7 d	n/a	n/a	n/a	n/a	(3)
	BMS	10, 20 mg/mL[k]	BWFI, NS[b]	n/a	n/a	48 hr	7 d	n/a	n/a	n/a	n/a	(3)
OTHER INFUSION CONTAINERS												
INFUSOR™ (Baxter)[j]	BMS	0.6 mg/mL	NS[e]	n/a	4.25-4.28	n/a	14 d	n/a	n/a	n/a	7 d[i]	(4)
	BMS	1.2 mg/mL	NS[f]	n/a	4.16-4.20	n/a	14 d	n/a	n/a	n/a	7 d[i]	(4)
	BMS	2 mg/mL	NS[g]	n/a	4.12-4.21	n/a	14 d	n/a	n/a	n/a	7 d[i]	(4)

Flush Compatibility: Sodium chloride 0.9%, heparin.[1]

Special Considerations: The phosphate ester, etoposide phosphate, is water soluble and is suitable for administration via multiple-day ambulatory infusion devices.[1]

Notes

[a] Storage temperature: 32°C.
[b] Bacteriostatic, preserved with benzyl alcohol.
[c] Protected from light.[2]
[d] Exposed to fluorescent light.[2]
[e] Also contains vinCRIStine sulfate 5 mcg/mL and DOXOrubicin HCl 120 mcg/mL.
[f] Also contains vinCRIStine sulfate 10 mcg/mL and DOXOrubicin HCl 240 mcg/mL.
[g] Also contains vinCRIStine sulfate 16 mcg/mL and DOXOrubicin HCl 400 mcg/mL.
[h] Storage temperature: 35-40°C.
[i] Tested at 35°C after 14 d at 4°C.
[j] INTERMATE™/INFUSOR™ Portable Elastomeric Infusion System devices are no longer available in the United States.
[k] Etoposide phosphate concentration expressed as etoposide equivalent.[3]

DOI 10.37573/9781585286720.084

REFERENCES

1. ASHP's Interactive Handbook on Injectable Drugs, 2020. Bethesda, MD: American Society of Health-System Pharmacists; Accessed August 2020.
2. Yuan P, Grimes GJ, Shankman SE, et al. Compatibility and stability of vincristine sulfate, doxorubicin hydrochloride, and etoposide phosphate in 0.9% sodium chloride injection. *Am J Health Syst Pharm*. 2001; 58(7):594-8.
3. Etopophos® (Etoposide Phosphate) Injection [package insert]. Princeton, NJ: E.R. Squibb & Sons, LLC; May 2019.
4. Svirskis D, Behera S, Naidoo N, et al. Stability of vincristine sulfate, doxorubicin hydrochloride and etoposide phosphate admixtures in polyisoprene elastomeric pump supporting transition of the EPOCH regimen to outpatient care. *J Oncol Pharm Pract*. 2019; 25(4):831-40.

Famotidine

Storage Conditions

	Drug Manufacturer	Concentration	Diluents	Osmolality (mOsm/kg)	pH	Temperature			Post-thaw Temp			
						Room	Refrig	Frozen	Room	Refrig	Body Temp	Refer.
CONTAINER												
Bag, Polyvinyl Chloride (PVC)	MSD	0.2 mg/mL	D5W, NS	[c]	[b]	n/a	n/a	28 d	n/a	14 d	n/a	(1)
	UN	0.2 mg/mL	D5W, NS	[c]	[b]	15 d	63 d	n/a	n/a	n/a	n/a	(1)
Syringe, Plastic (Unspecified)	MSD	2 mg/mL	D5W, NS, SWFI	[c]	[b]	n/a	14 d	n/a	n/a	n/a	n/a	(1)
Syringe, Polypropylene	ME	0.2 mg/mL	D5W, NS	[c]	[b]	15 d	n/a	n/a	n/a	n/a	n/a	(1)
	MSD	2 mg/mL	D5W, NS, SWFI	[c]	[b]	n/a	n/a	8 w	n/a	n/a	n/a	(1)
Unspecified	APP	0.2 mg/mL	D5W, NS, SWFI, D10W, LR	[c]	[b]	7 d	n/a	n/a	n/a	n/a	n/a	(3)
COMMERCIAL PREPARATIONS (RTU)												
GALAXY™ Plastic Container (Baxter)	BA	0.4 mg/mL	NS	iso	5.7-6.4	15 m[a]	n/a	n/a	n/a	n/a	n/a	(2)

Flush Compatibility: Sodium chloride 0.9%, heparin.[1]

Special Considerations: Store vials under refrigeration and protect from freezing; room temperature excursion statements support vial storage for 3 months to 26 weeks at controlled room temperature.[1]

Notes

[a] Expiration date per manufacturer's label when stored under the recommended conditions at controlled room temperature. Brief exposure to temperatures up to 35°C does not adversely affect the commercial premix product. Do not extrapolate commercial premix stability data to extemporaneously compounded solutions.[2]

[b] pH of undiluted solution is 5-5.6.[1]

[c] Osmolarity of the single and multiple dose products are 217 and 290 mOsm/L.[1]

REFERENCES

1. ASHP's Interactive Handbook on Injectable Drugs, 2020. Bethesda, MD: American Society of Health-System Pharmacists; Accessed June 2020.
2. Famotidine Injection in Galaxy Plastic Container (PL 2501) [package insert]. Deerfield, IL: Baxter Healthcare Corporation; May 2018.
3. Famotidine Injection [package insert]. Lake Zurich, IL: Fresenius Kabi USA, LLC; September 2019.

DOI 10.37573/9781585286720.085

FentaNYL Citrate

Storage Conditions

						Temperature			Post-thaw Temp			
	Drug Manufacturer	Concentration	Diluents	Osmolality (mOsm/kg)	pH	Room	Refrig	Frozen	Room	Refrig	Body Temp	Refer.
CONTAINER												
Bag, Ethylene Vinyl Acetate (EVA)	CUR	3 mcg/mL	NS[c]	n/a	[k]	51 d	51 d	n/a	n/a	n/a	n/a	(1)
Bag, Polyolefin	SZ	0.15, 25, 43 mcg/mL	NS[b]	n/a	4.0-5.6	n/a	28 d[h]	n/a	n/a	n/a	n/a	(8)
	SZ	10 mcg/mL	NS	n/a	[k]	93 d	93 d[h]	n/a	n/a	n/a	n/a	(3)
	SZ	50 mcg/mL	Undiluted	n/a	[k]	93 d	93 d[h]	n/a	n/a	n/a	n/a	(3)
Bag, Polypropylene	JN	1, 10 mcg/mL	NS[l]	n/a	[k]	30 d[f][h]	n/a	n/a	n/a	n/a	n/a	(1)(5)
Bag, Polyvinyl Chloride (PVC)	JN	2 mcg/mL	NS[j]	n/a	[k]	30 d	30 d	n/a	n/a	n/a	n/a	(1)
	UN	2 mcg/mL	NS[a][i]	n/a	[k]	30 d	30 d	n/a	n/a	n/a	n/a	(1)
	CUR	3 mcg/mL	NS[c]	n/a	[k]	7 d	7 d	n/a	n/a	n/a	n/a	(1)
	JN	5 mcg/mL	NS, D5W	n/a	[k]	48 hr	n/a	n/a	n/a	n/a	n/a	(1)
	DB	10 mcg/mL	NS[d]	n/a	[k]	30 d	30 d	n/a	n/a	n/a	n/a	(1)
	JN	20 mcg/mL	NS[m]	n/a	[k]	30 d	30 d	n/a	n/a	n/a	n/a	(1)
	JN	35 mcg/mL	NS	n/a	[k]	24 d[h]	28 d[h]	n/a	n/a	n/a	n/a	(1)
	AB	50 mcg/mL	Undiluted	n/a	5.43	28 d	28 d[h]	n/a	n/a	n/a	n/a	(1)(6)
Syringe, Polypropylene	SZ	0.15, 25, 43 mcg/mL	NS[b]	n/a	4.4-5.8	n/a	28 d[h]	n/a	n/a	n/a	n/a	(8)
	HOS	5 mcg/mL	NS	n/a	4.0-7.0	90 d[h]	n/a	n/a	n/a	n/a	n/a	(1)(7)
	DB	12.5, 33 mcg/mL	NS	n/a	[k]	7 d	7 d	n/a	n/a	n/a	7 d	(1)
	ES	16.7 mcg/mL	NS	n/a	[k]	24 hr[h]	24 hr[h]	n/a	n/a	n/a	n/a	(1)
	AB	50 mcg/mL	Undiluted	n/a	5.43	28 d	28 d	n/a	n/a	n/a	n/a	(1)(6)
Vial, Glass	CUR	3 mcg/mL	NS[c]	n/a	[k]	51 d	51 d	n/a	n/a	n/a	n/a	(1)
	JN	5 mcg/mL	NS, D5W	n/a	[k]	48 hr	n/a	n/a	n/a	n/a	n/a	(1)
	DB	10 mcg/mL	NS[d]	n/a	[k]	n/a	30 d	n/a	n/a	n/a	n/a	(1)

DOI 10.37573/9781585286720.086

Storage Conditions

	Drug Manufacturer	Concentration	Diluents	Osmolality (mOsm/kg)	pH	Temperature Room	Temperature Refrig	Temperature Frozen	Post-thaw Temp Room	Post-thaw Temp Refrig	Body Temp	Refer.
OTHER INFUSION CONTAINERS												
CADD® Cassette (Smiths Medical)	JN	1.25 mcg/mL	[e]	n/a	[k]	30 d	30 d	n/a	n/a	n/a	48 hr[g]	(1)
	JN	20 mcg/mL	NS	n/a	[k]	30 d	30 d	n/a	n/a	n/a	n/a	(2)
	ME	30, 50 mcg/mL	NS	n/a	[k]	14 d	14 d	n/a	n/a	n/a	n/a	(1)
	FK	2 mcg/mL	NS	n/a	[k]	184 d	184 d	n/a	n/a	n/a	n/a	(4)
Dosi-Fuser® (Leventon)	JN	1-5 mcg/mL	NS	n/a	[k]	30 d	60 d	n/a	n/a	n/a	n/a	(9)
	UN	10-50 mcg/mL	D5W, NS	n/a	n/a	30 d	90 d	n/a	n/a	n/a	7 d	(9)

Flush Compatibility: Sodium chloride 0.9%, heparin.[1]

Special Considerations: n/a

Notes

[a] Solution contained: bupivacaine (WI) 1.25 mg/mL.

[b] Solutions contained: fentaNYL 43 mcg/mL with bupivacaine (HOS) 0.01 mg/mL, fentaNYL 25 mcg/mL with bupivacaine (HOS) 20 mg/mL, and fentaNYL 0.15 mcg/mL with bupivacaine (HOS) 0.01, 20, and 37.5 mg/mL.[8]

[c] Solution contained: ropivacaine 1.5 mg/mL.[1]

[d] Solution contained: 50 mcg/mL droperidol (JN) and 1 mg/mL ketamine hydrochloride (JN).[1]

[e] Solution contained: bupivacaine 0.44 mg/mL and EPINEPHrine 0.69 mcg/mL.[1]

[f] Storage temperature: 30°C.

[g] Storage for 30 d at 3°C or 23°C, then 48 hr at 30°C.[1]

[h] Protected from light.

[i] Solution contained: bupivacaine 600 mcg/mL.[1]

[j] Solution contained: lidocaine (AST) 2.5 mg/mL.[1]

[k] pH range of undiluted solutions is 4-7.5.[1]

[l] Solutions contained: fentaNYL 10 mcg/mL with ropivacaine 2 mg/mL, fentaNYL 1 mcg/mL with ropivacaine 2 mg/mL or 1 mg/mL.[1,5]

[m] Solutions contained: fentaNYL as a single ingredient, or combined with bupivacaine (WI) 1.25 mg/mL.[1]

REFERENCES

1. ASHP's Interactive Handbook on Injectable Drugs, 2020. Bethesda, MD: American Society of Health-System Pharmacists; Accessed August 2020.
2. Allen LV, Jr., Stiles ML, Tu YH. Stability of fentanyl citrate in 0.9% sodium chloride solution in portable infusion pumps. *Am J Hosp Pharm*. 1990; 47(7):1572-4.
3. Donnelly RF. Stability of Fentanyl Citrate in Polyolefin Bags. *Int J Pharm Compd*. 2016; 20(6):514-16.

4. *Pharmaceutical report on chemical and physical stability of drugs commonly used with CADD® infusion pumps (IN193109GB-122019)*, 2019. Minneapolis, MN: Smiths Medical ASD, Inc.; Updated December 2019.
5. Oster Svedberg K, McKenzie J, Larrivee-Elkins C. Compatibility of ropivacaine with morphine, sufentanil, fentanyl, or clonidine. *J Clin Pharm Ther*. 2002; 27(1):39-45.
6. Donnelly RF. Chemical stability of fentanyl in polypropylene syringes and polyvinylchloride bags. *Int J Pharm Compd*. 2005; 9(6):482-3.
7. McCluskey SV, Graner KK, Kemp J, et al. Stability of fentanyl 5 microg/mL diluted with 0.9% sodium chloride injection and stored in polypropylene syringes. *Am J Health Syst Pharm*. 2009; 66(9):860-3.
8. Donnelly RF, Wong K, Spencer J. Physical compatibility of high-concentration bupivacaine with hydromorphone, morphine, and fentanyl. *Can J Hosp Pharm*. 2010; 63(2):154-5.
9. *Drug Stability Table - Dosi-Fuser® Elastomeric Pump (ES.H.00.73-10)*, 2015. Barcelona, Spain: Leventon SAU; Updated October 2015.

Ferric Carboxymaltose

						Storage Conditions						
						Temperature			Post-thaw Temp			
	Drug Manufacturer	Concentration	Diluents	Osmolality (mOsm/kg)	pH	Room	Refrig	Frozen	Room	Refrig	Body Temp	Refer.
CONTAINER												
Bag, Plastic (Unspecified)	AMR	2-4 mg/mL[a]	NS	isotonic	[b]	72 hr	n/a	n/a	n/a	n/a	n/a	(1)
Bag, Polypropylene	VFP	1, 2, 5 mg/mL	NS	n/a	n/a	72 hr	n/a	n/a	n/a	n/a	n/a	(3)

Flush Compatibility: Sodium chloride 0.9%.[1]

Special Considerations: Store vials at 20°C to 25°C; excursions permitted to 15°C to 30°C. Do not freeze. Dosage is expressed in mg of iron (elemental); product contains 50 mg/mL iron (elemental). May be administered undiluted as a slow IV push. Must be diluted for intravenous infusion. Avoid extravasation.[1,2]

Notes

[a] Dilute up to 750 mg iron (elemental) in no more than 250 mL NS; final iron (elemental) concentration must be at least 2 mg/mL.[1]

[b] pH of undiluted product is 5.0-7.0.[1]

REFERENCES

1. Injectafer® (Ferric Carboxymaltose) Injection [package insert]. Shirley, NY: American Regent, Inc.; September 2020.
2. ASHP's Interactive Handbook on Injectable Drugs, 2020. Bethesda, MD: American Society of Health-System Pharmacists; Accessed June 2020.
3. Philipp E, Braitsch M, Bichsel T, et al. Diluting ferric carboxymaltose in sodium chloride infusion solution (0.9% w/v) in polypropylene bottles and bags: effects on chemical stability. *Eur J Hosp Pharm*. 2016; 23(1):22-27.

DOI 10.37573/9781585286720.087

Ferric Gluconate

Storage Conditions

						Temperature			Post-thaw Temp			
	Drug Manufacturer	Concentration	Diluents	Osmolality (mOsm/kg)	pH	Room	Refrig	Frozen	Room	Refrig	Body Temp	Refer.
CONTAINER												
Bag, Plastic (Unspecified)	WAT	0.625 mg/mL[b]	NS	n/a	[a]	24 hr	7 d	n/a	n/a	n/a	n/a	(1)
	WAT	1.25 mg/mL[b]	NS	n/a	[a]	24 hr	7 d	n/a	n/a	n/a	n/a	(1)
Syringe, Unspecified	WAT	12.5 mg/mL	Undiluted	n/a	[a]	48 hr[c]	7 d	n/a	n/a	n/a	n/a	(1)
Unspecified	SAV	0.25 mg/mL[d]	NS	n/a	[a]	24 hr	n/a	n/a	n/a	n/a	n/a	(2)

Flush Compatibility: Sodium chloride 0.9%.[3]

Special Considerations: Do not freeze.[3]

Notes

[a] pH of undiluted solution is 7.7-9.7.[3]

[b] Diluted in 100 mL NS.[1]

[c] Iron concentration measured at 48 hours was 89.2% of initial concentration.[1]

[d] Concentration calculation: 62.5 mg ferric gluconate in 255 mL total volume equals 0.245 mg/mL; rounded.[2]

REFERENCES

1. Baribeault D. Short-term stability of a new generic sodium ferric gluconate in complex with sucrose. *Curr Med Res Opin*. 2011; 27(12):2241-3.
2. Ferrlecit® Medication Information Letter (Ref#: N/A) [personal communication]. Bridgewater, NJ: Sanofi-Aventis U.S., LLC; 2020:1.
3. Ferrlecit® (Sodium Ferric Gluconate) Injection [package insert]. Bridgewater, NJ: Sanofi-Aventis U.S., LLC; April 2020.

DOI 10.37573/9781585286720.088

Filgrastim

Storage Conditions

CONTAINER	Drug Manufacturer	Concentration	Diluents	Osmolality (mOsm/kg)	pH	Temperature: Room	Temperature: Refrig	Temperature: Frozen	Post-thaw Temp: Room	Post-thaw Temp: Refrig	Body Temp	Refer.
Bag, Polyvinyl Chloride (PVC)	AMG	5-15 mcg/mL[a][b]	D5W	n/a	[c]	24 hr	7 d	n/a	n/a	n/a	n/a	(1)
	AMG	>15 mcg/mL	D5W	n/a	[c]	24 hr	7 d	n/a	n/a	n/a	n/a	(1)
Syringe, Plastic (Unspecified)	AMG	5-15 mcg/mL[a][b]	D5W	n/a	[c]	24 hr	7 d	n/a	n/a	n/a	n/a	(1)
	AMG	>15 mcg/mL	D5W	n/a	[c]	24 hr	7 d	n/a	n/a	n/a	n/a	(1)
	AMG	300 mcg/mL	Undiluted	n/a	[c]	24 hr	7 d	n/a	n/a	n/a	n/a	(1)

Flush Compatibility: D5W. Incompatible with sodium chloride, incompatible with heparin.[1]

Special Considerations: When diluted in D5W or D5W plus human albumin, filgrastim is compatible with glass, PVC, polyolefin, and polypropylene containers. Store under refrigeration, protect from light, avoid freezing or shaking, discard if frozen more than once.[2]

Notes

[a] At filgrastim concentrations between 5 and 15 mcg/mL, add human albumin 2 mg/mL to minimize adsorption to containers.

[b] The manufacturer does not recommend dilutions less than 5 mcg/mL.[2]

[c] Stable at pH 3.8 to 4.2; stability is limited at neutral pH.[1]

REFERENCES

1. ASHP's Interactive Handbook on Injectable Drugs, 2020. Bethesda, MD: American Society of Health-System Pharmacists; Accessed December 2020.
2. Neupogen® (Filgrastim) Injection [package insert]. Thousand Oaks, CA: Amgen, Inc.; June 2018.

DOI 10.37573/9781585286720.089

Floxuridine

Storage Conditions

						Temperature			Post-thaw Temp			
	Drug Manufacturer	Concentration	Diluents	Osmolality (mOsm/kg)	pH	Room	Refrig	Frozen	Room	Refrig	Body Temp	Refer.
CONTAINER												
Syringe, Polypropylene	RC	1, 50 mg/mL	NS	n/a	[c]	n/a	n/a	n/a	n/a	n/a	21 d[a]	(2)
Unspecified	UN	5-10 mg/mL	D5W, NS	n/a	[c]	14 d	n/a	n/a	n/a	n/a	n/a	(1)
OTHER INFUSION CONTAINERS												
Implantable Pump (Fresenius Model VIP® 30)	UN	10 mg/mL	unspec.	n/a	[c]	n/a	n/a	n/a	n/a	n/a	6 wk	(1)
Infusaid® Model 400 Implantable Pump (Infusaid)	RC	2.58-12.2 mg/mL	NS[b]	n/a	[c]	n/a	n/a	n/a	n/a	n/a	4-12 d[d]	(3)
SMARTeZ® (Progressive Medical)	UN	10 mg/mL	NS	n/a	[c]	24 hr	14 d	n/a	n/a	n/a	n/a	(4)

Flush Compatibility: Sodium chloride 0.9%.[3]

Special Considerations: Store reconstituted solution under refrigeration and use within 14 days.[1] Caution: Used only for continuous regional intra-arterial infusion.[1,5]

Notes

[a] Storage temperature: 30°C.[2]

[b] Solution contained: 200 units/mL heparin sodium in bacteriostatic sodium chloride 0.9%.[3]

[c] pH of reconstituted preparation is 4-5.5.[1]

[d] At least 95% of initial concentration remained upon in vivo assessment of drug removed from devices after 8 different infusions for 5 patients (after 4, 7, 10, 11, and 12 days).[3]

DOI 10.37573/9781585286720.090

REFERENCES

1. ASHP's Interactive Handbook on Injectable Drugs, 2020. Bethesda, MD: American Society of Health-System Pharmacists; Accessed August 2020.
2. Stiles ML, Allen LV, Jr., Prince SJ. Stability of deferoxamine mesylate, floxuridine, fluorouracil, hydromorphone hydrochloride, lorazepam, and midazolam hydrochloride in polypropylene infusion-pump syringes. *Am J Health Syst Pharm*. 1996; 53(13):1583-8.
3. Keller JH, Ensminger WD. Stability of cancer chemotherapeutic agents in a totally implanted drug delivery system. *Am J Hosp Pharm*. 1982; 39(8):1321-3.
4. *SMARTeZ® - Stability Data for Drugs Using Elastomeric Infusion Pumps*, 2020. Fenton, MO: Progressive Medical, Inc.; Updated May 2020.
5. Floxuridine Injection, lyophilized [package insert]. Lake Zurich, IL: Fresenius Kabi USA, LLC; December 2019.

Fluconazole

Storage Conditions

	Drug Manufacturer	Concentration	Diluents	Osmolality (mOsm/kg)	pH	Temperature			Post-thaw Temp			
						Room	Refrig	Frozen	Room	Refrig	Body Temp	Refer.
CONTAINER												
Bag, Polyvinyl Chloride (PVC)	BA	1 mg/mL	D5W, LR	[a]	n/a	24 hr	n/a	n/a	n/a	n/a	n/a	(1)
OTHER INFUSION CONTAINERS												
Dosi-Fuser® (Leventon)	PF	2 mg/mL	NS	n/a	n/a	n/a	15 d	n/a	n/a	n/a	n/a	(6)
Easypump® ST/LT (B. Braun)	UN	2 mg/mL	RTU	n/a	[c]	48 hr[d]	7 d[d]	n/a	n/a	n/a	n/a	(5)
Homepump Eclipse® / Homepump® (Halyard)	UN	2 mg/mL	RTU	n/a	[c]	24 hr	14 d	n/a	n/a	n/a	n/a	(4)
SMARTeZ® (Progressive Medical)	UN	2 mg/mL	RTU	n/a	[c]	48 hr[b]	7 d[b]	n/a	n/a	n/a	n/a	(3)

Flush Compatibility: Sodium chloride 0.9%, heparin.[1]

Special Considerations: Do not freeze solutions containing fluconazole.[1]

Notes

[a] The infusion solution is iso-osmotic having an osmolarity of 300-315 mOsm/L.[1]

[b] Manufacturer(s) extrapolated data from other sources.

[c] pH of RTU solution is 3.5-6.5 in dextrose diluent; 4.0-8.0 in sodium chloride diluent.[2]

[d] Refrigerated 7 d followed by 48 hr room temperature.

REFERENCES

1. ASHP's Interactive Handbook on Injectable Drugs, 2020. Bethesda, MD: American Society of Health-System Pharmacists; Accessed June 2020.
2. Diflucan® (Fluconazole in Dextrose and Fluconazole in Sodium Chloride) Injection [package insert]. New York, NY: Roerig Div of Pfizer, Inc.; April 2020.

DOI 10.37573/9781585286720.091

3. *SMARTeZ® - Stability Data for Drugs Using Elastomeric Infusion Pumps*, 2020. Fenton, MO: Progressive Medical, Inc.; Updated May 2020.
4. *Stability Data for Drugs Using Homepump Disposable Ambulatory Infusion Systems (MK-00314 rev 3)*, 2015. Alpharetta, GA: Halyard Health; Updated June 2015.
5. *Drug Stability for Easypump® ST/LT*, 2020. Bethlehem, PA: B. Braun USA; Updated June 2020.
6. *Drug Stability Table - Dosi-Fuser® Elastomeric Pump (S-CL-00-001v16)*, 2021. Barcelona, Spain: Leventon SAU; Updated May 2021.

Fludarabine Phosphate

Storage Conditions

						Temperature			Post-thaw Temp			
	Drug Manufacturer	Concentration	Diluents	Osmolality (mOsm/kg)	pH	Room	Refrig	Frozen	Room	Refrig	Body Temp	Refer.
CONTAINER												
Bag, Polyethylene	TE	0.05 mg/mL	NS	n/a	n/a	15 d[c]	15 d[c]	n/a	n/a	n/a	n/a	(3)
Bag, Polyolefin	TE	0.04, 0.2, 1 mg/mL	NS	n/a	4.8-6.9	21 d	21 d	n/a	n/a	n/a	n/a	(4)
Bag, Polyvinyl Chloride (PVC)	UN	0.04 mg/mL	NS, D5W	n/a	[b]	48 hr	48 hr	n/a	n/a	n/a	n/a	(1)
Vial, Glass	UN	0.04 mg/mL	NS, D5W	n/a	[b]	48 hr	48 hr	n/a	n/a	n/a	n/a	(1)
	UN	1 mg/mL	NS, D5W	n/a	[b]	16 d[a]	n/a	n/a	n/a	n/a	n/a	(1)
	TE	25 mg/mL	Undiluted	n/a	4.8-6.9	21 d	21 d	n/a	n/a	n/a	n/a	(4)
	TE	25 mg/mL	Undiluted	n/a	[b]	15 d[c]	15 d[c]	n/a	n/a	n/a	n/a	(3)
OTHER INFUSION CONTAINERS												
INTERMATE™ (Baxter)[d]	SC	0.1-1.5 mg/mL	NS, D5W	n/a	[b]	5 wk	n/a	n/a	n/a	n/a	n/a	(2)

Flush Compatibility: Sodium chloride 0.9%, D5W.[5]

Special Considerations: n/a

Notes

[a] Exposed to light.[1]

[b] pH of reconstituted powder product is 7.2-8.2.[5] pH of liquid is 7.3-7.7.[1]

[c] Protected from light.[3]

[d] INTERMATE™/INFUSOR™ Portable Elastomeric Infusion System devices are no longer available in the United States.

DOI 10.37573/9781585286720.092

REFERENCES

1. ASHP's Interactive Handbook on Injectable Drugs, 2020. Bethesda, MD: American Society of Health-System Pharmacists; Accessed June 2020.
2. Stabforum - Stability Database: Fludarabine, Ontario, Canada: Baxter Healthcare; Accessed January 2021.
3. SzbBek E, KamjDska A, Urjasz H, et al. The stability of fludarabine phosphate in concentrate and diluted with sodium chloride 0.9. *Wspolczesna Onkologia-Contemporary Oncology*. 2011; 15:142-46.
4. Rainer T. New stability studies for fludarabine according to the European Pharmacopoeia 7.0. *Eur J Onc Pharm*. 2012; 6(1):14-5.
5. Fludarabine Phosphate Injection, lyophilized [package insert]. Lake Forest, IL: Hospira, Inc.; August 2020.

Fluorouracil

Storage Conditions

	Drug Manufacturer	Concentration	Diluents	Osmolality (mOsm/kg)	pH	Temperature Room	Temperature Refrig	Frozen	Post-thaw Temp Room	Post-thaw Temp Refrig	Body Temp	Refer.
CONTAINER												
Bag, Ethylene Vinyl Acetate (EVA)	RC	10 mg/mL	D5W, NS	n/a	[e]	28 d[a]	28 d[a]	n/a	n/a	n/a	28 d[a][g]	(8)(9)
	RC	15, 45 mg/mL	NS	n/a	[e]	72 hr[a]	n/a	n/a	n/a	n/a	n/a	(9)
	RC	50 mg/mL	Undiluted	n/a	[e]	28 d[a]	28 d[a]	n/a	n/a	n/a	28 d[a][g]	(8)(9)
Bag, Polyvinyl Chloride (PVC)	RC	1, 10 mg/mL	D5W, NS	n/a	[e]	14 d	14 d	n/a	n/a	n/a	n/a	(9)
	RC	1.5 mg/mL	D5W, NS	n/a	[e]	8 wk	n/a	n/a	n/a	n/a	n/a	(9)
	FA, RC	5, 50 mg/mL	NS, Undiluted	n/a	[e]	7 d[a]	13 wk[a][h]	n/a	n/a	n/a	n/a	(9)
	TE	8 mg/mL[l]	NS	n/a	[e]	n/a	n/a	79 d	n/a	28 d	n/a	(9)(11)
	RC	10 mg/mL	D5W	n/a	[e]	7 d	4 m	n/a	n/a	n/a	n/a	(9)
	DB	25 mg/mL	unspec.	n/a	[e]	n/a	14 d	n/a	n/a	n/a	14 d	(9)
	UN	50 mg/mL	Undiluted	n/a	[e]	14 d	n/a	n/a	n/a	n/a	n/a	(2)
Syringe, Plastic (Unspecified)	DB	24.04 mg/mL	[b]	n/a	[e]	14 d	n/a	n/a	n/a	n/a	7 d	(5)
Syringe, Polypropylene	ABI	10 mg/mL	NS	n/a	[e]	n/a	n/a	8 wk[d]	n/a	n/a	n/a	(9)
	RC	12, 40 mg/mL	D5W, NS	n/a	[e]	72 hr[a]	n/a	n/a	n/a	n/a	n/a	(9)
	UN	25 mg/mL	unspec.	n/a	[e]	28 d	28 d	n/a	n/a	n/a	n/a	(6)(9)
	RC	50 mg/mL	Undiluted	n/a	[e]	21 d[i]	n/a	n/a	n/a	n/a	n/a	(3)(9)
OTHER INFUSION CONTAINERS												
CADD® Cassette (Smiths Medical)	LY, RC, SO	50 mg/mL	Undiluted, D5W, NS	n/a	[e]	14 d[j]	5 d	n/a	n/a	n/a	7 d[j]	(12)
Dosi-Fuser® (Leventon)	EBE	1-10 mg/mL	NS	n/a	[e]	90 d	n/a	n/a	n/a	n/a	n/a	(7)
	UN	5-30 mg/mL	NS	n/a	[e]	30 d	n/a	n/a	n/a	n/a	n/a	(7)
	EBE	10 mg/mL	D5W	n/a	[e]	90 d	n/a	n/a	n/a	n/a	n/a	(7)
	UN	50 mg/mL	Undiluted	n/a	[e]	30 d	n/a	n/a	n/a	n/a	n/a	(7)
Easypump® ST/LT (B. Braun)	UN	5 mg/mL	D5W, NS	n/a	[e]	n/a	45 d	n/a	n/a	n/a	n/a	(13)
	UN	50 mg/mL	Undiluted	n/a	[e]	n/a	45 d	n/a	n/a	n/a	n/a	(13)
	ICN	25 mg/mL	D5W, NS	n/a	[e]	21 d	14 d	n/a	n/a	n/a	21 d[c]	(9)(10)
	ICN	50 mg/mL	Undiluted	n/a	[e]	21 d	n/a	n/a	n/a	n/a	21 d[c]	(10)

DOI 10.37573/9781585286720.093

Storage Conditions

	Drug Manufacturer	Concentration	Diluents	Osmolality (mOsm/kg)	pH	Temperature			Post-thaw Temp			
						Room	Refrig	Frozen	Room	Refrig	Body Temp	Refer.
OTHER INFUSION CONTAINERS												
Fresenius VIP 30 Implantable Pump	UN	50 mg/mL	Undiluted	n/a	[e]	n/a	n/a	n/a	n/a	n/a	8 wk	(9)
Homepump Eclipse® / Homepump® (Halyard)	UN	1-25 mg/mL	NS	n/a	[e]	45 d[m]	45 d[m]	n/a	n/a	n/a	n/a	(1)
	UN	50 mg/mL	Undiluted	n/a	[e]	8 wk[m]	n/a	n/a	n/a	n/a	n/a	(1)
	UN	50 mg/mL	Undiluted	n/a	[e]	45 d[m]	n/a	n/a	n/a	n/a	n/a	(1)
INFUSOR™ (Baxter)[k]	Various	0.1-25 mg/mL	D5W, NS	n/a	[e]	n/a	123 d[f]	n/a	n/a	n/a	7 d	(4)
	Various	0.1-50 mg/mL	D5W, NS	n/a	[e]	38 d[f]	n/a	n/a	n/a	n/a	7 d	(4)
	ACC	0.5-50 mg/mL	D5W, NS	n/a	[e]	61 d	n/a	n/a	n/a	n/a	8 d	(4)
	RC	10 mg/mL	D5W	n/a	[e]	n/a	4 m	n/a	n/a	n/a	n/a	(9)
	ACC	50 mg/mL	Undiluted	n/a	[e]	61 d	n/a	n/a	n/a	n/a	8 d	(4)
INTERMATE™ (Baxter)[k]	ACC	0.5-50 mg/mL	D5W, NS	n/a	[e]	61 d	n/a	n/a	n/a	n/a	n/a	(4)
	ACC	50 mg/mL	Undiluted	n/a	[e]	61 d	n/a	n/a	n/a	n/a	n/a	(4)
Medfusion Infumed 200	LY, RC, SO	50 mg/mL	Undiluted	n/a	[e]	7 d[j]	n/a	n/a	n/a	n/a	7 d[j]	(9)
Pancretec Provider 2000	LY, RC, SO	50 mg/mL	Undiluted	n/a	[e]	7 d[j]	n/a	n/a	n/a	n/a	7 d[j]	(9)
SMARTeZ® (Progressive Medical)	UN	5, 50 mg/mL	NS	n/a	[e]	45 d	45 d[n]	n/a	n/a	n/a	n/a	(14)

Flush Compatibility: Sodium chloride 0.9%, heparin.[9]

Special Considerations: n/a

Notes

[a] Protected from light.

[b] Diluted to a concentration of 961.54 units/mL of heparin.[5]

[c] Storage temperature: 31°C.[9,10]

[d] Stability was not affected by re-freezing and further storage at -20°C for 14 additional days (total of 10 wk).[9]

[e] pH of the undiluted solution is 8.6-9.4.[9]

[f] Followed by 7 d at 33°C.[4]

[g] Storage temperature: 35°C; concentrations increased due to water evaporation.[8,9]

[h] Followed by 7 d at 25°C in the dark.[9]

[i] Storage temperature: 30°C.[3,9]

[j] Fine precipitation was observed with the Roche product in the tubing and bags.[9,12]

[k] INTERMATE™/INFUSOR™ Portable Elastomeric Infusion System devices are no longer available in the United States.

[l] Due to commercial bag overfill, actual concentration was approximately 6.8 mg/mL.[9,11]

[m] Potential for drug precipitation depending on preparation, storage conditions, concentration, pH and diluent.[1]

[n] Manufacturer extrapolated data from other sources.

REFERENCES

1. *Stability Data for Drugs Using Homepump Disposable Ambulatory Infusion Systems (MK-00314 rev 3)*, 2015. Alpharetta, GA: Halyard Health; Updated June 2015.
2. Vyas HM, Baptista RJ, Mitrano FP, et al. Drug stability guidelines for a continuous infusion chemotherapy program. *Hosp Pharm*. 1987; 22(7):685-7.
3. Stiles ML, Allen LV, Jr., Prince SJ. Stability of deferoxamine mesylate, floxuridine, fluorouracil, hydromorphone hydrochloride, lorazepam, and midazolam hydrochloride in polypropylene infusion-pump syringes. *Am J Health Syst Pharm*. 1996; 53(13):1583-8.
4. Stabforum - Stability Database: 5-Fluorouracil, Ontario, Canada: Baxter Healthcare; Accessed January 2021.
5. Sewell GJ, Allsopp M, Collinson MP, et al. Stability studies on admixtures of 5-fluorouracil with carboplatin and 5-fluorouracil with heparin for administration in continuous infusion regimens. *J Clin Pharm Ther*. 1994; 19(2):127-33.
6. Adams P, Haines-Nutt R, Bradford E, et al. Pharmaceutical aspects of home infusion therapy for cancer patients. *Pharm J*. 1987; 238:476-78.
7. *Drug Stability Table - Dosi-Fuser® Elastomeric Pump (S-CL-00-001v16)*, 2021. Barcelona, Spain: Leventon SAU; Updated May 2021.
8. Rochard EB, Barthes DM, Courtois PY. Stability of fluorouracil, cytarabine, or doxorubicin hydrochloride in ethylene vinylacetate portable infusion-pump reservoirs. *Am J Hosp Pharm*. 1992; 49(3):619-23.
9. ASHP's Interactive Handbook on Injectable Drugs, 2020. Bethesda, MD: American Society of Health-System Pharmacists; Accessed September 2020.
10. Roberts S, Sewell GJ. Stability and compatibility of 5-fluorouracil infusions in the Braun Easypump®. *J Oncol Pharm Pract*. 2003; 9(2-3):109-12.
11. Galanti L, Lebitasy MP, Hecq JD, et al. Long-term stability of 5-Fluorouracil in 0.9% sodium chloride after freezing, microwave thawing, and refrigeration. *Can J Hosp Pharm*. 2009; 62(1):34-8.
12. *Pharmaceutical report on chemical and physical stability of drugs commonly used with CADD® infusion pumps (IN193109GB-122019)*, 2019. Minneapolis, MN: Smiths Medical ASD, Inc.; Updated December 2019.
13. *Drug Stability for Easypump® ST/LT*, 2020. Bethlehem, PA: B. Braun USA; Updated June 2020.
14. *SMARTeZ® - Stability Data for Drugs Using Elastomeric Infusion Pumps*, 2020. Fenton, MO: Progressive Medical, Inc.; Updated May 2020.

Foscarnet Sodium

Storage Conditions

	Drug Manufacturer	Concentration	Diluents	Osmolality (mOsm/kg)	pH	Temperature			Post-thaw Temp			
						Room	Refrig	Frozen	Room	Refrig	Body Temp	Refer.
CONTAINER												
Bag, Polyvinyl Chloride (PVC)	AST	12 mg/mL	D5W, NS	n/a	[d]	5 wk	5 wk	n/a	n/a	n/a	n/a	(1)
	AST	12 mg/mL	NS	n/a	[d]	30 d	30 d	n/a	n/a	n/a	n/a	(1)
OTHER INFUSION CONTAINERS												
Dosi-Fuser® (Leventon)	AST	12 mg/mL	NS	n/a	[d]	7 d[e]	14 d[e]	n/a	n/a	n/a	n/a	(3)
	AST	2-10 mg/mL	NS, D5W	n/a	[d]	4 d[e]	14 d[e]	n/a	n/a	n/a	n/a	(3)
	AST	24 mg/mL	Undiluted[a]	iso	7.4	48 hr[e]	14 d[e]	n/a	n/a	n/a	n/a	(3)
	AST	24 mg/mL	Undiluted[a]	iso	7.4	72 d[e]	72 d[e]	n/a	n/a	n/a	n/a	(3)
	AST	24 mg/mL	Undiluted[a]	iso	7.4	28 d[e]	28 d[e]	n/a	n/a	n/a	n/a	(3)
	AST	24 mg/mL	Undiluted[a]	iso	7.4	48 hr[e]	14 d[e]	n/a	n/a	n/a	n/a	(3)
Homepump Eclipse® / Homepump® (Halyard)	AST	12 mg/mL	NS, D5W	n/a	[d]	7 d	14 d	n/a	n/a	n/a	n/a	(4)
	AST	24 mg/mL	Undiluted[a]	iso	7.4	7 d	14 d	n/a	n/a	n/a	n/a	(4)
INTERMATE™ (Baxter)[b]	AST	12 mg/mL	NS, D5W	n/a	[d]	10 d[f]	16 d	n/a	n/a	n/a	n/a	(2)
	AST	12 mg/mL	NS, D5W	n/a	[d]	16 d	n/a	n/a	n/a	n/a	n/a	(2)
COMMERCIAL PREPARATIONS (RTU)												
Glass Bottle (Hospira)	HOS	24 mg/mL	Undiluted[a]	iso	7.4	[c]	n/a	n/a	n/a	n/a	n/a	(1)

Flush Compatibility: Sodium chloride 0.9%, heparin.[1]

Special Considerations: Administer IV at ≤ 60 mg/kg/hr. For peripheral administration, dilute to 12 mg/mL with D5W or NS. For central administration, the 24 mg/mL solution may be infused undiluted. Refrigerated products or products exposed to temperatures below freezing may exhibit precipitation; however, the precipitate can be dissolved by bringing bottle to room temperature and with repeated shaking. Incompatible with calcium-containing solutions such as LR or PN.[1]

DOI 10.37573/9781585286720.094

Notes

[a] Foscarnet is available as an isotonic 24 mg/mL solution.[1]

[b] INTERMATE™/INFUSOR™ Portable Elastomeric Infusion System devices are no longer available in the United States.

[c] Expiration date per manufacturer's label, and must be used within 24 hr of initial entry into the bottle.[1]

[d] pH of undiluted solution is 7.4.[1]

[e] Manufacturer extrapolated data from other source(s).

[f] Stored 16 days refrigerated followed by 10 days at room temperature.[2]

REFERENCES

1. ASHP's Interactive Handbook on Injectable Drugs, 2020. Bethesda, MD: American Society of Health-System Pharmacists; Accessed September 2020.
2. Stabforum - Stability Database: Foscarnet, Ontario, Canada: Baxter Healthcare; Accessed January 2021.
3. *Drug Stability Table - Dosi-Fuser® Elastomeric Pump (ES.H.00.73-10)*, 2015. Barcelona, Spain: Leventon SAU; Updated October 2015.
4. *Stability Data for Drugs Using Homepump Disposable Ambulatory Infusion Systems (MK-00314 rev 3)*, 2015. Alpharetta, GA: Halyard Health; Updated June 2015.

Fosphenytoin Sodium

Storage Conditions

						Temperature			Post-thaw Temp			
	Drug Manufacturer	Concentration	Diluents	Osmolality (mOsm/kg)	pH	Room	Refrig	Frozen	Room	Refrig	Body Temp	Refer.
CONTAINER												
Bag, Polyvinyl Chloride (PVC)	PD	1 mg PE/mL	D5W, NS	n/a	[b]	30 d	30 d	30 d	7 d	7 d	n/a	(2)
	PD	1 mg PE/mL	D5LR, LR, D5½NS, D10W	n/a	[b]	7 d	n/a	n/a	n/a	n/a	n/a	(1)
	PD	8 mg PE/mL	D5W, NS	n/a	[b]	30 d	30 d	30 d	7 d	7 d	n/a	(2)
	PD	8 mg PE/mL	D5LR, LR, D5½NS, D10W	n/a	[b]	7 d	n/a	n/a	n/a	n/a	n/a	(1)
	PD	20 mg PE/mL	D5W, NS	n/a	[b]	30 d	30 d	30 d	7 d	7 d	n/a	(2)
	PD	20 mg PE/mL	D5LR, LR, D5½NS, D10W	n/a	[b]	7 d	n/a	n/a	n/a	n/a	n/a	(1)
Syringe, Polypropylene	PD	50 mg PE/mL	Undiluted	n/a	[a]	30 d	30 d	30 d	7 d	7 d	n/a	(1)

Flush Compatibility: Sodium chloride 0.9%.[1]

Special Considerations: Concentrations expressed as phenytoin equivalent (PE).

Notes

[a] pH 8.6-9.0.[3]

[b] pH 8.6-9.0 or 8.3-9.3.[1]

REFERENCES

1. ASHP's Interactive Handbook on Injectable Drugs, 2020. Bethesda, MD: American Society of Health-System Pharmacists; Accessed June 2020.
2. Fischer JH, Cwik MJ, Luer MS, et al. Stability of fosphenytoin sodium with intravenous solutions in glass bottles, polyvinyl chloride bags, and polypropylene syringes. *Ann Pharmacother*. 1997; 31(5):553-9.
3. Cerebyx® (Fosphenytoin Sodium) Injection [package insert]. New York, NY: Pfizer Laboratories Div Pfizer Inc.; February 2020.

DOI 10.37573/9781585286720.095

Furosemide

Storage Conditions

	Drug Manufacturer	Concentration	Diluents	Osmolality (mOsm/kg)	pH	Temperature Room	Temperature Refrig	Frozen	Post-thaw Temp Room	Post-thaw Temp Refrig	Body Temp	Refer.
CONTAINER												
Bag, Polyvinyl Chloride (PVC)	HO	1 mg/mL	NS	[e]	[d]	24 hr	26 d[b]	n/a	n/a	n/a	n/a	(1)
	HO	1 mg/mL	LR	[e]	[d]	24 hr	n/a	n/a	n/a	n/a	n/a	(1)
	AB	1.2, 2.4, 3.2 mg/mL	NS	[e]	[d]	12 wk[c]	12 wk[c]	n/a	n/a	n/a	n/a	(1)
Syringe, Polypropylene	AB	1, 2, 4, 8 mg/mL	NS	[e]	[d]	12 wk[c]	12 wk[c]	n/a	n/a	n/a	n/a	(1)
	HO	3.33-10 mg/mL	NS[a]	[e]	[d]	5 d	5 d	n/a	n/a	n/a	n/a	(1)(3)
	HO	10 mg/mL	Undiluted	287	[d]	24 hr	n/a	n/a	n/a	n/a	n/a	(1)
	HOS	1 mg/mL	D5W	[e]	[d]	4 d[g]	n/a	n/a	n/a	n/a	n/a	(7)
	UN	5 mg/mL	unspec.	[e]	[h]	24 hr[i]	5 wk[i]	n/a	n/a	n/a	n/a	(5)
OTHER INFUSION CONTAINERS												
Easypump® ST/LT (B. Braun)	UN	10 mg/mL	NS	[e]	[d]	4 d	7 d	n/a	n/a	n/a	n/a	(6)
Homepump Eclipse® / Homepump® (Halyard)	UN	0.5-10 mg/mL	NS	[e]	[d]	4 d	7 d	n/a	n/a	n/a	n/a	(2)
INFUSOR™ (Baxter)[f]	SHP	0.5-10 mg/mL	NS	[e]	[d]	7 d	7 d	n/a	n/a	n/a	48 hr	(4)

Flush Compatibility: Sodium chloride 0.9%, heparin.[1]

Special Considerations: Refrigeration may result in precipitation or crystallization; resolubilization at room temperature will not affect drug stability. Protection from light is recommended. Do not use if solution has a yellow color.[1]

Notes

[a] Solution contained: dexAMETHasone sodium phosphate (ME) 0.33-3.33 mg/mL.

[b] 10% furosemide loss at 6°C.[1]

[c] Stored protected from light followed by 7 d at room temperature in fluorescent light.[1]

[d] pH of undiluted solution is 8-9.3.[1]

[e] Osmolality of 10 mg/mL (HO) is 287 mOsm/kg. Other unspecified brands ranged from 289-291 mOsm/kg.[1]

[f] INTERMATE™/INFUSOR™ Portable Elastomeric Infusion System devices are no longer available in the United States.

[g] Protected from light.

[h] pH of furosemide 5 mg/mL is 8.90-9.23.[5]

[i] Stored protected from light followed by 24 hr at 20°C not protected from light.[5]

DOI 10.37573/9781585286720.096

REFERENCES

1. ASHP's Interactive Handbook on Injectable Drugs, 2020. Bethesda, MD: American Society of Health-System Pharmacists; Accessed September 2020.
2. *Stability Data for Drugs Using Homepump Disposable Ambulatory Infusion Systems (MK-00314 rev 3)*, 2015. Alpharetta, GA: Halyard Health; Updated June 2015.
3. Negro S, Rendon AL, Azuara ML, et al. Compatibiliity and stability of furosemide and dexamethasone combined in infusion solutions. *Arzneimittelforschung*. 2006; 56(10):714-20.
4. Stabforum - Stability Database: Furosemide, Ontario, Canada: Baxter Healthcare; Accessed January 2021.
5. van der Schaar JAJ, Grouls R, Franssen EJF, et al. Stability of Furosemide 5 mg/mL in Polypropylene Syringes. *Int J Pharm Compd*. 2019; 23(5):414-17.
6. *Drug Stability for Easypump® ST/LT*, 2020. Bethlehem, PA: B. Braun USA; Updated June 2020.
7. Cies JJ, Moore WS, 2nd, Chopra A, et al. Stability of furosemide and chlorothiazide stored in syringes. *Am J Health Syst Pharm*. 2015; 72(24):2182-8.

Ganciclovir Sodium

Storage Conditions

						Temperature			Post-thaw Temp			
	Drug Manufacturer	Concentration	Diluents	Osmolality (mOsm/kg)	pH	Room	Refrig	Frozen	Room	Refrig	Body Temp	Refer.
CONTAINER												
Bag, Polyvinyl Chloride (PVC)	SY	0.28, 1.4 mg/mL	NS	n/a	[a]	7 d	80 d	13 m	n/a	n/a	n/a	(1)
	SY	1, 5 mg/mL	D5W, NS	n/a	[a]	5 wk	5 wk	n/a	n/a	n/a	n/a	(1)
	SY	1, 5, 10 mg/mL	D5W	n/a	[a]	n/a	5 wk[c]	n/a	n/a	n/a	n/a	(1)
	SY	2.44 mg/mL	D5W	n/a	[a]	5 d	5 d	n/a	n/a	n/a	n/a	(1)
	SY	2.59 mg/mL	NS	n/a	[a]	5 d	5 d	n/a	n/a	n/a	n/a	(1)
	SY	5, 10 mg/mL	NS, D5W	n/a	[a]	n/a	28 d	28 d	n/a	n/a	n/a	(3)
	APP	≤ 10 mg/mL	NS	n/a	[a]	24 hr	14 d	n/a	n/a	n/a	n/a	(10)
Syringe, Polypropylene	RC	0.25, 5 mg/mL	NS	n/a	[a]	185 d[c]	185 d[c]	n/a	n/a	n/a	n/a	(1)
	SY	1.4, 4, 7 mg/mL	NS	n/a	[a]	7 d	80 d	13 m	n/a	n/a	n/a	(1)
	SY	5.8 mg/mL	NS	n/a	[a]	12 hr	10 d	n/a	n/a	n/a	n/a	(1)
Unspecified	SY	2.2 mg/mL	NS	n/a	[a]	n/a	14 d	n/a	n/a	n/a	n/a	(1)
	CHE	≤ 10 mg/mL	NS, D5W, R, LR	n/a	[a]	24 hr	n/a	n/a	n/a	n/a	n/a	(6)
OTHER INFUSION CONTAINERS												
Dosi-Fuser® (Leventon)	RC	1-6 mg/mL	NS, D5W	n/a	[a]	42 d[b]	42 d[b]	n/a	n/a	n/a	n/a	(9)
Easypump® ST/LT (B. Braun)	UN	1, 10 mg/mL	NS, D5W	n/a	[a]	48 hr	14 d	n/a	n/a	n/a	n/a	(8)
Homepump Eclipse® / Homepump® (Halyard)	UN	2-5 mg/mL	NS	n/a	[a]	7 d	n/a	n/a	n/a	n/a	n/a	(5)
	UN	5 mg/mL	NS	n/a	[a]	24 hr	15 d	n/a	n/a	n/a	n/a	(5)

DOI 10.37573/9781585286720.097

Storage Conditions

						Temperature			Post-thaw Temp			
	Drug Manufacturer	Concentration	Diluents	Osmolality (mOsm/kg)	pH	Room	Refrig	Frozen	Room	Refrig	Body Temp	Refer.
OTHER INFUSION CONTAINERS												
INTERMATE™ (Baxter)[g]	SY	1 mg/mL	D5W	n/a	[a]	7 d[d]	28 d[f]	n/a	n/a	n/a	n/a	(2)
	RC	1, 5 mg/mL	NS	n/a	[a]	n/a	5 wk[c]	n/a	n/a	n/a	n/a	(1)
	SY	1-6 mg/mL	D5W, NS	n/a	[a]	n/a	n/a	9 wk	n/a	7 d[e]	n/a	(2)
	SY	1-6 mg/mL	D5W, NS	n/a	[a]	72 hr[d]	28 d[f]	n/a	n/a	n/a	n/a	(2)
	RC	1-6 mg/mL	D5W, NS	n/a	[a]	6 wk	6 wk[f]	n/a	n/a	n/a	n/a	(2)
SMARTeZ® (Progressive Medical)	UN	1, 10 mg/mL	NS	n/a	[a]	48 hr[b]	14 d[b]	n/a	n/a	n/a	n/a	(7)
COMMERCIAL PREPARATIONS (RTU)												
Flexible Plastic Container	EXL	2 mg/mL	RTU	n/a	7.5	[h]	n/a	n/a	n/a	n/a	n/a	(4)

Flush Compatibility: Sodium chloride 0.9%, heparin.[1]

Special Considerations: Do not use if discoloration is noted. Ganciclovir sodium is incompatible with diluents and solutions containing parabens. Administer by IV infusion only.[6]

Notes

[a] pH of 50 mg/mL reconstituted in SWFI is approximately 11.[6]

[b] Manufacturer extrapolated data from other sources.

[c] Protected from light.

[d] Following 28 d refrigerated.[2]

[e] Following 9 wk frozen.[2]

[f] Inspect for possible crystal formation in D5W; redissolves with gentle shaking and warming to ambient room temperature.[2]

[g] INTERMATE™/INFUSOR™ Portable Elastomeric Infusion System devices are no longer available in the United States.

[h] Crystals may form during storage at temperatures that are lower than recommended; bags should be gently shaken to redissolve such crystals and the solution must be clear at the time of use.[1,4]

REFERENCES

1. ASHP's Interactive Handbook on Injectable Drugs, 2020. Bethesda, MD: American Society of Health-System Pharmacists; Accessed July 2020.
2. Stabforum - Stability Database: Ganciclovir, Ontario, Canada: Baxter Healthcare; Accessed February 2021.
3. Mole L, Oliva C, O'Hanley P. Extended stability of ganciclovir for outpatient parenteral therapy for cytomegalovirus retinitis. *J Acquir Immune Defic Syndr*. 1992; 5(4):354-8.

4. Ganciclovir Injection [package insert]. Lenoir, NC: Exela Pharma Sciences, LLC; October 2017.
5. *Stability Data for Drugs Using Homepump Disposable Ambulatory Infusion Systems (MK-00314 rev 3)*, 2015. Alpharetta, GA: Halyard Health; Updated June 2015.
6. Cytovene®-IV (Ganciclovir) Injection, Lyophilized [package insert]. Montgomery, AL: H2-Pharma, LLC; June 2020.
7. *SMARTeZ® - Stability Data for Drugs Using Elastomeric Infusion Pumps*, 2020. Fenton, MO: Progressive Medical, Inc.; Updated May 2020.
8. *Drug Stability for Easypump® ST/LT*, 2020. Bethlehem, PA: B. Braun USA; Updated June 2020.
9. *Drug Stability Table - Dosi-Fuser® Elastomeric Pump (S-CL-00-001v16)*, 2021. Barcelona, Spain: Leventon SAU; Updated May 2021.
10. Ganciclovir Sodium Injection, Lyophilized [package insert]. Schaumburg, IL: APP Pharmaceuticals, LLC; November 2018.

Gemcitabine Hydrochloride

Storage Conditions

						Temperature			Post-thaw Temp			
	Drug Manufacturer	Concentration	Diluents	Osmolality (mOsm/kg)	pH	Room	Refrig	Frozen	Room	Refrig	Body Temp	Refer.
CONTAINER												
Bag, Polyvinyl Chloride (PVC)	LI	0.1, 10 mg/mL	D5W, NS	n/a	[c]	5 wk	5 wk[a][b]	n/a	n/a	n/a	n/a	(1)
	LI	0.1, 10, 38 mg/mL	D5W, NS	n/a	[c]	n/a	n/a	n/a	n/a	n/a	7 d[a][d]	(1)
	LI	7.5, 25 mg/mL	NS	n/a	[c]	27 d	n/a	n/a	n/a	n/a	n/a	(2)
Syringe, Polypropylene	LI	38 mg/mL	NS	n/a	[c]	5 wk	5 wk[a][b]	n/a	n/a	n/a	n/a	(1)
Vial, Glass	LI	38 mg/mL	NS, SWFI	n/a	[c]	5 wk	7 d[a][b]	n/a	n/a	n/a	n/a	(1)
	LI	7.5, 25 mg/mL	NS	n/a	[c]	27 d	n/a	n/a	n/a	n/a	n/a	(2)
OTHER INFUSION CONTAINERS												
INTERMATE™ (Baxter)[e]	LI	3-40 mg/mL	NS	n/a	[c]	7 d	n/a	n/a	n/a	n/a	n/a	(3)

Flush Compatibility: Sodium chloride 0.9%, heparin.[2]

Special Considerations: Avoid refrigeration of reconstituted solutions due to the potential for crystallization. Concentrate for injection should not be frozen.[2]

Notes

[a] Protected from light.[1]

[b] Reconstituted solution may develop non-redissolving crystals when stored at 4°C.[1,2]

[c] pH of reconstituted solution is 2.7-3.3.[1]

[d] Storage temperature: 32°C.[1]

[e] INTERMATE™/INFUSOR™ Portable Elastomeric Infusion System devices are no longer available in the United States.

REFERENCES

1. Xu Q, Zhang Y, Trissel LA. Physical and chemical stability of gemcitabine hydrochloride solutions. *J Am Pharm Assoc (Wash)*. 1999; 39(4):509-13.
2. ASHP's Interactive Handbook on Injectable Drugs, 2020. Bethesda, MD: American Society of Health-System Pharmacists; Accessed July 2020.
3. Stabforum - Stability Database: Gemcitabine, Ontario, Canada: Baxter Healthcare; Accessed August 2020.

DOI 10.37573/9781585286720.098

Gentamicin Sulfate

Storage Conditions

						Temperature			Post-thaw Temp			
	Drug Manufacturer	Concentration	Diluents	Osmolality (mOsm/kg)	pH	Room	Refrig	Frozen	Room	Refrig	Body Temp	Refer.
CONTAINER												
Bag, Polyvinyl Chloride (PVC)	SC	0.8 mg/mL	D5W	285	(c)	24 hr	n/a	30 d	24 hr	n/a	n/a	(1)
	SC	1 mg/mL	D5W, NS	(d)	(c)	24 hr	24 hr	30 d	n/a	n/a	n/a	(1)
	LY	1.2 mg/mL	D5W, NS	(d)	(c)	48 hr	48 hr	n/a	n/a	n/a	n/a	(1)
	ES	2.4 mg/mL	D5W, NS	(d)	(c)	n/a	n/a	28 d	n/a	n/a	n/a	(1)
Syringe, Glass	ES	10 mg/mL	NS	(d)	(c)	n/a	12 wk	n/a	n/a	n/a	n/a	(1)
Syringe, Polypropylene	ES	30 mg/mL	NS	(d)	(c)	48 hr	n/a	n/a	n/a	n/a	n/a	(1)
	UN	40 mg/mL	Undiluted	(d)	(c)	30 d	30 d	n/a	n/a	n/a	n/a	(1)
OTHER INFUSION CONTAINERS												
CADD® Cassette (Smiths Medical)	SC	5.45 mg/mL	D5W	(d)	(c)	n/a	n/a	30 d	n/a	4 d(f)	48 hr(f)	(1)
Dosi-Fuser® (Leventon)	HOS	5 mg/mL	D5W, NS	(d)	(c)	48 hr	17 d	30 d	n/a	n/a	n/a	(3)
	LY	0.5-5 mg/mL	D5W, NS	(d)	(c)	24 hr(a)	10 d(a)	30 d(a)	n/a	n/a	n/a	(3)
Easypump® ST/LT (B. Braun)	UN	0.5 mg/mL	NS	(d)	(c)	7 d	7 d	n/a	n/a	n/a	n/a	(4)
	UN	5 mg/mL	NS	(d)	(c)	7 d	14 d	n/a	n/a	n/a	n/a	(4)
Homepump Eclipse® / Homepump® (Halyard)	UN	0.8 mg/mL	NS	(d)	(c)	24 hr	n/a	n/a	n/a	n/a	n/a	(7)
	UN	1 mg/mL	D5W, NS	(d)	(c)	n/a	n/a	30 d(a)	n/a	n/a	n/a	(7)
	UN	4.8 mg/mL	NS	(d)	(c)	24 hr	28 d	n/a	n/a	n/a	n/a	(7)
INTERMATE™ (Baxter)(g)	LY	0.25 mg/mL	SWFI	(d)	(c)	n/a	10 d	n/a	n/a	n/a	n/a	(2)
	RS, ES	0.5 mg/mL	NS	(d)	(c)	48 hr	10 d	32 d	24 hr	n/a	n/a	(2)
	LY	0.5-5 mg/mL	D5W	(d)	(c)	24 hr	10 d	n/a	n/a	n/a	n/a	(2)
	LY	0.5-5 mg/mL	D5W, NS	(d)	(c)	n/a	n/a	30 d	24 hr	n/a	n/a	(2)
SMARTeZ® (Progressive Medical)	UN	0.5 mg/mL	NS	(d)	(c)	7 d(a)	7 d(a)	n/a	n/a	n/a	n/a	(5)
	UN	5 mg/mL	NS	(d)	(c)	7 d(a)	14 d(a)	n/a	n/a	n/a	n/a	(5)
	UN	10 mg/mL	NS	(d)	(c)	48 hr	28 d	n/a	n/a	n/a	n/a	(5)

DOI 10.37573/9781585286720.099

Storage Conditions

	Drug Manufacturer	Concentration	Diluents	Osmolality (mOsm/kg)	pH	Temperature			Post-thaw Temp			
						Room	Refrig	Frozen	Room	Refrig	Body Temp	Refer.
COMMERCIAL PREPARATIONS (RTU)												
ViaFlex™ Plus Container (Baxter)	BA	0.8, 1, 1.2, 1.6, 1, 2 mg/mL	NS	[b]	4.5	[e]	n/a	n/a	n/a	n/a	n/a	(6)

Flush Compatibility: Sodium chloride 0.9%. Incompatible with heparin.[1]

Special Considerations: n/a

Notes

[a] Manufacturer extrapolated data from other sources.

[b] The osmolarity of the premixed infusions in sodium chloride 0.9% is approximately 284 to 308 mOsm/L.[1]

[c] pH of undiluted injection is 3-5.5. pH of commercial solutions in NS is 4-4.5.[1]

[d] Undiluted gentamicin sulfate 40 mg/mL has an osmolality of 160 mOsm/kg. Gentamicin sulfate pediatric injection 10 mg/mL has an osmolality of 116 mOsm/kg by freezing-point depression or 212 mOsm/kg by vapor pressure. Gentamicin at 1 mg/mL has an osmolality of 262 and 278 mOsm/kg in D5W and NS respectively; at 2.5 mg/mL osmolality is 278 and 293 in D5W and NS respectively.[1]

[e] Expiration date per manufacturer's label. Do not extrapolate commercial premix stability data to extemporaneously compounded solutions.[6]

[f] Stored for 30 d at −20°C, followed by 4 d at 5°C, followed by 48 hr at 37°C.[1]

[g] INTERMATE™/INFUSOR™ Portable Elastomeric Infusion System devices are no longer available in the United States.

REFERENCES

1. ASHP's Interactive Handbook on Injectable Drugs, 2020. Bethesda, MD: American Society of Health-System Pharmacists; Accessed July 2020.
2. Stabforum - Stability Database: Gentamicin, Ontario, Canada: Baxter Healthcare; Accessed February 2021.
3. *Drug Stability Table - Dosi-Fuser® Elastomeric Pump (S-CL-00-001v16)*, 2021. Barcelona, Spain: Leventon SAU; Updated May 2021.
4. *Drug Stability for Easypump® ST/LT*, 2020. Bethlehem, PA: B. Braun USA; Updated June 2020.
5. *SMARTeZ® - Stability Data for Drugs Using Elastomeric Infusion Pumps*, 2020. Fenton, MO: Progressive Medical, Inc.; Updated May 2020.
6. Gentamicin Sulfate in Sodium Chloride Injection in VIAFLEX™ Plus Container [package insert]. Deerfield, IL: Baxter Healthcare Corporation; March 2019.
7. *Stability Data for Drugs Using Homepump Disposable Ambulatory Infusion Systems (MK-00314 rev 3)*, 2015. Alpharetta, GA: Halyard Health; Updated June 2015.

Glycopyrrolate

Storage Conditions

						Temperature			Post-thaw Temp			
	Drug Manufacturer	Concentration	Diluents	Osmolality (mOsm/kg)	pH	Room	Refrig	Frozen	Room	Refrig	Body Temp	Refer.
CONTAINER												
Syringe, Polypropylene	LEI	0.025 mg/mL	NS[a]	n/a	[f]	30 d[b]	30 d[b]	n/a	n/a	n/a	16 d[b][d]	(2)
	RB	0.2 mg/mL	Undiluted	n/a	[e]	90 d	90 d	n/a	n/a	n/a	n/a	(1)
	AMR	0.1 mg/mL	NS	n/a	n/a	24 hr	24 hr	n/a	n/a	n/a	n/a	(1)
Unspecified	RB	0.0008 mg/mL	D5W, NS, D5½NS	n/a	[c]	48 hr	n/a	n/a	n/a	n/a	n/a	(1)
OTHER INFUSION CONTAINERS												
CADD® Cassette (Smiths Medical)	LEI	0.025 mg/mL[a]	NS	n/a	[f]	30 d[b]	30 d[b]	n/a	n/a	n/a	9 d[b][d]	(2)

Flush Compatibility: Sodium chloride 0.9%.[1]

Special Considerations: Contains benzyl alcohol.[1] Because of the low pH of glycopyrrolate, admixture with alkaline drugs or solutions that result in an admixed pH above 6.0 will result in glycopyrrolate decomposition through hydrolysis.[1]

Notes

[a] Solution contained: buprenorphine (RKC) 0.084 mg/mL and haloperidol (ON) 0.104 mg/mL.[2]

[b] Protected from light.[2]

[c] pH range of 2.0-6.0.

[d] Storage temperature: 36°C.[2]

[e] pH of undiluted solution is 2-3.[1]

[f] pH of final admixture is 3.46.[2]

REFERENCES

1. ASHP's Interactive Handbook on Injectable Drugs, 2020. Bethesda, MD: American Society of Health-System Pharmacists; Accessed August 2020.
2. Jappinen A, Kokki H, Naaranlahti TJ, et al. Stability of buprenorphine, haloperidol and glycopyrrolate mixture in a 0.9% sodium chloride solution. *Pharm World Sci*. 1999; 21(6):272-4.

DOI 10.37573/9781585286720.100

Granisetron Hydrochloride

Storage Conditions

	Drug Manufacturer	Concentration	Diluents	Osmolality (mOsm/kg)	pH	Temperature: Room	Temperature: Refrig	Temperature: Frozen	Post-thaw Temp: Room	Post-thaw Temp: Refrig	Body Temp	Refer.
CONTAINER												
Bag, Polyvinyl Chloride (PVC)	SKB	0.008-0.053 mg/mL	D5W, NS[e]	n/a	[c]	5 wk	5 wk	n/a	n/a	n/a	n/a	(7)
	SKB	0.01, 0.04 mg/mL	D5W, NS[b]	n/a	[c]	14 d[d]	14 d[d]	n/a	n/a	n/a	n/a	(1)(2)
	BE	0.056 mg/mL	D5W, NS	n/a	[c]	n/a	n/a	30 d	72 hr[a]	7 d[a]	n/a	(1)
Syringe, Polypropylene	SKB	0.05, 0.07, 0.1 mg/mL	D5W, NS	n/a	[c]	14 d	14 d	n/a	n/a	n/a	n/a	(1)
	BE	0.15 mg/mL	D5W, NS	n/a	[c]	n/a	n/a	30 d	72 hr[a]	7 d[a]	n/a	(1)
	SKB	1 mg/mL	Undiluted	n/a	[c]	15 d[d]	15 d	n/a	n/a	n/a	n/a	(1)(3)
OTHER INFUSION CONTAINERS												
Dosi-Fuser® (Leventon)	UN	0.02 mg/mL	D5W	n/a	[c]	n/a	14 d[f]	n/a	n/a	n/a	n/a	(8)
	UN	0.02 mg/mL	NS	n/a	[c]	n/a	7 d[f]	n/a	n/a	n/a	n/a	(8)
Easypump® ST/LT (B. Braun)	UN	0.02, 0.5 mg/mL	NS	n/a	[c]	48 hr	7 d	n/a	n/a	n/a	n/a	(5)
	UN	0.02, 0.5 mg/mL	D5W	n/a	[c]	6 hr	72 hr	n/a	n/a	n/a	n/a	(5)
Homepump Eclipse® / Homepump® (Halyard)	SKB	0.02 mg/mL	D5W	n/a	[c]	n/a	14 d	n/a	n/a	n/a	n/a	(4)(6)
	SKB	0.02 mg/mL	NS	n/a	[c]	n/a	7 d	n/a	n/a	n/a	n/a	(4)(6)
SMARTeZ® (Progressive Medical)	UN	0.02, 0.5 mg/mL	NS	n/a	[c]	48 hr[f]	7 d[f]	n/a	n/a	n/a	n/a	(9)

Flush Compatibility: Sodium chloride 0.9%, heparin.[1]

Special Considerations: Protect intact vials from freezing and light.[1]

Notes

[a] Storage for 30 d frozen, followed by 7 d refrigerated, followed by 72 hr at 20°C.[1]

[b] Solution contained: 0.092 or 0.66 mg/mL dexAMETHasone sodium phosphate (AMR).[1,2]

[c] pH of undiluted product is 4-6.[1]

[d] Protected from light.

[e] Solution tested with and without dexAMETHasone (SAB) 0.05-0.35 mg/mL.[7]

[f] Manufacturer extrapolated data from other sources.

DOI 10.37573/9781585286720.101

REFERENCES

1. ASHP's Interactive Handbook on Injectable Drugs, 2020. Bethesda, MD: American Society of Health-System Pharmacists; Accessed September 2020.
2. Chin A, Moon YS, Chung KC, et al. Stability of granisetron hydrochloride with dexamethasone sodium phosphate for 14 days. *Am J Health Syst Pharm*. 1996; 53(10):1174-6.
3. Hourcade F, Sautou-Miranda V, Normand B, et al. Compatibility of granisetron towards glass and plastics and its stability under various storage conditions. *Int J Pharm*. 1997; 154(1):95-102.
4. *Stability Data for Drugs Using Homepump Disposable Ambulatory Infusion Systems (MK-00314 rev 3)*, 2015. Alpharetta, GA: Halyard Health; Updated June 2015.
5. *Drug Stability for Easypump® ST/LT*, 2020. Bethlehem, PA: B. Braun USA; Updated June 2020.
6. Chung KC, Chin A, Gill MA. Stability of granisetron hydrochloride in a disposable elastomeric infusion device. *Am J Health Syst Pharm*. 1995; 52(14):1541-3.
7. Walker S, Law S. Stability and Compatibility of Granisetron Alone and in Combination with Dexamethasone in 0.9% Sodium Chloride and 5% Dextrose in Water Solutions. *Can J Hosp Pharm*. 2002; 55(1):27-38.
8. *Drug Stability Table - Dosi-Fuser® Elastomeric Pump (ES.H.00.73-10)*, 2015. Barcelona, Spain: Leventon SAU; Updated October 2015.
9. *SMARTeZ® - Stability Data for Drugs Using Elastomeric Infusion Pumps*, 2020. Fenton, MO: Progressive Medical, Inc.; Updated May 2020.

Haloperidol Lactate

Storage Conditions

	Drug Manufacturer	Concentration	Diluents	Osmolality (mOsm/kg)	pH	Temperature: Room	Temperature: Refrig	Temperature: Frozen	Post-thaw Temp: Room	Post-thaw Temp: Refrig	Body Temp	Refer.
CONTAINER												
Bag, Polyvinyl Chloride (PVC)	MN	0.1 mg/mL	D5W	n/a	3-3.6	38 d	n/a	n/a	n/a	n/a	n/a	(1)
Syringe, Polypropylene	ON	0.104 mg/mL	NS[b]	n/a	3.46	30 d[a]	30 d[a]	n/a	n/a	n/a	16 d[d]	(3)
	EST	0.208, 0.416, 0.624 mg/mL	NS[f]	n/a	n/a	15 d[a]	15 d[a]	n/a	n/a	n/a	n/a	(4)
	SI	5 mg/mL	Undiluted	n/a	3.3-3.4	60 d[a]	n/a	n/a	n/a	n/a	n/a	(2)
Unspecified	EST	0.208, 0.416, 0.624 mg/mL	NS[e]	n/a	4.7-5.62	15 d[a]	n/a	n/a	n/a	n/a	n/a	(5)
Vial, Glass	MN	0.1 mg/mL	D5W	n/a	3-3.6	38 d	n/a	n/a	n/a	n/a	n/a	(1)
OTHER INFUSION CONTAINERS												
CADD® Cassette (Smiths Medical)	ON	0.104 mg/mL	NS[b]	n/a	3.46	30 d[a]	30 d[a]	n/a	n/a	n/a	9 d[d]	(3)
INFUSOR™ (Baxter)	EST	0.15, 0.3 mg/mL	NS[c]	n/a	n/a	72 hr[a]	n/a	n/a	n/a	n/a	72 hr[a]	(6)

Flush Compatibility: Sodium chloride 0.9%.[1]

Special Considerations: n/a

Notes

[a] Protected from light.

[b] Solution contained: buprenorphine 0.084 mg/mL (RKC) and glycopyrrolate 0.025 mg/mL (LEI).[3]

[c] Solution contained: morphine sulfate 0.8, 1.6, 3 mg/mL.[6]

[d] Storage temperature: 36°C.

[e] With traMADol HCl 8.8-33.3 mg/mL (GRU) and hyoscine N-butylbromide 3.33-6.67 mg/mL (BI).[5]

[f] With traMADol HCl 8.33, 16.67, 33.33 mg/mL (GRU).[4]

DOI 10.37573/9781585286720.102

REFERENCES

1. ASHP's Interactive Handbook on Injectable Drugs, 2020. Bethesda, MD: American Society of Health-System Pharmacists; Accessed May 2020.
2. Morrissey H, Ball P. Stability and Sterility Data in Pre-Filled Syringes for Zuclopenthixol Acetate and Haloperidol Used in Emergency Tranquilisation. *Primary Health Care*. 2015; 5(1):1-4.
3. Jappinen A, Kokki H, Naaranlahti TJ, et al. Stability of buprenorphine, haloperidol and glycopyrrolate mixture in a 0.9% sodium chloride solution. *Pharm World Sci*. 1999; 21(6):272-4.
4. Negro S, Martin A, Azuara ML, et al. Stability of tramadol and haloperidol for continuous subcutaneous infusion at home. *J Pain Symptom Manage*. 2005; 30(2):192-9.
5. Negro S, Martin A, Azuara L, et al. Compatibility and stability of ternary admixtures of tramadol, haloperidol, and hyoscine N-butyl bromide: retrospective clinical evaluation. *J Palliat Med*. 2010; 13(3):273-7.
6. Marìa EB, Fuensanta SnR, Catalina BO. Determination of compatibility and stability of haloperidol and morphine mixtures used in palliative care. *Braz J Pharm Sci*. 2018; 54(2):e17352.

Heparin Sodium

Storage Conditions

	Drug Manufacturer	Concentration	Diluents	Osmolality (mOsm/kg)	pH	Temperature Room	Temperature Refrig	Temperature Frozen	Post-thaw Temp Room	Post-thaw Temp Refrig	Body Temp	Refer.
CONTAINER												
Bag, Ethylene Vinyl Acetate (EVA)	FUJ	5 units/mL	NS	n/a	[a]	n/a	28 d	n/a	n/a	n/a	n/a	(3)
Bag, Polyvinyl Chloride (PVC)	UN	5,000 units/mL	Undiluted	n/a	[a]	10 d	7 d	n/a	n/a	n/a	n/a	(4)
	OR	20, 40 units/mL	D5W, NS	n/a	[a]	48 hr	n/a	n/a	n/a	n/a	n/a	(1)
	BRN	7 units/mL	D5W, NS	n/a	[a]	24 hr	24 hr	n/a	n/a	n/a	n/a	(1)
	UP	10 units/mL	LR, D5NS, D5LR	n/a	[a]	n/a	24 hr	n/a	n/a	n/a	n/a	(1)
Syringe, Polyethylene	UN	1 unit/mL	unspec.	n/a	[a]	n/a	n/a	n/a	n/a	n/a	1 yr	(1)
Syringe, Polypropylene	UN	500 units/mL	NS	n/a	[a]	21 d	21 d	n/a	n/a	n/a	n/a	(1)
	ES	1,000 units/mL	Undiluted	384	[a]	n/a	n/a	n/a	n/a	n/a	30 d[e]	(1)
	SCN	40,000 units/mL	Undiluted	n/a	[a]	n/a	n/a	n/a	n/a	n/a	30 d[e]	(1)
	HOS	100 units/mL	LR[b]	n/a	[a]	n/a	14 d	14 d	n/a	n/a	n/a	(2)
Unspecified	DB	1 unit/mL	D5W	n/a	[a]	7 d	n/a	n/a	n/a	n/a	n/a	(1)
	DB	1 unit/mL	NS	n/a	[a]	1 yr	n/a	n/a	n/a	n/a	n/a	(1)
	LY	5 units/mL	NS	n/a	[a]	n/a	28 d	n/a	n/a	n/a	n/a	(1)
	DB	10 units/mL	D5W	n/a	[a]	1 yr	n/a	n/a	n/a	n/a	n/a	(1)
	DB	10 units/mL	NS	n/a	[a]	1 yr	1 yr	n/a	n/a	n/a	n/a	(1)
	AH	35 units/mL	NS	n/a	[a]	24 hr	14 d	n/a	n/a	n/a	n/a	(1)
Vial, Glass	UP	10 units/mL	LR, D5NS, D5LR	n/a	[a]	n/a	24 hr	n/a	n/a	n/a	n/a	(1)
OTHER INFUSION CONTAINERS												
CADD® Cassette (Smiths Medical)	UN	5,000 units/mL	unspec.	n/a	[a]	n/a	7 d	n/a	n/a	n/a	10 d	(4)
Dosi-Fuser® (Leventon)	DIO	3,250 units/mL	NS	n/a	[a]	7 d[h]	14 d[h]	n/a	n/a	n/a	n/a	(10)

DOI 10.37573/9781585286720.103

Storage Conditions

	Drug Manufacturer	Concentration	Diluents	Osmolality (mOsm/kg)	pH	Temperature Room	Temperature Refrig	Temperature Frozen	Post-thaw Temp Room	Post-thaw Temp Refrig	Body Temp	Refer.
COMMERCIAL PREPARATIONS (RTU)												
Excel® Container (B. Braun)	BRN	2 units/mL	NS	360[g]	6.8-7.2	[f]	n/a	n/a	n/a	n/a	n/a	(8)(9)
	BRN	40, 50, 100 units/mL	D5W	315[g]	4.5-7.0	[f]	n/a	n/a	n/a	n/a	n/a	(7)(9)
Flexible Plastic (CR3) Container (Hospira)	HOS	50, 100 units/mL	D5W	304[g]	[a]	[d]	n/a	n/a	n/a	n/a	n/a	(5)(9)
Flexible Plastic (PVC) Container (Hospira)	HOS	2 units/mL	NS	378[g]	[a]	[c]	n/a	n/a	n/a	n/a	n/a	(6)(9)

Flush Compatibility: Sodium chloride 0.9%, heparin.[1]

Special Considerations: Do not freeze. Use care when adding to large volume parenteral solutions, especially flexible containers; repeated inversion and agitation after admixture provides an even distribution of heparin in the solution and a constant delivery concentration; it also eliminates the danger of overdosage due to pooling.[1]

Notes

[a] pH of undiluted injection and lock flush is adjusted to 5-7.5.[1]

[b] Solution contained: daptomycin 5 mg/mL.[2]

[c] Expiration date per manufacturer's label. Manufacturer recommends that premixed medications, in PVC containers, > 25 mL in volume should be used within 30 days after removal from overwrap.[6,9]

[d] Expiration date per manufacturer's label. Manufacturer recommends using within 7 days of removal of the overwrap.[5,9]

[e] Storage temperature: 30°C.[1]

[f] Expiration date per manufacturer's label. Manufacturer recommends that premixed medications, in Excel® containers, ≤ 250 mL in volume should be used within 2 months, and 500 mL and 100 mL in volume should be used within 3 months.[7-9]

[g] Expressed as mOsm/L.

[h] Manufacturer extrapolated data from other sources.

REFERENCES

1. ASHP's Interactive Handbook on Injectable Drugs, 2020. Bethesda, MD: American Society of Health-System Pharmacists; Accessed August 2020.
2. Ortega R, Salmeron-Garcia A, Cabeza J, et al. Stability of daptomycin 5 mg/mL and heparin sodium 100 units/mL combined in lactated Ringer's injection and stored in polypropylene syringes at 4 and -20 degrees C. *Am J Health Syst Pharm*. 2014; 71(11):956-9.
3. Hensrud DD, Burritt MF, Hall LG. Stability of heparin anticoagulant activity over time in parenteral nutrition solutions. *J Parenter Enteral Nutr*. 1996; 20(3):219-21.
4. *Pharmaceutical report on chemical and physical stability of drugs commonly used with CADD® infusion pumps (IN193109GB-122019)*, 2019. Minneapolis, MN: Smiths Medical ASD, Inc.; Updated December 2019.

5. Heparin Sodium and Dextrose Injection [package insert]. Lake Forest, IL: Hospira, Inc.; July 2020.
6. Heparin Sodium Injection [package insert]. Lake Forest, IL: Hospira, Inc.; June 2020.
7. Heparin Sodium in Dextrose Injection [package insert]. Bethlehem, PA: B. Braun Medical, Inc.; September 2020.
8. Heparin Sodium in Sodium Chloride Injection [package insert]. Bethlehem, PA: B. Braun Medical, Inc.; May 2016.
9. Cohen MR. Medication errors. 2nd ed. Washington, D.C.: American Pharmacists Association; 2007:142.
10. *Drug Stability Table - Dosi-Fuser® Elastomeric Pump (S-CL-00-001v16)*, 2021. Barcelona, Spain: Leventon SAU; Updated May 2021.

HydrALAZINE Hydrochloride

Storage Conditions

						Temperature			Post-thaw Temp			
	Drug Manufacturer	Concentration	Diluents	Osmolality (mOsm/kg)	pH[e]	Room	Refrig	Frozen	Room	Refrig	Body Temp	Refer.
CONTAINER												
Bag, Polyvinyl Chloride (PVC)	SI	0.015 mg/mL	NS	n/a	5.1	7 d[b][d]	n/a	n/a	n/a	n/a	n/a	(3)
	AMR	0.2 mg/mL	NS	n/a	4.1-4.9[a]	48 hr	n/a	n/a	n/a	n/a	n/a	(1)(2)
	UN	0.35 mg/mL	NS	n/a	[e]	52 d	n/a	n/a	n/a	n/a	n/a	(1)
Syringe, Polypropylene[c]	SI	0.027 mg/mL	NS	n/a	[e]	24 hr[d]	n/a	n/a	n/a	n/a	n/a	(4)

Flush Compatibility: Sodium chloride 0.9%, heparin.[1]

Special Considerations: HydrALAZINE reacts with various metals. Contact with metal parts (e.g., stainless steel needles) should be minimized. Store at controlled room temperature; refrigeration may cause crystallization.[1]

Notes

[a] pH of solution decreased from 4.9 on day 0 to 4.1 after 2 days.

[b] 10% loss due to sorption in Viaflex® sodium chloride 0.9% PVC bags (TR) at 0.015 mg/mL.[3]

[c] Syringes with polyethylene plungers.[1,4]

[d] Protected from light.

[e] pH of undiluted product is 3.4-4.4.[1]

REFERENCES

1. ASHP's Interactive Handbook on Injectable Drugs, 2020. Bethesda, MD: American Society of Health-System Pharmacists; Accessed July 2020.
2. Gupta VD. Chemical stability of hydralazine hydrochloride after reconstitution in 0.9% sodium chloride injection or 5% dextrose injection for infusion. *Int J Pharm Compd*. 2005; 9(5):399-401.
3. Kowaluk EA, Roberts MS, Blackburn HD, et al. Interactions between drugs and polyvinyl chloride infusion bags. *Am J Hosp Pharm*. 1981; 38(9):1308-14.
4. Kowaluk EA, Roberts MS, Polack AE. Interactions between drugs and intravenous delivery systems. *Am J Hosp Pharm*. 1982; 39(3):460-7.

DOI 10.37573/9781585286720.104

Hydrocortisone Sodium Succinate

Storage Conditions

	Drug Manufacturer	Concentration	Diluents	Osmolality (mOsm/kg)	pH	Temperature Room	Temperature Refrig	Temperature Frozen	Post-thaw Temp Room	Post-thaw Temp Refrig	Body Temp	Refer.
CONTAINER												
Bag, Polyolefin	UN	1 mg/mL	NS	[d]	6.3-7.3	6 d[c]	48 d	n/a	n/a	n/a	n/a	(3)
Bag, Polyvinyl Chloride (PVC)	UN	1 mg/mL	NS	[d]	6.3-7.3	7 d[c]	41 d	n/a	n/a	n/a	n/a	(3)
Syringe, Polypropylene	UP	10 mg/mL	NS	[d]	[a]	7 d	21 d	n/a	n/a	n/a	n/a	(1)(2)
	PH	50 mg/mL	SWFI	[d]	6.3-7.6	6 d	81 d	n/a	n/a	n/a	n/a	(1)(3)
Vial, Glass	UP	125 mg/mL	SWFI, NS[b]	[d]	[a]	n/a	n/a	28 d	n/a	n/a	n/a	(1)
	PH	50, 125 mg/mL	SWFI, BWFI, BNS[f]	[d]	7-8	72 hr[e]	n/a	n/a	n/a	n/a	n/a	(4)

Flush Compatibility: Sodium chloride 0.9%, heparin.[1]

Special Considerations: n/a

Notes

[a] pH of reconstituted solution is 7-8.[1]

[b] Reconstituted vial.

[c] Stability increased to 8 days, when protected from light.[3]

[d] 50 mg/mL solution (AB) is 260-292 mOsm/kg.[1]

[e] Protected from light.

[f] Bacteriostatic Sodium Chloride Injection.[4]

REFERENCES

1. ASHP's Interactive Handbook on Injectable Drugs, 2020. Bethesda, MD: American Society of Health-System Pharmacists; Accessed November 2020.
2. Gupta VD, Ling J. Stability of hydrocortisone sodium succinate after reconstitution in 0.9% sodium chloride injection and storage in polypropylene syringes for pediatric use. *Int J Pharm Compd*. 2000; 4(5):396-7.
3. Rigge DC, Jones MF. Shelf lives of aseptically prepared medicines–stability of hydrocortisone sodium succinate in PVC and non-PVC bags and in polypropylene syringes. *J Pharm Biomed Anal*. 2005; 38(2):332-6.
4. Solu-Cortef® (Hydrocortisone Sodium Succinate) Injection [package insert]. New York, NY: Pharmacia & Upjohn Company LLC; September 2020.

DOI 10.37573/9781585286720.105

HYDROmorphone Hydrochloride

Storage Conditions

	Drug Manufacturer	Concentration	Diluents	Osmolality (mOsm/kg)	pH	Temperature: Room	Temperature: Refrig	Temperature: Frozen	Post-thaw Temp: Room	Post-thaw Temp: Refrig	Body Temp	Refer.
CONTAINER												
Bag, Polyolefin	SZ	0.01 mg/mL	NS[j][k][l]	n/a	4.0-5.1	n/a	28 d[a]	n/a	n/a	n/a	n/a	(5)
	SZ	25 mg/mL	NS[k]	n/a	4.6-4.8	n/a	28 d[a]	n/a	n/a	n/a	n/a	(5)
	SZ	43 mg/mL	NS[l]	n/a	4.6-4.8	n/a	28 d[a]	n/a	n/a	n/a	n/a	(5)
Bag, Polyvinyl Chloride (PVC)	KN	0.02, 0.1 mg/mL	NS	n/a	[f]	72 hr[b]	n/a	n/a	n/a	n/a	n/a	(1)
	SZ	0.2 mg/mL	NS[i]	n/a	[f]	7 d[a]	n/a	n/a	n/a	n/a	n/a	(4)
	KN	1, 5 mg/mL	D5W, NS	n/a	[f]	6 wk	6 wk	n/a	n/a	n/a	n/a	(1)
	UN	10, 50 mg/mL	unspec.	n/a	[f]	6 wk	6 wk	n/a	n/a	n/a	n/a	(1)
Syringe, Plastic (Unspecified)	SZ	0.2 mg/mL	NS[i]	n/a	[f]	7 d[a]	n/a	n/a	n/a	n/a	n/a	(4)
Syringe, Polypropylene	SZ	0.01 mg/mL	NS[j][k][l]	n/a	4.6-5.4	n/a	28 d[a]	n/a	n/a	n/a	n/a	(5)
	SAB	0.02, 0.04 mg/mL	NS[g]	n/a	[f]	13 wk[b]	13 wk[a]	n/a	n/a	n/a	n/a	(3)
	KN	0.1 mg/mL	NS	n/a	[f]	30 d	n/a	n/a	n/a	n/a	n/a	(1)
	UN[d]	1.5, 80 mg/mL	NS	n/a	[f]	60 d	60 d[a]	n/a	n/a	n/a	n/a	(1)
	KN	10 mg/mL	Undiluted	n/a	[f]	30 d	n/a	n/a	n/a	n/a	n/a	(1)
	SZ	25 mg/mL	NS[k]	n/a	4.6-4.8	n/a	28 d[a]	n/a	n/a	n/a	n/a	(5)
	SZ	43 mg/mL	NS[l]	n/a	4.5-4.7	n/a	28 d[a]	n/a	n/a	n/a	n/a	(5)
Vial, Glass	UN[d]	10, 50 mg/mL	unspec.	n/a	[f]	6 wk	6 wk	n/a	n/a	n/a	n/a	(1)
	SZ	0.2 mg/mL	NS[i]	n/a	[f]	7 d[a]	n/a	n/a	n/a	n/a	n/a	(4)
OTHER INFUSION CONTAINERS												
Dosi-Fuser® (Leventon)	KN	1 mg/mL	D5W	n/a	[f]	7 d[e]	32 d[c][e]	n/a	n/a	n/a	n/a	(2)
	KN	1-10 mg/mL	NS	n/a	[f]	7 d[e]	32 d[c][e]	n/a	n/a	n/a	n/a	(2)
SynchroMed® EL Implantable Pump (Medtronic)	KN	2, 10 mg/mL	Undiluted	n/a	[f]	n/a	n/a	n/a	n/a	n/a	4 m[h]	(6)

DOI 10.37573/9781585286720.106

Flush Compatibility: Sodium chloride 0.9%, heparin.[1]

Special Considerations: n/a

Notes

[a] Protected from light.
[b] Exposed to fluorescent light.[1,3]
[c] 32 d refrigerated, followed by 72 hr at room temperature.[2]
[d] Compounded using HYDROmorphone hydrochloride powder.[1]
[e] Manufacturer extrapolated data from other sources.[2]
[f] pH range of undiluted product is 4-5.5.[1]
[g] Solution contained: bupivacaine (AST) 2.5 mg/mL.[3]
[h] Storage temperature: 37°C.[6]
[i] Solution contained: ketamine (SZ) 0.2, 0.6, and 1 mg/mL.[4]
[j] Solution contained: bupivacaine (HOS) 37.5 mg/mL.[5]
[k] Solution contained: bupivacaine (HOS) 20 mg/mL.[5]
[l] Solution contained: bupivacaine (HOS) 0.01 mg/mL.[5]

REFERENCES

1. ASHP's Interactive Handbook on Injectable Drugs, 2020. Bethesda, MD: American Society of Health-System Pharmacists; Accessed September 2020.
2. *Drug Stability Table - Dosi-Fuser® Elastomeric Pump (ES.H.00.73-10)*, 2015. Barcelona, Spain: Leventon SAU; Updated October 2015.
3. Donnelly RF. Physical Compatibility and Chemical Stability of Bupivacaine and Hydromorphone in Polypropylene Syringes. *Can J Hosp Pharm*. 2004; 57(4):230.
4. Ensom MH, Decarie D, Leung K, et al. Stability of Hydromorphone-Ketamine Solutions in Glass Bottles, Plastic Syringes, and IV Bags for Pediatric Use. *Can J Hosp Pharm*. 2009; 62(2):112-8.
5. Donnelly RF, Wong K, Spencer J. Physical compatibility of high-concentration bupivacaine with hydromorphone, morphine, and fentanyl. *Can J Hosp Pharm*. 2010; 63(2):154-5.
6. Hildebrand KR, Elsberry DE, Anderson VC. Stability and compatibility of hydromorphone hydrochloride in an implantable infusion system. *J Pain Symptom Manage*. 2001; 22(6):1042-7.

HydrOXYzine Hydrochloride

Storage Conditions

						Temperature			Post-thaw Temp			
	Drug Manufacturer	Concentration	Diluents	Osmolality (mOsm/kg)	pH	Room	Refrig	Frozen	Room	Refrig	Body Temp	Refer.
CONTAINER												
Syringe, Glass	PF	12.5 mg/mL[b]	[b]	n/a	n/a	12 m[c]	12 m[c]	n/a	n/a	n/a	n/a	(1)
Syringe, Plastic (Unspecified)	PF	12.5 mg/mL[b]	[b]	n/a	n/a	12 m[c]	12 m[c]	n/a	n/a	n/a	n/a	(1)
	NF	50 mg/mL[d]	[d]	n/a	[a]	10 d	10 d	n/a	n/a	n/a	n/a	(1)

Flush Compatibility: Sodium chloride 0.9%. Incompatible with heparin.[2]

Special Considerations: n/a

Notes

[a] pH of undiluted solution is 3.5-6.[1]

[b] Solution contained: chlorproMAZINE HCl 6.25 mg/mL (ES) and meperidine HCl 25 mg/mL (WI).

[c] Protected from light.

[d] Solution contained: atropine sulfate USP 1 mg/mL.

REFERENCES

1. ASHP's Interactive Handbook on Injectable Drugs, 2020. Bethesda, MD: American Society of Health-System Pharmacists; Accessed December 2020.
2. Misgen R. Compatibilities and incompatibilities of some intravenous solution admixtures. *Am J Health Syst Pharm*. 1965; 22:92-4.

DOI 10.37573/9781585286720.107

Ibuprofen

Storage Conditions

	Drug Manufacturer	Concentration	Diluents	Osmolality (mOsm/kg)	pH	Temperature			Post-thaw Temp			
						Room	Refrig	Frozen	Room	Refrig	Body Temp	Refer.
CONTAINER												
Bag, Plastic (Unspecified)	CMB	≤4 mg/mL[b]	NS, D5W, LR	n/a	[a]	24 hr	n/a	n/a	n/a	n/a	n/a	(1)
	CMB	≤4 mg/mL[c]	NS, D5W, LR	n/a	[a]	7 d	7 d	n/a	n/a	n/a	n/a	(2)

Flush Compatibility: Sodium chloride 0.9%. [(1)(2)]

Special Considerations: Caldolor® contains arginine; vial stopper is latex free. Dilute to a final concentration of 4 mg/mL or less prior to infusion.[(1,2)]
Do not confuse ibuprofen (Caldolor®) with ibuprofen LYSINE (LYSINATE) (NeoProfen®); these have different physicochemical properties and clinical indications.[(3)]

Notes

[a] pH of 100 mg/mL (undiluted) is approximately 7.4.[(1)]

[b] Recommended minimum dilution volume of 100 mL of appropriate diluent for fixed doses of 100, 200 and 400 mg. Minimum dilution volume of 200 mL for fixed doses of 800 mg. For weight-based dosing (e.g., pediatrics), dilute to a concentration of 4 mg/mL or less.[(1)]

[c] Dilute contents of 400 mg or 800 mg vials into a 250 mL bag of appropriate diluent per manufacturer recommendations.[(2)]

REFERENCES

1. Caldolor® (Ibuprofen) Injection [package insert]. Nashville, TN: Cumberland Pharmaceuticals, Inc.; January 2020.
2. Caldolor® Medication Information Letter (Ref#: N/A) [personal communication]. Nashville, TN: Cumberland Pharmaceuticals, Inc; 2011:1.
3. Cada DJ, Levien TL, Baker DE. Ibuprofen Lysine Injection. *Hosp Pharm*. 2006; 41(10):970-78.

DOI 10.37573/9781585286720.108

Ibuprofen LYSINATE

Storage Conditions

						Temperature			Post-thaw Temp			
	Drug Manufacturer	Concentration	Diluents	Osmolality (mOsm/kg)	pH	Room	Refrig	Frozen	Room	Refrig	Body Temp	Refer.
CONTAINER												
Unspecified, Plastic	RL	1, 4 mg/mL	D5W, NS, SWFI	n/a	6.18	15 d	n/a	n/a	n/a	n/a	n/a	(2)
	RL	27.5 mg/mL	SWFI	n/a	[a]	15 d[b]	n/a	n/a	n/a	n/a	n/a	(2)

Flush Compatibility: Sodium chloride 0.9%, D5W.[(1)]

Special Considerations: The manufacturer recommends storing vials in original carton until ready for use. Protect from light.[(1)] Stability should not be extrapolated between ibuprofen salt forms.

Notes

[a] pH of undiluted product is adjusted to 7.[(1)]

[b] Exposed to light.[(2)]

REFERENCES

1. Neoprofen® (Ibuprofen Lysine) Injection [package insert]. Lebanon, NJ: Recordati Rare Diseases, Inc.; January 2021.
2. Volonte MG, Valora PD, Cingolani A, et al. Stability of ibuprofen in injection solutions. *Am J Health Syst Pharm*. 2005; 62(6):630-3.

DOI 10.37573/9781585286720.109

Ifosfamide

Storage Conditions

	Drug Manufacturer	Concentration	Diluents	Osmolality (mOsm/kg)	pH	Temperature			Post-thaw Temp			
						Room	Refrig	Frozen	Room	Refrig	Body Temp	Refer.
CONTAINER												
Bag, Polyvinyl Chloride (PVC)	UN	0.6-20 mg/mL	D5NS, D5W, LR, NS	n/a	[e]	7 d	6 wk	n/a	n/a	n/a	n/a	(4)
	SIC	10, 20, 30 mg/mL	NS[l]	n/a	n/a	14 d	n/a	n/a	n/a	n/a	n/a	(7)
Bag, Polyolefin	UN	0.6-20 mg/mL	D5NS, D5W, LR, NS	n/a	[e]	7 d	6 wk	n/a	n/a	n/a	n/a	(4)
Syringe, Polypropylene	UN	0.6, 20 mg/mL	D5W, LR, NS	n/a	n/a	24 hr	n/a	n/a	n/a	n/a	n/a	(4)
	UN	50 mg/mL	NS[a][f]	n/a	[e]	28 d	28 d	n/a	n/a	n/a	n/a	(1)(4)
Unspecified	UN	0.6, 16 mg/mL	D5LR, D5NS, D5W, LR, NS, ½NS	n/a	n/a	7 d	6 wk	n/a	n/a	n/a	n/a	(4)
Vial, Glass	BI	80 mg/mL	NS[b]	n/a	[e]	9 d	n/a	n/a	n/a	n/a	9 d[c]	(3)(4)
	UN	0.6-20 mg/mL	D5NS, D5W, LR, NS	n/a	n/a	7 d	6 wk	n/a	n/a	n/a	n/a	(4)
OTHER INFUSION CONTAINERS												
CADD® Cassette (Smiths Medical)	FL	20, 40, 80 mg/mL	NS	n/a	[e]	n/a	n/a	n/a	n/a	n/a	8 d[g]	(2)(4)
	FL	80 mg/mL	SWFI	n/a	[e]	n/a	n/a	n/a	n/a	n/a	8 d[g]	(2)
	FL	10 mg/mL	NS	n/a	[e]	8 d	8 d[c]	n/a	n/a	n/a	n/a	(2)(4)
Dosi-Fuser® (Leventon)	BA	100 mg/mL	NS[i]	n/a	n/a	10 d[m]	14 d[m]	n/a	n/a	n/a	n/a	(8)
Easypump® ST/LT (B. Braun)	UN	0.6, 40 mg/mL	NS, D5W	n/a	n/a	24 hr[m]	72 hr[m]	n/a	n/a	n/a	n/a	(9)
	UN	0.6 mg/mL	D5W	n/a	n/a	7 d[m]	n/a	n/a	n/a	n/a	n/a	(9)
	UN	40 mg/mL	D5W	n/a	n/a	72 hr[m]	n/a	n/a	n/a	n/a	n/a	(9)
Graseby™ 9000 Cassette (Graseby Medical)	AM	20 mg/mL	SWFI[d]	n/a	[e]	n/a	14 d[c]	n/a	n/a	n/a	7 d[c]	(4)(5)
INFUSOR™ (Baxter)[k]	AM	0.8-100 mg/mL	NS[h]	n/a	n/a	n/a	7 d[j]	n/a	n/a	n/a	48 hr[j]	(6)
SMARTeZ® (Progressive Medical)	UN	0.06, 40 mg/mL	NS, D5W	n/a	n/a	24 hr[m]	72 hr[m]	n/a	n/a	n/a	n/a	(10)

DOI 10.37573/9781585286720.110

Flush Compatibility: Sodium chloride 0.9%.[4]

Special Considerations: Do not reconstitute ifosfamide with BWFI containing benzyl alcohol.

Notes

[a] Solution contained: mesna 40 mg/mL.
[b] Solution contained: mesna (BI) 76 mg/mL or ifosfamide alone. Mesna stability not tested.
[c] Protected from light.
[d] Solution contained: mesna (AM) 20 mg/mL.
[e] pH of solution is approximately 6.0.[1]
[f] Solution contained: epiRUBicin 1 mg/mL.
[g] Storage temperature: 35°C.
[h] Solution contained: mesna (AM) 0.4-100 mg/mL.
[i] Solution contained: mesna 100 mg/mL.
[j] 7 d refrigerated, followed by 48 hr at 33°C.
[k] INTERMATE™/INFUSOR™ Portable Elastomeric Infusion System devices are no longer available in the United States.
[l] Solution contained: mesna 1:1 respectively (10, 20 and 30 mg/mL).[7]
[m] Manufacturer extrapolated data from other sources.

REFERENCES

1. Adams P, Haines-Nutt R, Bradford E, et al. Pharmaceutical aspects of home infusion therapy for cancer patients. *Pharm J*. 1987; 238:476-78.
2. Munoz M, Girona V, Pujol M, et al. Stability of ifosfamide in 0.9% sodium chloride solution or water for injection in a portable i.v. pump cassette. *Am J Hosp Pharm*. 1992; 49(5):1137-9.
3. Radford JA, Margison JM, Swindell R, et al. The stability of ifosfamide in aqueous solution and its suitability for continuous 7-day infusion by ambulatory pump. *Cancer Chemother Pharmacol*. 1990; 26(2):144-46.
4. ASHP's Interactive Handbook on Injectable Drugs, 2020. Bethesda, MD: American Society of Health-System Pharmacists; Accessed September 2020.
5. Priston M, Sewell G. Stability of three cytotoxic drug infusions in the Graseby 9000 ambulatory infusion pump. *J Oncol Pharm Pract*. 1998; 4(3):143-49.
6. Stabforum - Stability Database: Ifosfamide, Ontario, Canada: Baxter Healthcare; Accessed January 2021.
7. Zhang Y, Kawedia JD, Myers AL, et al. Physical and chemical stability of high-dose ifosfamide and mesna for prolonged 14-day continuous infusion. *J Oncol Pharm Pract*. 2014; 20(1):51-7.
8. *Drug Stability Table - Dosi-Fuser® Elastomeric Pump (S-CL-00-001v16)*, 2020. Barcelona, Spain: Leventon SAU; Updated October 2020.
9. *Drug Stability for Easypump® ST/LT*, 2020. Bethlehem, PA: B. Braun USA; Updated June 2020.
10. *SMARTeZ® - Stability Data for Drugs Using Elastomeric Infusion Pumps*, 2020. Fenton, MO: Progressive Medical, Inc.; Updated May 2020.

Imipenem – Cilastatin Sodium

Storage Conditions

						Temperature			Post-thaw Temp			
	Drug Manufacturer	Concentration	Diluents	Osmolality (mOsm/kg)	pH	Room	Refrig	Frozen	Room	Refrig	Body Temp	Refer.
CONTAINER												
Bag, Ethylene Vinyl Acetate (EVA)	MSD	2.5, 5 mg/mL	NS	[b]	[a]	8 hr	72 hr	n/a	n/a	n/a	n/a	(5)
Bag, Polyvinyl Chloride (PVC)	MSD	5 mg/mL	D5W	[b]	7.4	6 hr	48 hr	n/a	n/a	n/a	n/a	(4)
Vial, Glass	MSD	2.5 mg/mL	D5W, D10W	[b]	[a]	6 hr	24 hr	n/a	n/a	n/a	n/a	(1)
	MSD	2.5 mg/mL	D5NS	[b]	[a]	9 hr	24 hr	n/a	n/a	n/a	n/a	(1)
	MSD	2.5 mg/mL	D5LR	[b]	[a]	3 hr	24 hr	n/a	n/a	n/a	n/a	(1)
	MSD	2.5 mg/mL	NS	[b]	[a]	9 hr	72 hr	n/a	n/a	n/a	n/a	(1)
	MSD	2.5 mg/mL	D5¼NS, D5½NS, LR	[b]	[a]	6 hr	48 hr	n/a	n/a	n/a	n/a	(1)
	MSD	5 mg/mL	NS	[b]	[a]	9 hr	48 hr	n/a	n/a	n/a	n/a	(1)
	MSD	5 mg/mL	D5¼NS, D5½NS, D5NS, D5W, D10W, LR	[b]	[a]	3 hr	24 hr	n/a	n/a	n/a	n/a	(1)
OTHER INFUSION CONTAINERS												
Dosi-Fuser® (Leventon)	MSD	5 mg/mL	NS	[b]	[a]	10 hr[e]	48 hr[e]	n/a	n/a	n/a	n/a	(8)
	MSD	5 mg/mL	NS	[b]	[a]	24 hr[e]	72 hr[e]	n/a	n/a	n/a	n/a	(8)
	MSD	5 mg/mL	D5W	[b]	[a]	4 hr[e]	24 hr[e]	n/a	n/a	n/a	n/a	(8)
Easypump® ST/LT (B. Braun)	UN	5 mg/mL	NS	[b]	[a]	24 hr	72 hr	n/a	n/a	n/a	n/a	(6)
Homepump Eclipse® / Homepump® (Halyard)	UN	5 mg/mL	NS	[b]	[a]	n/a	24 hr	n/a	n/a	n/a	n/a	(2)
	UN	5 mg/mL	NS	[b]	[a]	10 hr[e]	48 hr[e]	n/a	n/a	n/a	n/a	(2)
INTERMATE™ (Baxter)[d]	MSD	2.5 mg/mL	D5W	[b]	[a]	7 hr	24 hr[c]	n/a	n/a	n/a	n/a	(3)
	MSD	2.5 mg/mL	NS	[b]	[a]	7 hr	48 hr[c]	n/a	n/a	n/a	n/a	(3)
	MSD	5 mg/mL	D5W	[b]	[a]	7 hr	n/a	n/a	n/a	n/a	n/a	(3)
	MSD	5 mg/mL	NS	[b]	[a]	7 hr	24 hr[c]	n/a	n/a	n/a	n/a	(3)
SMARTeZ® (Progressive Medical)	UN	5 mg/mL	NS	[b]	[a]	24 hr[e]	72 hr[e]	n/a	n/a	n/a	n/a	(7)

DOI 10.37573/9781585286720.111

Flush Compatibility: Sodium chloride 0.9%, heparin.[1]

Special Considerations: Concentrations are reported as the imipenem component of a fixed combination of equal quantities of both imipenem and cilastatin. Stability applies to both components. Reconstitute vial with 10-mL diluent, shake well, and transfer resulting suspension to infusion solution container. Repeat with additional 10 mL of diluent to ensure complete transfer of vial contents to the infusion solution. Agitate resulting mixture until clear.[1]

Notes

[a] pH of the IV product is buffered to 6.5-8.5.[1]

[b] When reconstituted and diluted as directed by the manufacturer, the osmolality of the mixture approximates that of the diluent.[1]

[c] Followed by 7 hours at room temperature.[3]

[d] INTERMATE™/INFUSOR™ Portable Elastomeric Infusion System devices are no longer available in the United States.

[e] Manufacturer extrapolated data from other sources.

REFERENCES

1. ASHP's Interactive Handbook on Injectable Drugs, 2020. Bethesda, MD: American Society of Health-System Pharmacists; Accessed July 2020.
2. *Stability Data for Drugs Using Homepump Disposable Ambulatory Infusion Systems (MK-00314 rev 3)*, 2015. Alpharetta, GA: Halyard Health; Updated June 2015.
3. Stabforum - Stability Database: Cilastatin + Imipenem, Ontario, Canada: Baxter Healthcare; Accessed February 2021.
4. Walker SE, Walshaw PR, Grad H. Imipenem Stability and Staining of Teeth. *Can J Hosp Pharm*. 1997; 50(2):61-7.
5. Trissel LA, Xu QA. Stability of Imipenem-Cilastatin Sodium in AutoDose Infusion System Bags. *Hosp Pharm*. 2003; 38(2):130-34.
6. *Drug Stability for Easypump® ST/LT*, 2020. Bethlehem, PA: B. Braun USA; Updated June 2020.
7. *SMARTeZ® - Stability Data for Drugs Using Elastomeric Infusion Pumps*, 2020. Fenton, MO: Progressive Medical, Inc.; Updated May 2020.
8. *Drug Stability Table - Dosi-Fuser® Elastomeric Pump (ES.H.00.73-10)*, 2015. Barcelona, Spain: Leventon SAU; Updated October 2015.

Immune Globulin (Human)

Storage Conditions

CONTAINER	Drug Manufacturer	Concentration	Diluents	Osmolality (mOsm/kg)	pH	Temperature Room	Temperature Refrig	Temperature Frozen	Post-thaw Temp Room	Post-thaw Temp Refrig	Body Temp	Refer.
Bag, Ethylene Vinyl Acetate (EVA)	BAX[d]	5%, 10%	SWFI[k]	636, 1250	6.4-7.2	72 hr	14 d	n/a	n/a	n/a	n/a	(1)(24)
	BAX[c]	10%	RTU	240-300	4.6-5.1	7 d	21 d	n/a	n/a	n/a	n/a	(3)(24)
	BPL[h]	5%	RTU	420-500	4.8-5.1	14 d	n/a	n/a	n/a	n/a	n/a	(9)(25)
Bag, Plastic (Unspecified)	CBH[a]	3%, 6%, 9%, 12%	D5W, NS, SWFI	[j]	6.4-6.8	n/a	24 hr	n/a	n/a	n/a	n/a	(1)(2)
	BPL[h]	5%, 10%	RTU	420-500	4.8-5.1	[q]	n/a	n/a	n/a	n/a	n/a	(1)(9)
	GRI[f]	10%	RTU	258	4-4.5	8 hr	n/a	n/a	n/a	n/a	n/a	(5)
	KED[t]	10%	RTU	258	4-4.5	8 hr	n/a	n/a	n/a	n/a	n/a	(20)
	OCT[g]	5%, 10%	RTU	310-380	4.5-6	8 hr	n/a	n/a	n/a	n/a	n/a	(6)(23)
	ADM[s]	10%	RTU	≤ 510	4-4.6	[q]	n/a	n/a	n/a	n/a	n/a	(22)(26)
	OCT[m]	10%	RTU	240-404	4.5-5	8 hr	n/a	n/a	n/a	n/a	n/a	(8)
Bag, Polyolefin	BAX[d]	5%, 10%	SWFI[k]	636, 1250	6.4-7.2	72 hr	14 d	n/a	n/a	n/a	n/a	(1)(24)
	BAX[c]	10%	RTU	240-300	4.6-5.1	7 d	21 d	n/a	n/a	n/a	n/a	(3)(24)
	BPL[h]	5%	RTU	420-500	4.8-5.1	14 d	n/a	n/a	n/a	n/a	n/a	(9)(25)
Bag, Polyvinyl Chloride (PVC)	GRI[b]	5%	RTU	240-370	5-6	10 d	10 d	n/a	n/a	n/a	n/a	(1)(17)
	KED[t]	10%	RTU[i]	258	4-4.5	15 d	15 d	n/a	n/a	n/a	n/a	(16)(20)
	BAX[d]	5%, 10%	SWFI[k]	636, 1250	6.4-7.2	2 hr	24 hr	n/a	n/a	n/a	n/a	(4)(24)
	BAX[d]	5%, 10%	SWFI	n/a	6.4-7.2	12 hr	48 hr	n/a	n/a	n/a	n/a	(1)
	GRI[l]	10%	RTU	280-404	4.1-4.8	8 hr	n/a	n/a	n/a	n/a	n/a	(7)
Syringe, Unspecified	CBH[u]	20%	RTU	380	4.6-5.2	[q]	n/a	n/a	n/a	n/a	n/a	(19)(21)
	BAX[n]	20%	RTU	280-292	4.6-5.1	2 hr	n/a	n/a	n/a	n/a	n/a	(10)
Unspecified	GRI[b]	5%, 10%	RTU	240-370	5-6	[q]	n/a	n/a	n/a	n/a	n/a	(13)(18)
	CBH[e]	10%	RTU	240-440	4.6-5	8 hr	n/a	n/a	n/a	n/a	n/a	(14)
Vial, Glass	CBH[a]	3%, 6%, 9%, 12%	D5W, NS, SWFI	[j]	6.4-6.8	n/a	24 hr	n/a	n/a	n/a	n/a	(1)(2)
	BAX[d]	5%, 10%	SWFI[k]	636, 1250	6.4-7.2	2 hr	24 hr	n/a	n/a	n/a	n/a	(4)(24)
	GRI[f]	10%	RTU	258	4-4.5	8 hr	n/a	n/a	n/a	n/a	n/a	(5)

DOI 10.37573/9781585286720.112

Storage Conditions

						Temperature			Post-thaw Temp			
	Drug Manufacturer	Concentration	Diluents	Osmolality (mOsm/kg)	pH	Room	Refrig	Frozen	Room	Refrig	Body Temp	Refer.
OTHER INFUSION CONTAINERS												
Dosi-Fuser® (Leventon)	UN	5-10%	SWFI	n/a	n/a	12 hr[o]	24 hr[o]	n/a	n/a	n/a	n/a	(12)
	UN	5-10%	SWFI	n/a	n/a	n/a	12 hr[r][o]	n/a	n/a	n/a	n/a	(12)
Easypump® ST/LT (B. Braun)	CBH[u]	20%	RTU	n/a	4.6-5.2	7 d	n/a	n/a	n/a	n/a	n/a	(27)
INTERMATE™ (Baxter)[p]	BA	5-10%	SWFI	n/a	n/a	n/a	12 hr[r]	n/a	n/a	n/a	n/a	(15)
	BA	5-10%	SWFI	n/a	n/a	12 hr	24 hr	n/a	n/a	n/a	n/a	(15)

Flush Compatibility: D5W, sodium chloride 0.9% unless noted as incompatible with sodium chloride diluents. Incompatible with heparin.[1]

Special Considerations: The optimal pH for immune globulin in solution is 4.0-4.5; preparations with higher (e.g., physiologic) pH contain stabilizing agents.[11] Due to the difference in stabilizers and Ig production methods, clinicians should use the data that is specific to the brand. Do not freeze. Do not shake.[1]

Notes

[a] Carimune® NF (CBH).
[b] Flebogamma® DIF (GRI).
[c] Gammagard Liquid® (BAX).
[d] Gammagard S/D® (BAX).
[e] Privigen® (CBH).
[f] Gamunex®-C (GRI).
[g] Octagam® (OCT).
[h] Gammaplex® (BPL).
[i] May dilute with D5W if necessary.
[j] Osmolality: 3%: 444, 498, 192; 6%: 636, 690, 384; 9%: 828, 882, 576; 12%: 1020, 1074, 768.[1,2]
[k] Manufacturer of lyophilized immune globulin product provides diluent (SWFI) for initial reconstitution and/or infusion. Diluent should be at room temperature prior to reconstitution.[4]
[l] Xembify® (GRI).
[m] Panzyga® (OCT).
[n] Cuvitru® (BAX).
[o] Manufacturer extrapolated data from other sources.
[p] INTERMATE™/INFUSOR™ Portable Elastomeric Infusion System devices are no longer available in the United States.
[q] Manufacturer recommends to use promptly after a vial is entered.
[r] Followed by 12 hours at 25°C.[12,15]
[s] Bivigam® (ADM).
[t] Gammaked™ (KED).
[u] Hizentra® (CBH).

REFERENCES

1. ASHP's Interactive Handbook on Injectable Drugs, 2020. Bethesda, MD: American Society of Health-System Pharmacists; Accessed December 2020.
2. Carimune® NF (Human Immunoglobulin G) Injection, Lyophilized [package insert]. Kankakee, IL: CSL Behring LLC; February 2020.
3. Gammaguard Liquid® (Immune Globulin Infusion (Human)) Injection [package insert]. Lexington, MA: Baxalta US, Inc.; October 2020.
4. Gammaguard S/D® (Immune Globulin Intravenous (Human)) Injection [package insert]. Lexington, MA: Baxalta US, Inc.; November 2020.
5. Gamunex-C® (Immune Globulin (Human)) Injection [package insert]. Research Triangle Park, NC: Grifols USA, LLC; January 2020.
6. Octagam® 5% (Immune Globulin (Human)) Injection [package insert]. Hoboken, NJ: Octapharma USA, Inc.; February 2020.
7. Xembify® 20% (Immune Globulin Subcutaneous (Human)) Injection [package insert]. Research Triangle Park, NC: Grifols USA, LLC; July 2019.
8. Panzyga® (Immune Globulin Intravenous (Human)) Injection [package insert]. Hoboken, NJ: Octapharma USA, Inc.; January 2019.
9. Gammaplex 5%® (Immune Globulin Intravenous (Human), 5%) Injection [package insert]. Durham, NC: Bio Products Laboratory, Inc.; September 2019.
10. Cuvitru® (Immune Globulin Subcutaneous (Human)) Injection [package insert]. Lexington, MA: Baxalta US, Inc.; November 2020.
11. Shah S. Pharmacy considerations for the use of IGIV therapy. *Am J Health Syst Pharm*. 2005; 62(16 Suppl 3):S5-11.
12. *Drug Stability Table - Dosi-Fuser® Elastomeric Pump (S-CL-00-001v16)*, 2021. Barcelona, Spain: Leventon SAU; Updated May 2021.
13. Flebogamma® 5% DIF (Immune Globulin (Human)) Injection [package insert]. Research Triangle Park, NC: Grifols USA, LLC; November 2019.
14. Privigen® (Immune Globulin Intravenous (Human), 10%) Injection [package insert]. Kankakee, IL: CSL Behring LLC; September 2020.
15. Stabforum - Stability Database: Human Immunoglobulin IG G, Ontario, Canada: Baxter Healthcare; Accessed February 2021.
16. Gammaked™ Medication Information Letter (Ref#: N/A) [personal communication]. Fort Lee, NJ: Kedrion Biopharma, Inc.; 2016:2.
17. Lopez M, Costa M, Jorquera JI. Compatibility Study of Two Intravenous Immunoglobulins Preparations with Plastic Containers [poster]. FOCIS 5th Annual Meeting. Boston, MA; 2005.
18. Flebogamma® 10% DIF (Immune Globulin (Human)) Injection [package insert]. Research Triangle Park, NC: Grifols USA, LLC; November 2019.
19. Hizentra® Osmolality Information Letter (Ref#: 1-1044069098) [personal communication]. King of Prussia, PA: CSL Behring; 2016:1.
20. Gammaked™ 10% (Immune Globulin (Human), 10% Caprylate/Chromatography Purified) Injection [package insert]. Fort Lee, NJ: Kedrion Biopharma, Inc.; January 2014.
21. Hizentra® 20% (Immune Globulin Subcutaneous (Human), 20%) Injection [package insert]. Kankakee, IL: CSL Behring; April 2020.
22. Bivigam® 10% (Immune Globulin Intravenous (Human), 10%) Injection [package insert]. Boca Raton, FL: ADMA Biologics, Inc.; November 2020.
23. Octagam® 10% (Immune Globulin (Human)) Injection [package insert]. Hoboken, NJ: Octapharma USA, Inc.; February 2020.
24. Gammagard S/D® IgA Medication Information Letter (Ref#: N/A) [personal communication]. Deerfield, IL: Baxter Healthcare Corporation; 2014:3.
25. Gammaplex® Medication Information Letter (Ref#: N/A) [personal communication]. Durham, NC: Bio Products Laboratory, Inc.; 2016:3.
26. Bivigam® Medication Information Letter (Ref#: N/A) [personal communication]. Boca Raton, FL: Biotest Pharmaceuticals; 2016:2.
27. *Drug Stability for Easypump® ST/LT*, 2020. Bethlehem, PA: B. Braun USA; Updated June 2020.

InFLIXimab

Storage Conditions

						Temperature			Post-thaw Temp			
	Drug Manufacturer	Concentration	Diluents	Osmolality (mOsm/kg)	pH	Room	Refrig	Frozen	Room	Refrig	Body Temp	Refer.
CONTAINER												
Bag, Ethylene Vinyl Acetate (EVA)	JN	0.4-4 mg/mL	NS	n/a	[b]	24 hr	n/a	n/a	n/a	n/a	n/a	(5)
Bag, Polyethylene	JN	0.4-4 mg/mL	NS	n/a	[b]	24 hr	n/a	n/a	n/a	n/a	n/a	(5)
Bag, Polyolefin	JN, CEL	0.4 mg/mL	NS	n/a	[b]	n/a	14 d[d]	n/a	n/a	n/a	n/a	(1)
Bag, Polyvinyl Chloride (PVC)	CEN	0.4 mg/mL	NS	n/a	[b]	n/a	14 d[c]	n/a	n/a	n/a	n/a	(4)
Bag, Unspecified	JN	0.4-4 mg/mL	NS	n/a	[b]	24 hr[a]	28 d[a]	n/a	n/a	n/a	n/a	(2)
Vial, Glass	JN	0.4-4 mg/mL	NS	n/a	[b]	24 hr	n/a	n/a	n/a	n/a	n/a	(5)
	JN, CEL	2 mg/mL	NS	n/a	[b]	n/a	14 d[d]	n/a	n/a	n/a	n/a	(1)
	JN, CEL	10 mg/mL	SWFI	n/a	[b]	n/a	14 d[d]	n/a	n/a	n/a	n/a	(1)
OTHER INFUSION CONTAINERS												
INTERMATE™ (Baxter)[e]	HOS	0.4-4 mg/mL	NS	n/a	[b]	48 hr	9 wk	n/a	n/a	n/a	n/a	(6)

Flush Compatibility: Sodium chloride 0.9%.[3]

Special Considerations: Intravenous administration requires an infusion set with an in-line, sterile, non-pyrogenic, low-protein-binding filter (pore size of 1.2 μm or less).[3,5]

Notes

[a] Chemical and physical in use stability of the diluted solution has been demonstrated for up to 28 days at 2°C to 8°C and for an additional 24 hours at 25°C after removal from refrigeration.[2]

[b] pH of reconstituted solution 10 mg/mL in SWFI is approximately 7.2.[3]

[c] No loss of biological activity as measured by an indirect ELISA method.[4]

[d] Protected from light.[1]

[e] INTERMATE™/INFUSOR™ Portable Elastomeric Infusion System devices are no longer available in the United States.

DOI 10.37573/9781585286720.113

REFERENCES

1. Hermosilla J, Sanchez-Martin R, Perez-Robles R, et al. Comparative Stability Studies of Different Infliximab and Biosimilar CT-P13 Clinical Solutions by Combined Use of Physicochemical Analytical Techniques and Enzyme-Linked Immunosorbent Assay (ELISA). *BioDrugs*. 2019; 33(2):193-205.
2. European Medicines Agency. Remicade® - Annex 1: Summary of Product Characteristics. https://www.ema.europa.eu/documents/product-information/remicade-epar-product-information_en.pdf (accessed 2020 September).
3. Remicade® (Infliximab) Injection, Lyophilized [package insert]. Horsham, PA: Janssen Biotech, Inc.; May 2020.
4. Ikeda R, Vermeulen LC, Lau E, et al. Stability of infliximab in polyvinyl chloride bags. *Am J Health Syst Pharm*. 2012; 69(17):1509-12.
5. ASHP's Interactive Handbook on Injectable Drugs, 2020. Bethesda, MD: American Society of Health-System Pharmacists; Accessed September 2020.
6. Stabforum - Stability Database: Infliximab Biosimilar, Ontario, Canada: Baxter Healthcare; Accessed January 2021.

Insulin, Regular

Storage Conditions

						Temperature			Post-thaw Temp			
	Drug Manufacturer	Concentration	Diluents	Osmolality (mOsm/kg)	pH	Room	Refrig	Frozen	Room	Refrig	Body Temp	Refer.
CONTAINER												
Bag, Polypropylene	NVN	0.05-1 units/mL	NS, D5W, D10W[f]	n/a	n/a	24 hr[e]	n/a	n/a	n/a	n/a	n/a	(3)
Bag, Polyvinyl Chloride (PVC)	LI	0.1-1 units/mL	NS	n/a	n/a	48 hr[d][e]	48 hr[d][e]	n/a	n/a	n/a	n/a	(2)(6)
Syringe, Plastic (Unspecified)	UN	100 units/mL	Undiluted	n/a	[h]	n/a	7 d[g]	n/a	n/a	n/a	n/a	(1)
Syringe, Polypropylene	BP	0.8 units/mL[i]	NS	n/a	n/a	18 hr	n/a	n/a	n/a	n/a	n/a	(1)
	LI	100 units/mL[j]	Undiluted	n/a	[h]	n/a	14 d	n/a	n/a	n/a	n/a	(1)
	LI, NVN	100 units/mL[j]	Undiluted	n/a	[h]	29 d	29 d	n/a	n/a	n/a	n/a	(1)
	LI	100 units/mL[k]	Undiluted	n/a	[h]	28 d[l]	28 d	n/a	n/a	n/a	n/a	(1)
Vial, Unspecified	LI	100 units/mL	Undiluted	n/a	[h]	31 d[a]	31 d[a]	n/a	n/a	n/a	n/a	(2)
	NVN	100 units/mL	Undiluted	n/a	[h]	6 wk[b]	6 wk[b]	n/a	n/a	n/a	n/a	(3)
	NVN	100 units/mL	Undiluted	n/a	[h]	28 d[b]	28 d[b]	n/a	n/a	n/a	n/a	(3)
	NVN	100 units/mL	Undiluted	n/a	[h]	5 d[c]	5 d[c]	n/a	n/a	n/a	n/a	(4)

Flush Compatibility: Sodium chloride 0.9%, heparin[1]

Special Considerations: Protect from heat and light. Do not freeze or use previously frozen product. Avoid vigorous shaking.[1,2,3] Regular insulin, containing 100 units/mL (U-100), is clear and colorless. Discoloration, turbidity, or unusual viscosity indicates deterioration or contamination.[1] Repeated drawing of insulin into disposable siliconized syringes and then expulsion of insulin back into the vials introduces silicone oil, contaminating the vial, and resulting in white precipitate formation, and impairment of biological effect, thus not recommended.[1] Regular insulin 500 units/mL (U-500) is not intended for intravenous or intramuscular administration.[5]

DOI 10.37573/9781585286720.114

Notes

[a] Not in-use (unopened) 3mL and 10mL multiple-dose vials stored refrigerated (2-8°C) may be used until the expiration date. In-use (opened) 3mL and 10mL multiple-dose vials, stored refrigerated or at room temperature, may be used for 31 days. Not in-use (unopened) 3mL and 10mL multiple-dose vials stored at room temperature may be used for 31 days.[2]

[b] Not in-use (unopened) 3mL and 10mL multiple-dose vials stored refrigerated (2-8°C) may be used until the expiration date. In-use (opened) or not in-use (unopened) 3 mL and 10 mL multiple-dose vials stored at room temperature may be used for 28 days and 6 weeks, respectively.[3] In-use (opened) vials are not to be refrigerated.[3]

[c] Regular insulin (NVN) packaged in both non-insulated mailers and insulated containers with frozen gel packs exposed to simulated summer and winter temperatures, maintained stability regardless of shipping condition or packaging. Mean kinetic temperature of 5.7°C and 33.1°C at 5 days for non-insulated winter and summer simulated transit conditions, respectively.[4]

[d] Humulin R® U-100 prepared at concentrations from 0.1-1 unit/mL with NS in polyvinyl chloride infusion bags is stable when stored in refrigeration for 48 hours, then may be used at room temperature for up to an additional 48 hours.[2,6]

[e] Priming of IV infusion sets to accommodate adsorption of insulin is recommended. For standard polypropylene IV infusion set, a priming volume of 20 mL (1 unit/mL) was sufficient to minimize the effect of insulin adsorption losses to the IV infusion set.[7]

[f] Solution contained: potassium chloride 40 mmol/L.[3]

[g] Regular insulin can be stored for 5 to 7 days under refrigeration in plastic syringes.[1]

[h] All regular insulin products have a neutral pH of approximately 7-7.8.[1]

[i] Regular insulin, 0.8 units/mL diluted in NS stored for 18 hours at room temperature with no significant loss due to sorption in the following plastic syringes: Brunswick (Sherwood Medical) and Plastipak™ (BD) syringes with polypropylene barrel, and Sabre (Gillette U.K.) syringe with a polypropylene-polystyrene barrel.[1]

[j] 1-mL polypropylene syringe (BD).[1]

[k] 1-mL polypropylene syringe (BD) and 1-mL polypropylene-ethylene copolymer syringe (Terumo).[1]

[l] Storage under refrigeration recommended due to accelerated loss of antibacterial preservative with polypropylene syringes stored at room temperature.[1]

REFERENCES

1. ASHP's Interactive Handbook on Injectable Drugs, 2020. Bethesda, MD: American Society of Health-System Pharmacists; Accessed August 2020.
2. Humulin® R (Insulin Human) Injection [package insert]. Indianapolis, IN: Eli Lilly and Company; March 2020.
3. Novolin® R (Insulin Human) Injection [package insert]. Plainsboro, NJ: Novo Nordisk, Inc.; November 2019.
4. Chandler C, Gryniewicz CM, Pringle T, et al. Insulin temperature and stability under simulated transit conditions. *Am J Health Syst Pharm*. 2008; 65(10):953-63.
5. Humulin® R U-500 (Insulin Human) Injection [package insert]. Indianapolis, IN: Eli Lilly and Company; November 2020.
6. Eli Lilly and Company. Humulin® R U-100 (Insulin Human) Injection 100 units/mL: Intravenous Use. https://www.lillymedical.com/en-us/answers/humulin-r-u-100-insulin-human-injection-100-units-ml-intravenous-use-4939 (accessed 2020 August 8).
7. Goldberg PA, Kedves A, Walter K, et al. "Waste not, want not": determining the optimal priming volume for intravenous insulin infusions. *Diabetes Technol Ther*. 2006; 8(5):598-601.

Interferon Alfa-2b

Storage Conditions

						Temperature			Post-thaw Temp			
	Drug Manufacturer	Concentration	Diluents	Osmolality (mOsm/kg)	pH	Room	Refrig	Frozen	Room	Refrig	Body Temp	Refer.
CONTAINER												
Syringe, Polypropylene	MSD	2 million International Units/mL	SWFI[c]	[a]	[e]	n/a	21 d[b]	n/a	n/a	n/a	n/a	(2)
	MSD	2 million International Units/mL	SWFI	[a]	[e]	n/a	6 wk	n/a	n/a	n/a	n/a	(3)
	MSD	3, 6 million International Units/mL	SWFI, BWFI	[a]	[e]	n/a	6 wk[d]	n/a	n/a	n/a	n/a	(1)(3)
Vial, Glass	UN	3, 10 million International Units/mL	SWFI	[a]	[e]	30 d	30 d	n/a	n/a	n/a	n/a	(5)

Flush Compatibility: Sodium chloride 0.9%. Incompatible with dextrose-containing solutions.[1]

Special Considerations: Product is labeled in International Units (I.U.) The single-use vial powder for injection is be reconstituted with the provided vial of SWFI; each vial also contains human albumin, resulting in a final concentration of 1 mg/mL albumin. The multidose vials for injection are albumin-free. Refrigerate, and do not freeze product.[4]

Notes

[a] Reconstituted vial, 10 million International Units in 1 mL SWFI, results in an isotonic solution.[1]

[b] Tested in polypropylene centrifuge tubes.[2]

[c] Solution contained: albumin 1 mg/mL.[2]

[d] Solutions tested with and without albumin 1 mg/mL.[3]

[e] Interferon alfa-2b is most stable between pH 6.8 and 7.5.[1]

REFERENCES

1. ASHP's Interactive Handbook on Injectable Drugs, 2020. Bethesda, MD: American Society of Health-System Pharmacists; Accessed August 2020.
2. Schepart BS, Burns BA, Evans S, et al. Long-term stability of interferon alfa-2b diluted to 2 million units/mL. *Am J Health Syst Pharm*. 1995; 52(19):2128-30.
3. Appenheimer MM, Schepart BS, Poleon GP, et al. Stability of albumin-free interferon alfa-2b for 42 days. *Am J Health Syst Pharm*. 1998; 55(15):1602-5.
4. Intron® A (Interferon Alfa-2b) Injection [package insert]. Whitehouse Station, NJ: Merck Sharp & Dohme Corp.; December 2020.
5. Ruiz L, Reyes N, Sotolongo J, et al. Long-term stabilization of a new freeze-dried and albumin-free formulation of recombinant human interferon alpha 2b. *PDA J Pharm Sci Technol*. 2006; 60(1):72-8.

DOI 10.37573/9781585286720.115

Irinotecan Hydrochloride (Conventional)

Storage Conditions

						Temperature			Post-thaw Temp			
CONTAINER	Drug Manufacturer	Concentration	Diluents	Osmolality (mOsm/kg)	pH	Room	Refrig	Frozen	Room	Refrig	Body Temp	Refer.
Bag, Polyethylene	PF[d]	Various	D5W, NS	n/a	[c]	28 d[a]	n/a	n/a	n/a	n/a	n/a	(3)
Bag, Polyvinyl Chloride (PVC)	RPR	0.4, 1 mg/mL	NS	n/a	[c]	7 d	n/a	n/a	n/a	n/a	n/a	(1)(2)
	RPR	0.4, 1, 2.8 mg/mL	D5W, NS	n/a	[c]	28 d[a]	28 d[a][b]	n/a	n/a	n/a	n/a	(1)(2)
	RPR	2 mg/mL	D5W, NS	n/a	[c]	2 hr	4 d[b]	n/a	n/a	n/a	n/a	(2)
	RPR	0.12 - 2.8 mg/mL	D5W, NS	n/a	[c]	24 hr[a]	48 hr[a][b]	n/a	n/a	n/a	n/a	(2)
	RPR	2.8 mg/mL	NS	n/a	[c]	14 d	n/a	n/a	n/a	n/a	n/a	(1)(2)

Flush Compatibility: Sodium chloride 0.9%.[(1)]

Special Considerations: Precipitation may result from freezing irinotecan hydrochloride concentrate for injection and diluted solutions for infusion; freezing should be avoided.[(2)]

Notes

[a] Protected from light.

[b] Refrigerated storage of irinotecan hydrochloride in sodium chloride 0.9% is not recommended because of occasional visible precipitation.[(2)]

[c] pH of undiluted solution is 3-4.[(2)]

[d] Pfizer, United Kingdom

REFERENCES

1. Thiesen J, Krämer I. Physicochemical stability of irinotecan injection concentrate and diluted infusion solutions in PVC bags. *J Oncol Pharm Pract*. 2000; 6(3):115-21.
2. ASHP's Interactive Handbook on Injectable Drugs, 2020. Bethesda, MD: American Society of Health-System Pharmacists; Accessed July 2020.
3. Camptosar® Medication Information Letter (Ref#: US20-030801) [personal communication]. New York, NY: Pfizer; 2020:4.

DOI 10.37573/9781585286720.116

Iron Sucrose

Storage Conditions

						Temperature			Post-thaw Temp			
	Drug Manufacturer	Concentration	Diluents	Osmolality (mOsm/kg)	pH	Room	Refrig	Frozen	Room	Refrig	Body Temp	Refer.
CONTAINER												
Bag, Polyvinyl Chloride (PVC)	AMR	1-2 mg/mL	NS	n/a	[a]	7 d	n/a	n/a	n/a	n/a	n/a	(1)
Bag, Unspecified	AMR	1-2 mg/mL	NS	n/a	[a]	7 d	n/a	n/a	n/a	n/a	n/a	(1)
Syringe, Plastic (Unspecified)	AMR	2-10 mg/mL	NS	n/a	[a]	7 d	7 d	n/a	n/a	n/a	n/a	(1)
OTHER INFUSION CONTAINERS												
Easypump® ST/LT (B. Braun)	AMR	1 mg/mL	NS	n/a	[a]	24 hr	24 hr	n/a	n/a	n/a	n/a	(2)
	VFP	2, 5 mg/mL	NS	n/a	[a]	72 hr	n/a	n/a	n/a	n/a	n/a	(2)
SMARTeZ® (Progressive Medical)	UN	1 mg/mL	NS	n/a	[a]	24 hr[b]	24 hr[b]	n/a	n/a	n/a	n/a	(3)
	UN	2, 5 mg/mL	NS	n/a	[a]	72 hr	n/a	n/a	n/a	n/a	n/a	(3)

Flush Compatibility: Sodium chloride 0.9%.[1]

Special Considerations: Concentration of iron sucrose is stated as mg/mL of elemental iron. Do not dilute below 1 mg/mL. Do not mix with other medications or parenteral nutrition.[1]

Notes

[a] pH range is 10.5-11.[1]

[b] Manufacturer extrapolated data from other sources.

REFERENCES

1. Venofer® (Iron Sucrose) Injection [package insert]. Shirley, NY: American Regent, Inc.; September 2020.
2. *Drug Stability for Easypump® ST/LT*, 2020. Bethlehem, PA: B. Braun USA; Updated June 2020.
3. *SMARTeZ® - Stability Data for Drugs Using Elastomeric Infusion Pumps*, 2020. Fenton, MO: Progressive Medical, Inc.; Updated May 2020.

DOI 10.37573/9781585286720.117

Isoproterenol

Storage Conditions

						Temperature			Post-thaw Temp			
	Drug Manufacturer	Concentration	Diluents	Osmolality (mOsm/kg)	pH	Room	Refrig	Frozen	Room	Refrig	Body Temp	Refer.
CONTAINER												
Bag, Polyvinyl Chloride (PVC)	WI	4 mcg/mL	D5W	n/a	4	30 m	n/a	n/a	n/a	n/a	n/a	(3)
Unspecified	UN	5 mcg/mL	D5W	n/a	3.7-5.7[b]	24 hr	n/a	n/a	n/a	n/a	n/a	(2)
	BN	2 mcg/mL	D5W	n/a	n/a	24 hr[c]	n/a	n/a	n/a	n/a	n/a	(2)
	BN	2 mcg/mL	D5W	n/a	n/a	10 d[a]	n/a	n/a	n/a	n/a	n/a	(2)
	WI	2 mcg/mL	D5W, NS, LR	n/a	n/a	12 hr	n/a	n/a	n/a	n/a	n/a	(2)
	WI	4 mcg/mL	D5W, NS	n/a	n/a	8 hr	n/a	n/a	n/a	n/a	n/a	(2)

Flush Compatibility: Sodium chloride 0.9%.

Special Considerations: Protect from light. The drug should not be used if the solution is pinkish or slightly darker than yellow or if a precipitate is present.(1) Isoproterenol hydrochloride 2 mcg/mL displayed no significant reduction when tested for binding to 5-µm stainless steel depth filter (Argyle Filter Connector), a 0.22-µm cellulose ester membrane filter (Ivex-2 Filter Set) and a 0.22-µm polycarbonate membrane filter (In-Sure Filter Set).(2) Isoproterenol hydrochloride did not display significant sorption to a 0.45-µm cellulose membrane filter (Abbott S-A-I-F) during an 8-hour simulated infusion.(2)

Notes

[a] Protected from light.

[b] Isoproterenol hydrochloride displayed significant decomposition at a pH value above approximately 6. If drugs that may raise the pH above 6 are mixed, they should be administered immediately after preparation, or, preferably, administered separately.(2)

[c] Exposed to light.

REFERENCES

1. Isuprel™ (Isoproterenol Hydrochloride) Injection [package insert]. Lake Forest, IL: Hospira, Inc.; January 2021.
2. ASHP's Interactive Handbook on Injectable Drugs, 2020. Bethesda, MD: American Society of Health-System Pharmacists; Accessed August 2020.
3. Leach JK, Strickland RD, Millis DL, et al. Biological activity of dilute isoproterenol solution stored for long periods in plastic bags. *Am J Hosp Pharm*. 1977; 34(7):709-12.
4. Rusmin S, Welton S, DeLuca P, et al. Effect of inline filtration on the potency of drugs administered intravenously. *Am J Hosp Pharm*. 1977; 34(10):1071-4.

DOI 10.37573/9781585286720.118

Ketamine Hydrochloride

Storage Conditions

						Temperature			Post-thaw Temp			
	Drug Manufacturer	Concentration	Diluents	Osmolality (mOsm/kg)	pH	Room	Refrig	Frozen	Room	Refrig	Body Temp	Refer.
CONTAINER												
Bag, Polyolefin	QI	1, 2, 4 mg/mL	NS[m]	[f]	[g]	15 d[n]	15 d[n]	n/a	n/a	n/a	15 d[n]	(1)
	QI	0.5, 1, 2 mg/mL	NS[r]	[f]	[g]	14 d[n]	14 d[n]	n/a	n/a	n/a	n/a	(1)
	PAN	0.123 mg/mL	NS[o]	[f]	[g]	24 hr	n/a	n/a	n/a	n/a	n/a	(1)
Bag, Polyvinyl Chloride (PVC)	SZ	0.2, 0.6, 1 mg/mL	NS[h]	[f]	4.5-4.8	7 d	n/a	n/a	n/a	n/a	n/a	(1)(4)
	PAN	1 mg/mL	NS	[f]	[g]	28 d	7 d	n/a	n/a	n/a	n/a	(1)
	PAN	40 mg/mL	NS[p]	[f]	[g]	7 d	n/a	n/a	n/a	n/a	n/a	(1)
	PAN	0.1 mg/mL	NS[q]	[f]	[g]	7 d	n/a	n/a	n/a	n/a	n/a	(1)
	PAN	40 mg/mL	NS[q]	[f]	[g]	7 d	n/a	n/a	n/a	n/a	n/a	(1)
	JN	1 mg/mL	NS[i]	[f]	[g]	30 d	30 d	n/a	n/a	n/a	n/a	(1)
	PD	1 mg/mL	NS[b]	[f]	[g]	6 d	n/a	n/a	n/a	n/a	n/a	(1)
	PD	25 mg/mL	NS[c]	[f]	[g]	6 d	n/a	n/a	n/a	n/a	n/a	(1)
Syringe, Plastic	SZ	0.2, 0.6, 1 mg/mL	NS[h]	[f]	4.5-4.8	7 d	n/a	n/a	n/a	n/a	n/a	(4)
	PD	2 mg/mL	NS[k]	[f]	[g]	48 hr	n/a	n/a	n/a	n/a	n/a	(1)
	PD	1 mg/mL	NS[d]	[f]	[g]	6 d	n/a	n/a	n/a	n/a	n/a	(1)
	PD	10, 25 mg/mL	NS[e]	[f]	[g]	6 d	n/a	n/a	n/a	n/a	n/a	(1)
	PF	50 mg/mL	Undiluted	[f]	[g]	50 d	n/a	n/a	n/a	n/a	n/a	(1)
Syringe, Polypropylene	FGN	1 mg/mL	NS	[f]	[g]	1 yr	1 yr	n/a	n/a	n/a	1 yr[j]	(1)
	PF	50 mg/mL	Undiluted	[f]	[g]	180 d[n]	n/a	n/a	n/a	n/a	n/a	(1)
	PF	1 mg/mL	NS[s]	[f]	[g]	4 d	n/a	n/a	n/a	n/a	n/a	(1)
	REN	62.5 mg/mL	NS[t]	[f]	[g]	48 hr[n]	n/a	n/a	n/a	n/a	n/a	(1)
	SZ	2 mg/mL	NS[l]	[f]	[g]	13 wk	13 wk	n/a	n/a	n/a	n/a	(1)
	AB	10 mg/mL	SWFI	[f]	4.2	30 d	n/a	n/a	n/a	n/a	n/a	(1)(2)
Unspecified	PD	1.33 mg/mL	NS[a]	[f]	5.5-7.5	4 d	n/a	n/a	n/a	n/a	n/a	(1)(3)
Vial, Glass	SZ	0.2, 0.6, 1 mg/mL	NS[h]	[f]	4.5-4.8	7 d[n]	n/a	n/a	n/a	n/a	n/a	(1)(4)
	JN	1 mg/mL	NS[i]	[f]	[g]	30 d	n/a	n/a	n/a	n/a	n/a	(1)
	SZ	10 mg/mL	SWFI	[f]	4.90	26 wk	n/a	n/a	n/a	n/a	n/a	(1)(8)

DOI 10.37573/9781585286720.119

Storage Conditions

	Drug Manufacturer	Concentration	Diluents	Osmolality (mOsm/kg)	pH	Temperature			Post-thaw Temp			
						Room	Refrig	Frozen	Room	Refrig	Body Temp	Refer.
OTHER INFUSION CONTAINERS												
CADD® Cassette (Smiths Medical)	PD	25 mg/mL	NS[c]	[f]	[g]	6 d	n/a	n/a	n/a	n/a	n/a	(1)
Dosi-Fuser® (Leventon)	MOL	4 mg/mL	NS	[f]	[g]	14 d	30 d	n/a	n/a	n/a	n/a	(7)
Easypump® ST/LT (B. Braun)	UN	1, 2 mg/mL	NS	[f]	[g]	48 hr	n/a	n/a	n/a	n/a	n/a	(6)

Flush Compatibility: Sodium chloride 0.9%.[1]

Special Considerations: Available in concentrations of 10, 50, or 100 mg/mL. The 100 mg/mL injection is a concentrate, and must be diluted with an equal volume of either Sterile Water for Injection, Sodium chloride 0.9%, or 5% Dextrose in Water.[1,5]

Notes

[a] Solution contained: morphine sulfate (AB) 2 mg/mL.[1,3]
[b] Solution contained: morphine sulfate (SAB) 1 mg/mL.[1]
[c] Solution contained: morphine sulfate (SAB) 25 mg/mL.[1]
[d] Solution contained: morphine sulfate (SX) 1 or 10 mg/mL.[1]
[e] Solution contained: morphine sulfate (SX) 1, 10, or 25 mg/mL.[1]
[f] Undiluted 10 mg/mL solution is 300 mOsm/kg, and undiluted 50 mg/mL solution is 387 mOsm/kg.[1]
[g] pH of undiluted solution is 3.5-5.5.[1]
[h] Solution contained: HYDROmorphone (SZ) 0.2 mg/mL.[4]
[i] Solution contained: fentaNYL (DB) 10 mcg/mL and droperidol (JN) 50 mcg/mL.[1]
[j] Storage temperature: 40°C.[1]
[k] Solution contained: meperidine HCl (DB) 12 mg/mL.[1]
[l] Solution contained: morphine sulfate (SZ) 2, 5 or 10 mg/mL.[1]
[m] Solution contained: butorphanol tartrate (HE) 50, 100 or 150 mcg/mL.[1]
[n] Protected from light.[1]
[o] Solution contained: acetaminophen (BMS) 8.2 mg/mL.[1]
[p] Solution contained: oxyCODONE HCl (MUN) 0.4 mg/mL.[1]
[q] Solution contained: oxyCODONE HCl (MUN) 10 mg/mL.[1]
[r] Solution contained: traMADol HCl (GRU) 5 mg/mL.[1]
[s] Solution contained: fentaNYL citrate (unspecified) 40 mcg/mL.[1]
[t] Solution contained: lidocaine HCl (APN) 50 mg/mL.[1]

REFERENCES

1. ASHP's Interactive Handbook on Injectable Drugs, 2020. Bethesda, MD: American Society of Health-System Pharmacists; Accessed December 2020.
2. Gupta VD. Stability of Ketamine Hydrochloride Injection After Reconstitution in Water for Injection and Storagein 1-mL Tuberculin Polypropylene Syringes for Pediatric Use. *Int J Pharm Compd*. 2002; 6(4):316-7.
3. Schmid R, Koren G, Klein J, et al. The stability of a ketamine-morphine solution. *Anesth Analg*. 2002; 94(4):898-900.
4. Ensom MH, Decarie D, Leung K, et al. Stability of Hydromorphone-Ketamine Solutions in Glass Bottles, Plastic Syringes, and IV Bags for Pediatric Use. *Can J Hosp Pharm*. 2009; 62(2):112-8.
5. Ketamine Hydrochloride Injection, USP [package insert]. Lake Forest, IL: Hospira, Inc.; June 2020.
6. *Drug Stability for Easypump® ST/LT*, 2020. Bethlehem, PA: B. Braun USA; Updated June 2020.
7. *Drug Stability Table - Dosi-Fuser® Elastomeric Pump (S-CL-00-001v16)*, 2021. Barcelona, Spain: Leventon SAU; Updated May 2021.
8. Donnelly RF. Stability of diluted ketamine packaged in glass vials. *Can J Hosp Pharm*. 2013; 66(3):198.

Ketorolac Tromethamine

Storage Conditions

	Drug Manufacturer	Concentration	Diluents	Osmolality (mOsm/kg)	pH	Temperature: Room	Temperature: Refrig	Temperature: Frozen	Post-thaw Temp: Room	Post-thaw Temp: Refrig	Body Temp	Refer.
CONTAINER												
Bag, Polyolefin	RC	0.1, 0.3 mg/mL	D5W	[i]	[a]	n/a	n/a	15 d[b]	n/a	5 wk[b]	n/a	(4)
	RC	0.2 mg/mL	D5W	[i]	5.5-5.7	n/a	n/a	12 wk	n/a	60 d	n/a	(3)
Bag, Polyvinyl Chloride (PVC)	RC	0.3 mg/mL	NS	[i]	6.1-6.7	5 wk	50 d	n/a	n/a	n/a	n/a	(2)
	RC	0.3 mg/mL	D5W	[i]	5.3-6.6	7 d	50 d	n/a	n/a	n/a	n/a	(2)
	RC	0.3, 0.6 mg/mL	NS, D5W	[i]	5.66-6.84	21 d	21 d	n/a	n/a	n/a	n/a	(1)
	RC	0.6 mg/mL	D5W	[i]	[a]	7 d	50 d	n/a	n/a	n/a	n/a	(4)
	SY	0.06 mg/mL	R	[i]	[a]	48 hr	n/a	n/a	n/a	n/a	n/a	(4)
	SY	0.6 mg/mL	D5NS, D5W, NS, R	[i]	[a]	48 hr	n/a	n/a	n/a	n/a	n/a	(4)
Vial, Glass	SY	0.06 mg/mL	R	[i]	[a]	48 hr	n/a	n/a	n/a	n/a	n/a	(4)
	SY	0.6 mg/mL	NS, D5W	[i]	[a]	48 hr	n/a	n/a	n/a	n/a	n/a	(4)
OTHER INFUSION CONTAINERS												
INFUSOR™ (Baxter)[c]	REC	0.5-1.5 mg/mL	NS, D5W[e]	[i]	[a]	17 d[h]	n/a	n/a	n/a	n/a	7 d[h]	(5)
	REC	0.5-8 mg/mL	NS, D5W	[i]	[a]	n/a	28 d[f]	n/a	n/a	n/a	7 d[f]	(5)
	REC	1.5-8 mg/mL	NS, D5W[d]	[i]	[a]	28 d[g]	n/a	n/a	n/a	n/a	7 d[g]	(5)
	REC	1.5-8 mg/mL	NS, D5W[e]	[i]	[a]	28 d[g]	n/a	n/a	n/a	n/a	7 d[g]	(5)

Flush Compatibility: Sodium chloride 0.9%.[4]

Special Considerations: Protect from light.[4]

Notes

[a] pH of undiluted solutions is 6.9-7.9.[4]

[b] Storage temperature: -20°C for 15 days, followed by 5 weeks refrigerated.[4]

[c] INTERMATE™/INFUSOR™ Portable Elastomeric Infusion System devices are no longer available in the United States.

[d] Solution contained: morphine HCl (STE) 0.1-1.6 mg/mL.[5]

DOI 10.37573/9781585286720.120

[e] Solution contained: traMADol HCl (SE) 1.6-35 mg/mL.[5]

[f] Storage temperature: 5°C for 28 days, followed by 7 days at 33°C.[5]

[g] Storage temperature: 25°C for 28 days, followed by 7 days at 33°C.[5]

[h] Storage temperature: 25°C for 17 days, followed by 7 days at 33°C.[5]

[i] Undiluted solutions (15 mg/mL and 30 mg/mL) are isotonic.[4]

REFERENCES

1. Shi A, Walker S, Law S. Stability of Ketorolac Tromethamine in IV Solutions and Waste Reduction. *Can J Hosp Pharm*. 2000; 53(4):263-9.
2. Gupta VD, Maswoswe J, Bailey RE. Stability of ketorolac tromethamine in 5% dextrose injection and 0.9% sodium chloride injections. *Int J Pharm Compd*. 1997; 1(3):206-7.
3. Hecq JD, Boitquin LP, Vanbeckbergen DF, et al. Effect of freezing, long-term storage, and microwave thawing on the stability of ketorolac tromethamine. *Ann Pharmacother*. 2005; 39(10):1654-8.
4. ASHP's Interactive Handbook on Injectable Drugs, 2020. Bethesda, MD: American Society of Health-System Pharmacists; Accessed July 2020.
5. Stabforum - Stability Database: Ketorolac, Ketorolac+Morphine, Ketorolac+Tramadol, Ontario, Canada: Baxter Healthcare; Accessed February 2021.

Lacosamide

Storage Conditions

						Temperature			Post-thaw Temp			
	Drug Manufacturer	Concentration	Diluents	Osmolality (mOsm/kg)	pH	Room	Refrig	Frozen	Room	Refrig	Body Temp	Refer.
CONTAINER												
Bag, Non-DEHP Polyvinyl Chloride (PVC)	UCB	unspec.	[a]	n/a	[b]	24 hr	24 hr	n/a	n/a	n/a	n/a	(3)
Bag, Polyvinyl Chloride (PVC)	UCB	unspec.	[a]	n/a	[b]	24 hr	24 hr	n/a	n/a	n/a	n/a	(2)(3)
Vial, Glass	UCB	unspec.	[a]	n/a	[b]	24 hr	24 hr	n/a	n/a	n/a	n/a	(2)

Flush Compatibility: D5W, Sodium chloride 0.9%.[1]

Special Considerations: Store at 20°C to 25°C with excursions permitted between 15°C and 30°C. Do not freeze.[1,3]

Notes

[a] Compatible diluents per the manufacturer include: NS, D5W, and LR.[1,3]

[b] VIMPAT injection contains hydrochloric acid for pH adjustment. VIMPAT injection has a pH of 3.5 to 5.0.[1]

REFERENCES

1. VIMPAT® (Lacosamide) Injection [package insert]. Smyrna, GA: UCB, Inc.; January 2021.
2. VIMPAT® - Summary of Product Characteristics [package insert]. Smyrna, GA: UCB, Inc.; February 2008.
3. VIMPAT® Compatibility, Stability and Storage Information Response Letter (Ref#: US20-008285) [personal communication]. Smyrna, GA: UCB, Inc.; 2020:8.

DOI 10.37573/9781585286720.121

Leucovorin Calcium

Storage Conditions

						Temperature			Post-thaw Temp			
	Drug Manufacturer	Concentration	Diluents	Osmolality (mOsm/kg)	pH	Room	Refrig	Frozen	Room	Refrig	Body Temp	Refer.
CONTAINER												
Bag, Polyethylene	TE	0.12 mg/mL	NS	n/a	[d]	30 d[a]	30 d[a]	n/a	n/a	n/a	n/a	(1)
Bag, Polyolefin	LE	1 mg/mL	NS	n/a	[d]	7 d[a]	7 d[a]	n/a	n/a	n/a	n/a	(3)
Bag, Polyvinyl Chloride (PVC)	LE	0.1, 0.5, 1, 1.5 mg/mL	D5W	n/a	[d]	4 d[a]	4 d[a]	n/a	n/a	n/a	n/a	(3)
	LE	1, 1.5 mg/mL	NS	n/a	[d]	4 d[a]	4 d[a]	n/a	n/a	n/a	n/a	(3)
Vial, Glass	LE	0.1, 0.5, 1, 1.5 mg/mL	D5W, NS	n/a	[d]	4 d[a]	4 d[a]	n/a	n/a	n/a	n/a	(3)
	LE	1 mg/mL	NS	n/a	[d]	7 d[a]	7 d[a]	n/a	n/a	n/a	n/a	(3)
	TE	10 mg/mL	Undiluted	n/a	[d]	30 d[a]	30 d[a]	n/a	n/a	n/a	n/a	(1)
OTHER INFUSION CONTAINERS												
Dosi-Fuser® (Leventon)	LE	0.2-2 mg/mL	D5W, NS, SWFI	n/a	[d]	n/a	48 hr[e]	n/a	n/a	n/a	24 hr[e]	(7)
	LE	10-20 mg/mL	D5W, NS, SWFI	n/a	[d]	n/a	48 hr[e]	n/a	n/a	n/a	7 d[e]	(7)
Easypump® ST/LT (B. Braun)	UN	4 mg/mL	NS	n/a	[d]	48 hr	14 d	n/a	n/a	n/a	n/a	(6)
Homepump Eclipse® / Homepump® (Halyard)	UN	4 mg/mL	NS	n/a	[d]	7 d	7 d	n/a	n/a	n/a	n/a	(5)
INFUSOR™ (Baxter)[b]	MED	0.5-1 mg/mL	D5W, NS	n/a	[d]	n/a	7 d	n/a	n/a	n/a	n/a	(4)
	MED	1-6 mg/mL	D5W, NS	n/a	[d]	n/a	14 d	n/a	n/a	n/a	n/a	(4)
	MED	6 mg/mL	D5W, NS	n/a	[d]	n/a	14 d	n/a	n/a	n/a	72 hr[c]	(4)
SMARTeZ® (Progressive Medical)	UN	4 mg/mL	NS	n/a	[d]	48 hr[e]	14 d[e]	n/a	n/a	n/a	n/a	(2)

Flush Compatibility: Sodium chloride 0.9%, heparin.[3]

Special Considerations: Leucovorin is also referred to as Folinic Acid or Folinate.[2,4,5]

DOI 10.37573/9781585286720.122

Notes

[a] Protected from light.

[b] INTERMATE™/INFUSOR™ Portable Elastomeric Infusion System devices are no longer available in the United States.

[c] 14 days refrigerated followed by 72 hours at 33°C.[4]

[d] pH is 6.5-8.5.[3]

[e] Manufacturer extrapolated data from other sources.

REFERENCES

1. Karbownik A, Szalek E, Urjasz H, et al. Stability of calcium folinate (Teva) in concentrate after re-use and in dilute infusions in 0.9% NaCl in polyethylene bags. *Acta Pol Pharm*. 2013; 70(2):301-7.
2. *SMARTeZ® - Stability Data for Drugs Using Elastomeric Infusion Pumps*, 2020. Fenton, MO: Progressive Medical, Inc.; Updated May 2020.
3. ASHP's Interactive Handbook on Injectable Drugs, 2020. Bethesda, MD: American Society of Health-System Pharmacists; Accessed July 2020.
4. Stabforum - Stability Database: Folinate, Ontario, Canada: Baxter Healthcare; Accessed January 2021.
5. *Stability Data for Drugs Using Homepump Disposable Ambulatory Infusion Systems (MK-00314 rev 3)*, 2015. Alpharetta, GA: Halyard Health; Updated June 2015.
6. *Drug Stability for Easypump® ST/LT*, 2020. Bethlehem, PA: B. Braun USA; Updated June 2020.
7. *Drug Stability Table - Dosi-Fuser® Elastomeric Pump (S-CL-00-001v16)*, 2021. Barcelona, Spain: Leventon SAU; Updated May 2021.

LevETIRAcetam

Storage Conditions

						Temperature			Post-thaw Temp			
	Drug Manufacturer	Concentration	Diluents	Osmolality (mOsm/kg)	pH	Room	Refrig	Frozen	Room	Refrig	Body Temp	Refer.
CONTAINER												
Bag, Polyolefin	HOS	40 mg/mL	NS	[a]	5.5	n/a	14 d	n/a	n/a	n/a	n/a	(1)
Bag, Polyvinyl Chloride (PVC)	HOS	40 mg/mL	NS	[a]	5.5	4 hr	14 d	n/a	n/a	n/a	n/a	(1)(3)
Syringe, Polypropylene	HOS	40 mg/mL	NS	[a]	5.5	n/a	14 d	n/a	n/a	n/a	n/a	(1)

Flush Compatibility: Sodium chloride 0.9%.[2]

Special Considerations: n/a

Notes

[a] 100 mg/mL has an osmolality of approximately 950 mOsm/kg; 5 mg/mL diluted with sodium chloride 0.9% has an osmolality of approximately 430 mOsm/kg.[3]

REFERENCES

1. Raphael CD, Zhao F, Hughes SE, et al. A Pilot Chemical and Physical Stability Study of Extemporaneously Compounded Levetiracetam Intravenous Solution. *J Pain Palliat Care Pharmacother*. 2015; 29(4):370-3.
2. ASHP's Interactive Handbook on Injectable Drugs, 2020. Bethesda, MD: American Society of Health-System Pharmacists; Accessed August 2020.
3. Keppra® (Levetiracetam) Injection [package insert]. Smyrna, GA: UCB, Inc.; October 2020.

DOI 10.37573/9781585286720.123

LevoFLOXacin

Storage Conditions

	Drug Manufacturer	Concentration	Diluents	Osmolality (mOsm/kg)	pH	Temperature Room	Temperature Refrig	Temperature Frozen	Post-thaw Temp Room	Post-thaw Temp Refrig	Body Temp	Refer.
CONTAINER												
Bag, Polyvinyl Chloride (PVC)	OMJ	0.5, 5 mg/mL	D5LR, D5NS, D5W, NS	n/a	[d]	3 d[a]	14 d[a]	26 wk[a]	n/a	n/a	n/a	(1)
OTHER INFUSION CONTAINERS												
Easypump® ST/LT (B. Braun)	UN	0.5, 5 mg/mL	D5W, NS	n/a	[d]	7 d	14 d	n/a	n/a	n/a	n/a	(5)
Homepump Eclipse® / Homepump® (Halyard)	UN	5 mg/mL	D5W, NS	n/a	[d]	72 hr[b]	14 d[b]	6 m[b]	n/a	n/a	n/a	(2)
SMARTeZ® (Progressive Medical)	UN	0.5, 5 mg/mL	D5W, NS	n/a	[d]	7 d	14 d	n/a	n/a	n/a	n/a	(3)
COMMERCIAL PREPARATIONS (RTU)												
Single-Use Flexible Container	BA	5 mg/mL	D5W	iso	[d]	[c]	n/a	n/a	n/a	n/a	n/a	(4)

Flush Compatibility: Sodium chloride 0.9%.[1]

Special Considerations: Protect from light and freezing; avoid excessive heat.[1]

Notes

[a] Protected from light.
[b] Manufacturer(s) extrapolated data from other sources.
[c] Expiration date per manufacturer's label. Do not extrapolate commercial premix stability data to extemporaneously prepared solutions.
[d] pH range of diluted solutions is 3.8-5.8; pH of 5 mg/mL in NS or D5W is 4.6-4.7.[1]

REFERENCES

1. ASHP's Interactive Handbook on Injectable Drugs, 2020. Bethesda, MD: American Society of Health-System Pharmacists; Accessed September 2020.
2. *Stability Data for Drugs Using Homepump Disposable Ambulatory Infusion Systems (MK-00314 rev 3)*, 2015. Alpharetta, GA: Halyard Health; Updated June 2015.
3. *SMARTeZ® - Stability Data for Drugs Using Elastomeric Infusion Pumps*, 2020. Fenton, MO: Progressive Medical, Inc.; Updated May 2020.
4. Levofloxacin Injection in 5% Dextrose [package insert]. Deerfield, IL: Baxter Healthcare Corporation; March 2019.
5. *Drug Stability for Easypump® ST/LT*, 2020. Bethlehem, PA: B. Braun USA; Updated June 2020.

DOI 10.37573/9781585286720.124

LEVOleucovorin Calcium

						Storage Conditions						
						Temperature			Post-thaw Temp			
	Drug Manufacturer	Concentration	Diluents	Osmolality (mOsm/kg)	pH	Room	Refrig	Frozen	Room	Refrig	Body Temp	Refer.
CONTAINER												
Bag, Polyethylene	TE	1.67, 1.68 mg/mL	D5W, NS	n/a	6.3-6.5	n/a	14 d[a]	n/a	n/a	n/a	n/a	(2)
Bag, Polyolefin	WY	1.6 mg/mL	D5W	n/a	6.5	n/a	n/a	95 d	n/a	30 d[h]	n/a	(1)
Syringe, Plastic (Unspecified)	TE	10 mg/mL	Undiluted	n/a	7.4-7.9	n/a	14 d[a]	n/a	n/a	n/a	n/a	(2)
OTHER INFUSION CONTAINERS												
INFUSOR™ (Baxter)[c]	WY	0.5-0.75 mg/mL	D5W, NS	n/a	n/a	n/a	14 d	n/a	n/a	n/a	72 hr[b]	(3)
	WY	1 mg/mL	D5W, NS	n/a	n/a	7 d[d]	14 d	n/a	n/a	n/a	7 d[b][e]	(3)
	WY	5-10 mg/mL	D5W, NS, SWFI	n/a	n/a	14 d	14 wk	n/a	n/a	n/a	7 d[b][f][g]	(3)

Flush Compatibility: Sodium chloride 0.9%.

Special Considerations: Do not extrapolate stability between LEVOleucovorin and leucovorin. LEVOleucovorin is also referred to as LEVOfolinate.

Notes

[a] Protected from light.[2]

[b] Storage temperature: 33°C.[3]

[c] INTERMATE™/INFUSOR™ Portable Elastomeric Infusion System devices are no longer available in the United States.

[d] Followed by 24 hours at 33°C.[3]

[e] Following 14 days refrigerated.[3]

[f] Following 14 weeks refrigerated.[3]

[g] Following 14 days at room temperature.[3]

[h] Following 95 days frozen.[1]

REFERENCES

1. Lebitasy M, Hecq JD, Athanassopoulos A, et al. Effect of freeze-thawing on the long-term stability of calcium levofolinate in 5% dextrose stored on polyolefin infusion bags. *J Clin Pharm Ther*. 2009; 34(4):423-8.
2. Sanogo S, Silimbani P, Gaggeri R, et al. Stability of calcium levofolinate reconstituted in syringes and diluted in NaCl 0.9% and glucose 5% polyolefin/polyamide infusion bags. *J Oncol Pharm Pract*. 2020: 1078155220918025.
3. Stabforum - Stability Database: Levofolinate, Ontario, Canada: Baxter Healthcare; Accessed August 2020.

DOI 10.37573/9781585286720.125

Levothyroxine Sodium

Storage Conditions

						Temperature			Post-thaw Temp			
	Drug Manufacturer	Concentration	Diluents	Osmolality (mOsm/kg)	pH	Room	Refrig	Frozen	Room	Refrig	Body Temp	Refer.
CONTAINER												
Bag, Polyolefin	PP	1 mcg/mL	D5W	n/a	[c]	24 hr[d]	n/a	n/a	n/a	n/a	n/a	(4)
Bag, Polyvinyl Chloride (PVC)	PP	1 mcg/mL	D5W	n/a	[c]	24 hr[d]	n/a	n/a	n/a	n/a	n/a	(4)
	PP	0.4 mcg/mL	NS	n/a	[e]	16.9 hr[i] 18.3 hr[b]	n/a	n/a	n/a	n/a	n/a	(5)
	PP	2 mcg/mL	NS	n/a	[e]	6.5 hr[i] 12.3 hr[b]	n/a	n/a	n/a	n/a	n/a	(5)
Syringe, Polypropylene	APP	100 mcg/mL	NS	n/a	[a]	n/a	7 d	n/a	n/a	n/a	n/a	(7)
Vial, Glass	FRK	20, 40 mcg/mL	NS	n/a	n/a	4 hr	n/a	n/a	n/a	n/a	n/a	(2)
	FRK	20, 40, 100 mcg/mL	Undiluted	n/a	[f]	24 hr[g]	n/a	48 hr[h]	n/a	n/a	48 hr[h]	(3)(6)
	PP	1 mcg/mL	D5W	n/a	[c]	24 hr[d]	n/a	n/a	n/a	n/a	n/a	(4)

Flush Compatibility: Sodium chloride 0.9%.[1]

Special Considerations: Store intact vials at room temperature protected from light.

Notes

[a] pH of diluted solution after 7 days of storage is 10.2.[7]

[b] Time predicted to maintain at least 90% of initial drug concentration when protected from light.[5]

[c] pH of diluted solution is between 6.25-6.97.[4]

[d] 24 hour simulated infusion of drug through PVC tubing resulted in 13% loss of drug in glass and polyolefin containers, and 18% loss of drug in PVC containers over the first hour due to sorption of drug to the PVC material. Drug concentration greater than 90% of the initial concentration by 3 hours and thereafter remained above 90% in all 3 container types for the duration of the 24-hour study period. Use of polyolefin tubing or flushing the PVC tubing with drug solution prior to administration is recommended to minimize sorption.[4]

[e] Mean pH values were 6.10 and 6.12 for levothyroxine 0.4 mcg/mL exposed to ambient light and protected from light, respectively, and 6.96 and 6.98 for levothyroxine 2 mcg/mL exposed to ambient light and protected from light, respectively.[5]

[f] pH of undiluted solution is 9.5-10.8.[3]

[g] The unopened vial may be stored up to 24 hours exposed to indoor lighting outside of the carton.[3]

[h] Intact single dose vials of levothyroxine sodium injection, solution, USP subjected to 3 consecutive freeze/thaw cycles. Test samples exposed to freezing temperatures of -25°C to -10°C for 48 hours followed by accelerated storage conditions at 38°C to 42°C for 48 hours met finished product specifications with no significant difference in test results.[6]

[i] Time predicted to maintain at least 90% of initial drug concentration when exposed to light.[5]

DOI 10.37573/9781585286720.126

REFERENCES

1. ASHP's Interactive Handbook on Injectable Drugs, 2020. Bethesda, MD: American Society of Health-System Pharmacists; Accessed August 2020.
2. Levothyroxine Sodium Injection, Lyophilized [package insert]. Lake Zurich, IL: Fresenius Kabi USA, LLC; December 2019.
3. Levothyroxine Sodium Injection [package insert]. Lake Zurich, IL: Fresenius Kabi USA, LLC; April 2019.
4. Frenette AJ, MacLean RD, Williamson D, et al. Stability of levothyroxine injection in glass, polyvinyl chloride, and polyolefin containers. *Am J Health Syst Pharm*. 2011; 68(18):1723-8.
5. Strong DK, Decarie D, Ensom MH. Stability of Levothyroxine in Sodium Chloride for IV Administration. *Can J Hosp Pharm*. 2010; 63(6):437-43.
6. Levothyroxine Sodium Stability Medication Information Letter (Ref#: N/A) [personal communication]. Lake Zurich, IL: Fresenius Kabi USA, LLC; 2020:4.
7. Gupta VD. Stability of levothyroxine sodium injection in polypropylene syringes. *Int J Pharm Compd*. 2000; 4(6):482-3.

Lidocaine

Storage Conditions

	Drug Manufacturer	Concentration	Diluents	Osmolality (mOsm/kg)[n]	pH	Temperature Room	Temperature Refrig	Temperature Frozen	Post-thaw Temp Room	Post-thaw Temp Refrig	Body Temp	Refer.
CONTAINER												
Bag, Polyvinyl Chloride (PVC)	AST	1 mg/mL	NS, D5LR, D5NS, D5W, LR	n/a	[a]	n/a	24 hr	n/a	n/a	n/a	n/a	(1)
	AST	2 mg/mL	NS, D5LR, LR, D5W, D5½NS, ½NS	n/a	[a]	14 d	n/a	n/a	n/a	n/a	n/a	(1)(6)
	ES	0.515 mg/mL	D5W, NS[c]	n/a	[a]	21 d	n/a	n/a	n/a	n/a	n/a	(1)(7)
	ES	4 mg/mL	D5W	n/a	[a]	120 d[d]	120 d[d]	n/a	n/a	n/a	n/a	(1)(8)
	AST	1, 8 mg/mL	D5W, NS	n/a	[a]	48 hr	n/a	n/a	n/a	n/a	n/a	(1)
	AST	4 mg/mL	D5W[m]	n/a	[a]	24 hr	n/a	n/a	n/a	n/a	n/a	(1)
	AST	2.5 mg/mL	NS[p]	n/a	[a]	30 d	30 d	n/a	n/a	n/a	n/a	(1)
Bag, Unspecified	AST	4 mg/mL	D5W, NS[e]	n/a	[a]	24 hr	n/a	n/a	n/a	n/a	n/a	(1)
	AST	2 mg/mL	D5W, LR, NS [f][g][i][k][m][s]	n/a	[a]	24 hr	n/a	n/a	n/a	n/a	n/a	(1)
	UN	2 mg/mL	D5W[h]	n/a	[a]	24 hr	24 hr	n/a	n/a	n/a	n/a	(1)
	UN	1, 1.5 mg/mL	NS[j]	n/a	[a]	24 hr	n/a	n/a	n/a	n/a	n/a	(1)
	AST	4, 10 mg/mL	D5W, NS[l]	n/a	[a]	24 hr	n/a	n/a	n/a	n/a	n/a	(1)
	UN	2 mg/mL	unspec.[o]	n/a	[a]	24 hr	n/a	n/a	n/a	n/a	n/a	(1)
	ANT	2 mg/mL	NS[q][r]	n/a	[a]	72 hr	n/a	n/a	n/a	n/a	n/a	(1)
Syringe, Unspecified	ES	10, 20 mg/mL	unspec.[t]	n/a	[a]	48 hr	n/a	n/a	n/a	n/a	n/a	(1)
	ES	10 mg/mL	unspec.[u]	n/a	[a]	48 hr	n/a	n/a	n/a	n/a	n/a	(1)
	UN	20 mg/mL	unspec.[w]	n/a	[a]	66 d	n/a	n/a	n/a	n/a	n/a	(1)
	ASZ	10, 20 mg/mL	unspec.[x]	n/a	[a]	n/a	7 d	n/a	n/a	n/a	n/a	(1)
Vial, Glass	AST	1 mg/mL	NS, D5LR, D5NS, D5W, LR	n/a	[a]	n/a	24 hr	n/a	n/a	n/a	n/a	(1)
	AST	2 mg/mL	NS, D5LR, LR, D5W, D5½NS, ½NS	n/a	[a]	14 d	n/a	n/a	n/a	n/a	n/a	(1)(6)
	ES	0.515 mg/mL	D5W, NS[c]	n/a	[a]	21 d	n/a	n/a	n/a	n/a	n/a	(1)(7)
	AST	1, 8 mg/mL	D5W	n/a	[a]	48 hr	n/a	n/a	n/a	n/a	n/a	(1)

DOI 10.37573/9781585286720.127

Storage Conditions

						Temperature			Post-thaw Temp			
	Drug Manufacturer	Concentration	Diluents	Osmolality (mOsm/kg)[n]	pH	Room	Refrig	Frozen	Room	Refrig	Body Temp	Refer.
OTHER INFUSION CONTAINERS												
Easypump® ST/LT (B. Braun)	UN	5, 20 mg/mL	NS	n/a	[a]	30 d	n/a	n/a	n/a	n/a	n/a	(12)
INFUSOR™ (Baxter)[aa]	AST	2.4-40 mg/mL	D5W, NS, SWFI	n/a	[a]	15 d	13 wk[v]	n/a	n/a	n/a	n/a	(11)
	AST	2.4-40 mg/mL	D5W, NS, SWFI	n/a	[a]	5 wk	22 wk	n/a	n/a	n/a	n/a	(11)
SMARTeZ® (Progressive Medical)	UN	5, 20 mg/mL	NS	n/a	[a]	30 d	n/a	n/a	n/a	n/a	n/a	(2)
COMMERCIAL PREPARATIONS (RTU)												
ViaFlex™ Plus Container (Baxter)	BA	4, 8 mg/mL	D5W	n/a	[b]	30 d[z]	n/a	n/a	n/a	n/a	n/a	(3)(10)
Excel® Container (B. Braun)	BRN	4, 8 mg/mL	D5W	n/a	[b]	30 d[z]	n/a	n/a	n/a	n/a	n/a	(4)(9)

Flush Compatibility: Sodium chloride 0.9%, D5W.[1]

Special Considerations: Products containing 40, 100, or 200 mg/mL should not be administered by direct intravenous injection without prior dilution to 1-2 mg/mL solution. Lidocaine hydrochloride products containing preservatives should not be given intravenously.[1]

Notes

[a] pH of the injection is 6.5, and ranges from 5.0-7.0.[1]

[b] Premixed infusion solutions in D5W have a pH of 3.0-7.0.[3,4]

[c] Cardioplegic solutions contained: potassium chloride, sodium bicarbonate, dextrose, and sodium chloride.[1,7]

[d] Storage temperature: 4°C and 30°C.[1,8]

[e] Solution contained: alteplase (GEN) 0.5 mg/mL.[1]

[f] Solution contained: aminophylline (AQ) 1 mg/mL.[1]

[g] Solution contained: amiodarone hydrochloride (LZ) 1.8 mg/mL.[1]

[h] Solution contained: atracurium besylate (BW) 0.5 mg/mL.[1]

[i] Solution contained: calcium gluconate (ES) 2 mg/mL.[1]

[j] Solution contained: ciprofloxacin (MI) 2 mg/mL.[1]

[k] Solution contained: digoxin (ES) 1 mcg/mL.[1]

[l] Solution contained: DOBUTamine hydrochloride (LI) 1 mg/mL at 21°C.[1]

[m] Solution contained: DOPamine hydrochloride (AS)(ACC) 0.8 mg/mL.[1]

[n] The osmolalities of lidocaine hydrochloride products were determined to be 296 mOsm/kg for the 10 mg/mL concentration and 352 mOsm/kg for the 20 mg/mL concentration.[1,5]

[o] Solution contained: eptifibatide (ME) 0.75 mg/mL.[(1)]

[p] Solution contained: fentaNYL citrate 2 mcg/mL at 4°C and 23°C.[(1)]

[q] Solution contained: floxacillin sodium (BE) 20 mg/mL at 15°C and 30°C.[(1)]

[r] Solution contained: furosemide (HO) 1 mg/mL at 15°C and 30°C.[(1)]

[s] Solution contained: procainamide hydrochloride (SQ) 1 mg/mL.[(1)]

[t] Solution contained: glycopyrrolate (RB) 0.2 mg/mL.[(1)]

[u] Solution contained: metoclopramide hydrochloride (RB) 5 mg/mL.[(1)]

[v] Storage temperature: Refrigerated for 13 weeks, followed by 15 days at room temperature.

[w] Solution contained: phenylephrine 2.5 mg/mL.[(1)]

[x] Solution contained: sodium bicarbonate (HOS) 84 mg/mL. Protected from light. [(1)]

[z] Storage once removed from overwrap.[(9,10)]

[aa] INTERMATE™/INFUSOR™ Portable Elastomeric Infusion System devices are no longer available in the United States.

REFERENCES

1. ASHP's Interactive Handbook on Injectable Drugs, 2020. Bethesda, MD: American Society of Health-System Pharmacists; Accessed August 2020.
2. *SMARTeZ® - Stability Data for Drugs Using Elastomeric Infusion Pumps*, 2020. Fenton, MO: Progressive Medical, Inc.; Updated May 2020.
3. Lidocaine Hydrochloride and 5% Dextrose Injection, USP in VIAFLEX™ Plus Container [package insert]. Deerfield, IL: Baxter Healthcare Corporation; February 2017.
4. Lidocaine Hydrochloride and 5% Dextrose Injection, USP [package insert]. Bethlehem, PA: B. Braun Medical, Inc.; May 2020.
5. Bretschneider H. Osmolalities of commercially supplied drugs often used in anesthesia. *Anesth Analg*. 1987; 66(4):361-2.
6. Kirschenbaum HL, Aronoff W, Perentesis GP, et al. Stability and compatibility of lidocaine hydrochloride with selected large-volume parenterals and drug additives. *Am J Hosp Pharm*. 1982; 39(6):1013-5.
7. Lackner TE, Baldus D, Butler CD, et al. Lidocaine stability in cardioplegic solution stored in glass bottles and polyvinyl chloride bags. *Am J Hosp Pharm*. 1983; 40(1):97-101.
8. Smith FM, Nuessle NO. Stability of lidocaine hydrochloride in 5% dextrose injection in plastic bags. *Am J Hosp Pharm*. 1981; 38(11):1745-7.
9. Lidocaine and 5% Dextrose Stability Medication Information Response (Ref#: N/A) [personal communication]. Bethlehem, PA: B. Braun Medical, Inc.; 2020:1.
10. Lidocaine Hydrochloride and 5% Dextrose Injection, USP in VIAFLEX™ Plus Container Stability Medication Information Letter (Ref#: US2020-07512) [personal communication]. Deerfield, IL: Baxter Healthcare Corporation; 2020:2.
11. Stabforum - Stability Database: Lidocaine, Ontario, Canada: Baxter Healthcare; Accessed February 2021.
12. *Drug Stability for Easypump® ST/LT*, 2020. Bethlehem, PA: B. Braun USA; Updated June 2020.

Linezolid

Storage Conditions

						Temperature			Post-thaw Temp			
	Drug Manufacturer	Concentration	Diluents	Osmolality (mOsm/kg)	pH	Room	Refrig	Frozen	Room	Refrig	Body Temp	Refer.
CONTAINER												
Unspecified	PF	2 mg/mL	D5W, D10W, NS	n/a	n/a	34 d	n/a	n/a	n/a	n/a	n/a	(3)
OTHER INFUSION CONTAINERS												
Easypump® ST/LT (B. Braun)	UN	0.15, 2 mg/mL	NS	n/a	n/a	24 hr	13 d	n/a	n/a	n/a	n/a	(5)
SMARTeZ® (Progressive Medical)	UN	0.15, 2 mg/mL	NS	n/a	n/a	24 hr[e]	13 d[e]	n/a	n/a	n/a	n/a	(2)
COMMERCIAL PREPARATIONS (RTU)												
Flexible Plastic Bag (Pfizer)	PF	2 mg/mL	RTU[a]	iso	4.8	[b][c]	n/a	n/a	n/a	n/a	[d]	(1)(3)(4)

Flush Compatibility: Sodium chloride 0.9%, heparin.[3]

Special Considerations: Administer IV over 30 minutes to 2 hours. Yellow color may intensify over time without affecting stability.[1,3] The manufacturers state that linezolid RTU solutions for infusion are compatible with NS, D5W, and LR.[3]

Notes

[a] RTU sterile isotonic solution. Inactive ingredients include sodium citrate, citric acid, and dextrose. Do not use the RTU bag in series connections.[1]

[b] Expiration date per manufacturer's label. Use within 30 d of foil overwrap removal. Studies support storage out of the overwrap for less than 30 d in a pharmacy exposed to ambient room light.[4]

[c] Protected from light and freezing.[1,3]

[d] Linezolid (PF) 2 mg/mL remained stable without noticeable degradation for 72 hr when stored at 70°C.[6]

[e] Manufacturer extrapolated data from other sources.

DOI 10.37573/9781585286720.128

REFERENCES

1. Zyvox® (Linezolid) Injection [package insert]. New York, NY: Pharmacia & Upjohn Co; September 2020.
2. SMARTeZ® - Stability Data for Drugs Using Elastomeric Infusion Pumps, 2020. Fenton, MO: Progressive Medical, Inc.; Updated May 2020.
3. ASHP's Interactive Handbook on Injectable Drugs, 2020. Bethesda, MD: American Society of Health-System Pharmacists; Accessed September 2020.
4. Pfizer Medical Information. *Zyvox® – Stability Out Of Overwrap*. https://www.pfizermedicalinformation.com/en-us/document/208449. Accessed September 23, 2020.
5. Drug Stability for Easypump® ST/LT, 2020. Bethlehem, PA: B. Braun USA; Updated June 2020.
6. Taylor R, Sunderland B, Luna G, et al. Evaluation of the stability of linezolid in aqueous solution and commonly used intravenous fluids. *Drug Des Devel Ther*. 2017; 11:2087-97.

Lipid Emulsion

Storage Conditions

						Temperature			Post-thaw Temp			
	Drug Manufacturer	Concentration	Diluents	Osmolality (mOsm/kg)	pH	Room	Refrig	Frozen	Room	Refrig	Body Temp	Refer.
CONTAINER												
Bag, Ethylene Vinyl Acetate (EVA)	FRK[a]	0.1 gm/mL (10%)	Undiluted	342	6-9	24 hr	6 d[c]	n/a	n/a	n/a	n/a	(1)(2)
	FRK[b]	0.2 gm/mL (20%)	Undiluted	380	6-9	48 hr	7 d[d]	n/a	n/a	n/a	n/a	(3)(4)
Syringe, Plastic (Unspecified)	FRK[a]	0.1 gm/mL (10%)	Undiluted	342	6-9	12 hr	7 d	n/a	n/a	n/a	n/a	(1)(2)
Syringe, Polypropylene	FRK[b]	0.2 gm/mL (20%)	Undiluted	380	6-9	24 hr	6 d[c]	n/a	n/a	n/a	n/a	(3)(4)
	BA[e]	0.2 gm/mL (20%)	Undiluted	350	6-8.9	30 d	30 d	n/a	n/a	n/a	21 d[g]	(5)(6)
	BA[f]	0.2 gm/mL (20%)	Undiluted	340	6-9	30 d	30 d	n/a	n/a	n/a	21 d[g]	(5)(7)
	FRK[a]	0.1 gm/mL (10%)	Undiluted	342	6-9	30 d	30 d	n/a	n/a	n/a	21 d[g]	(1)(5)
	FRK[b]	0.2 gm/mL (20%)	Undiluted	380	6-9	30 d	30 d	n/a	n/a	n/a	21 d[g]	(3)(5)

Flush Compatibility: Sodium chloride 0.9%.

Special Considerations: n/a

Notes

[a] Omegaven® (fish oil triglycerides) (FRK).(1,2,5)
[b] SMOFlipid® (lipid injectable emulsion) (FRK).(3–5)
[c] 6 days at 2-8°C, followed by 24 hours at 20-25°C.(2)
[d] 7 days at 2-8°C, followed by 48 hours at 20-25°C.(4)
[e] Intralipid® (lipid injectable emulsion) (BA).(5,6)
[f] Clinolipid® (Clinoleic outside the USA) (BA).(5,7)
[g] Storage temperature: 40°C.

DOI 10.37573/9781585286720.129

REFERENCES

1. Omegaven® (Fish Oil Triglycerides) Injectable Emulsion [package insert]. Lake Zurich, IL: Fresenius Kabi USA, LLC; December 2020.
2. Omegaven® Stability - Internal Data (Ref#: N/A) [personal communication]. Lake Zurich, IL: Fresenius Kabi USA, LLC; 2018:2.
3. SMOFlipid® (Lipid Injectable Emulsion, USP) [package insert]. Lake Zurich, IL: Fresenius Kabi USA, LLC; January 2021.
4. SMOFlipid® Stability - Internal Data (Ref#: N/A) [personal communication]. Lake Zurich, IL: Fresenius Kabi USA, LLC; 2020:3.
5. Watrobska-Swietlikowska D. Stability of commercial parenteral lipid emulsions repacking to polypropylene syringes. PLoS One. 2019; 14(4):e0214451.
6. Intralipid® 20% (I.V. Fat Emulsion) [package insert]. Deerfield, IL: Baxter Healthcare Corporation; January 2019.
7. Clinolipid® (Olive Oil and Soybean Oil Lipid Injectable Emulsion) [package insert]. Deerfield, IL: Baxter Healthcare Corporation; November 2020.

LORazepam

Storage Conditions

CONTAINER	Drug Manufacturer	Concentration	Diluents	Osmolality (mOsm/kg)	pH	Temperature Room	Temperature Refrig	Temperature Frozen	Post-thaw Temp Room	Post-thaw Temp Refrig	Body Temp	Refer.
Bag, Polyolefin	WY	0.1 mg/mL	D5W, NS	n/a	n/a	7 d	7 d	n/a	n/a	n/a	72 hr	(1)
	WY	0.1 mg/mL	D5W	n/a	n/a	n/a	n/a	7 d[d]	n/a	n/a	n/a	(1)
	AB	0.91 mg/mL[e]	NS	n/a	n/a	5 wk[a]	5 wk[a]	5 wk[a]	n/a	n/a	5 d[a]	(1)(2)
	WY	0.1 mg/mL	LR	n/a	n/a	7 d	7 d	n/a	n/a	n/a	72 hr	(1)
Syringe, Polypropylene	WAY	0.2, 0.5, 1 mg/mL[e][h]	D5W, NS	n/a	n/a	24 hr[b]	n/a	n/a	n/a	n/a	n/a	(1)
	WY	1 mg/mL[e]	D5W, NS	n/a	n/a	28 hr	n/a	n/a	n/a	n/a	n/a	(1)
	PF	0.16 mg/mL[d]	NS	n/a	[c]	48 hr	n/a	n/a	n/a	n/a	n/a	(3)
Vial, Glass	WY	1 mg/mL	BWFI	n/a	n/a	n/a[g]	7 d	n/a	n/a	n/a	n/a	(1)
	WY	1 mg/mL[e]	D5W	n/a	n/a	28 hr	n/a	n/a	n/a	n/a	n/a	(1)
	WY	2 mg/mL[f]	D5W	n/a	n/a	28 hr	n/a	n/a	n/a	n/a	n/a	(1)

Flush Compatibility: Sodium chloride 0.9%, heparin.[1]

Special Considerations: Store product under refrigeration and protect from light and freezing. Both the 2- and 4-mg/mL products contain the same concentration of solubilizing agents. Use of the 4 mg/mL concentration may result in over-dilution of the solubilizing agent, increasing the potential for precipitation of an admixture; compounding procedures should be consistent for demonstrated results.[1]

Notes

[a] Protected from light.

[b] Physically stable over 24 hr and chemically stable for 48 hr at room temperature.[1]

[c] pH of diluted solution was 7.06-7.54.[3]

[d] Physical stability only. Chemical stability of reconstituted solutions not performed.[3]

[e] Prepared from 2 mg/mL commercial preparation.

[f] Prepared from 4 mg/mL commercial preparation.

[g] 12% loss at 22°C in 7 d.

[h] When prepared from 4 mg/mL commercial preparation, consistently precipitated.

DOI 10.37573/9781585286720.130

REFERENCES

1. ASHP's Interactive Handbook on Injectable Drugs, 2020. Bethesda, MD: American Society of Health-System Pharmacists; Accessed August 2020.
2. Norenberg JP, Achusim LE, Steel TH, et al. Stability of lorazepam in 0.9% sodium chloride stored in polyolefin bags. *Am J Health Syst Pharm*. 2004; 61(10):1039-41.
3. Closset M, Hecq JD, Soumoy L, et al. Physical stability of highly concentrated injectable drugs solutions used in intensive care units. *Ann Pharm Fr*. 2017; 75(3):185-88.

Magnesium Sulfate

Storage Conditions

	Drug Manufacturer	Concentration	Diluents	Osmolality (mOsm/kg)	pH	Temperature: Room	Temperature: Refrig	Temperature: Frozen	Post-thaw Temp: Room	Post-thaw Temp: Refrig	Body Temp	Refer.
CONTAINER												
Bag, Polyvinyl Chloride (PVC)	AMR	37 mg/mL	LR, NS	[a]	[b]	3 m	n/a	n/a	n/a	n/a	n/a	(1)
	SZ	40, 100 mg/mL	D5W, NS[d]	[a]	[b]	7 d[e]	7 d[e]	n/a	n/a	n/a	n/a	(2)
Syringe, Plastic (Unspecified)	ES	500 mg/mL	Undiluted[g]	[a]	[b]	48 hr	n/a	n/a	n/a	n/a	n/a	(1)
Unspecified	AB	40 mg/mL	D5W	[a]	[b]	n/a	60 d[c]	n/a	n/a	n/a	n/a	(1)
	DB	39 mg/mL	D5W, NS[f]	[a]	[b]	24 hr	n/a	n/a	n/a	n/a	n/a	(4)
Vial, Glass	AMR	37 mg/mL	LR, NS	[a]	[b]	3 m	n/a	n/a	n/a	n/a	n/a	(1)
OTHER INFUSION CONTAINERS												
Dosi-Fuser® (Leventon)	MCO	8-20 mg/mL	NS	[a]	[b]	30 d	n/a	n/a	n/a	n/a	14 d	(5)
Easypump® ST/LT (B. Braun)	UN	20 mg/mL	NS	[a]	[b]	24 hr	29 d	n/a	n/a	n/a	n/a	(3)

Flush Compatibility: Sodium chloride 0.9%, heparin.[(1)]

Special Considerations: Store intact vials at controlled room temperature. Refrigeration of intact vials may result in precipitation or crystallization. Do not freeze.[(1)]

Notes

[a] Magnesium sulfate 4% (40 mg/mL) and 8% (80 mg/mL) solutions in SWFI for injection have osmolarities of 325 and 649 mOsm/L, respectively. Magnesium sulfate 1% (10 mg/mL) and 2% (20 mg/mL) solutions in D5W have osmolarities of 333 and 415 mOsm/L, respectively. Magnesium sulfate 50% (500 mg/mL) solution has calculated osmolarity of 4050 mOsm/L.[(1)]

[b] Magnesium sulfate injection has a pH adjusted to 5.5-7. Premixed solutions have pH values in the range of 3.5-6.5.[(1)]

[c] Storage temperature: 0°C.[(1)]

[d] Solution contained: calcium gluconate 40 mg/mL (PP) and 100 mg/mL (PP).[(2)]

[e] Protected from light.[(2)]

[f] Solution contained: potassium chloride 80 mEq/L (BRN).[(4)]

[g] Solution contained: metoclopramide hydrochloride 2 mg/mL (RB) and 5 mg/mL (RB).[(1)]

DOI 10.37573/9781585286720.131

REFERENCES

1. ASHP's Interactive Handbook on Injectable Drugs, 2020. Bethesda, MD: American Society of Health-System Pharmacists; Accessed August 2020.
2. Beauregard N, Bertrand N, Dufour A, et al. Physical compatibility of calcium gluconate and magnesium sulfate injections. *Am J Health Syst Pharm*. 2012; 69(2):98.
3. *Drug Stability for Easypump® ST/LT*, 2020. Bethlehem, PA: B. Braun USA; Updated June 2020.
4. Quay I, Tan E. Compatibility and stability of potassium chloride and magnesium sulfate in 0.9% sodium chloride injection and 5% dextrose injection solutions. *Int J Pharm Compd*. 2001; 5(4):323-4.
5. *Drug Stability Table - Dosi-Fuser® Elastomeric Pump (S-CL-00-001v16)*, 2021. Barcelona, Spain: Leventon SAU; Updated May 2021.

Meperidine Hydrochloride

Storage Conditions

	Drug Manufacturer	Concentration	Diluents	Osmolality (mOsm/kg)	pH	Temperature Room	Temperature Refrig	Temperature Frozen	Post-thaw Temp Room	Post-thaw Temp Refrig	Body Temp	Refer.
CONTAINER												
Bag, Polyvinyl Chloride (PVC)	WI	1.2 mg/mL	D5W	n/a	[a]	36 hr	n/a	n/a	n/a	n/a	n/a	(1)
	UN	2.5 mg/mL	NS	n/a	[a]	24 d	n/a	n/a	n/a	n/a	n/a	(1)
Syringe, Glass	WI	25 mg/mL	[b]	n/a	[a]	12 m[c]	12 m[c]	n/a	n/a	n/a	n/a	(1)
Syringe, Plastic (Unspecified)	WY	5, 10 mg/mL	D5W, NS	n/a	[a]	12 wk	12 wk[c]	12 wk[c]	n/a	n/a	n/a	(1)(3)
	WI	25 mg/mL	[b]	n/a	[a]	12 m[c]	12 m[c]	n/a	n/a	n/a	n/a	(1)
Syringe, Polypropylene	AB[d]	0.25, 1, 10, 20, 30 mg/mL	D5W, NS	n/a	[a]	28 d[c]	28 d[c]	n/a	n/a	n/a	n/a	(1)
OTHER INFUSION CONTAINERS												
CADD® Cassette (Smiths Medical)	REN	5, 20 mg/mL	NS	n/a	n/a	21 d[c]	n/a	n/a	n/a	n/a	n/a	(2)
	AGT	1, 40 mg/mL	NS	n/a	n/a	30 d[c]	n/a	n/a	n/a	n/a	n/a	(1)
	UN	15 mg/mL	SWFI	n/a	n/a	n/a	14 d	n/a	n/a	n/a	9 d[e]	(4)
	UN	8 mg/mL	NS[f]	n/a	n/a	21 d	n/a	n/a	n/a	n/a	n/a	(4)
Implantable Pump (Infusaid)	SW	10 mg/mL	NS	n/a	[a]	n/a	n/a	n/a	n/a	n/a	90 d	(1)

Flush Compatibility: Sodium chloride 0.9%.[1]

Special Considerations: Protect solutions from light, do not freeze.[1] Meperidine is known internationally as pethidine.[3]

Notes

[a] pH of undiluted solution is 3.5-6.[1]

[b] Solution contained: chlorproMAZINE HCl 6.25 mg/mL and hydrOXYzine HCl 12.5 mg/mL.

[c] Protected from light.

[d] Preservative free product (AB).

[e] Storage temperature: 35°C.[4]

[f] Solution contained: cloNIDine 3 mcg/mL.[4]

DOI 10.37573/9781585286720.132

REFERENCES

1. ASHP's Interactive Handbook on Injectable Drugs, 2020. Bethesda, MD: American Society of Health-System Pharmacists; Accessed August 2020.
2. Laville I, Mercier L, Chachaty E, et al. [Shelf-lives of morphine and pethidine solutions stored in patient-controlled analgesia devices: physico-chemical and microbiological stability study]. *Pathol Biol (Paris)*. 2005; 53(4):210-6.
3. Strong ML, Schaaf LJ, Pankaskie MC, et al. Shelf-lives and factors affecting the stability of morphine sulphate and meperidine (pethidine) hydrochloride in plastic syringes for use in patient-controlled analgesic devices. *J Clin Pharm Ther*. 1994; 19(6):361-9.
4. *Pharmaceutical report on chemical and physical stability of drugs commonly used with CADD® infusion pumps (IN193109GB-122019)*, 2019. Minneapolis, MN: Smiths Medical ASD, Inc.; Updated December 2019.

Meropenem

Storage Conditions

						Temperature			Post-thaw Temp			
	Drug Manufacturer	Concentration	Diluents	Osmolality (mOsm/kg)	pH	Room	Refrig	Frozen	Room	Refrig	Body Temp	Refer.
CONTAINER												
Bag, Polypropylene	FRK	4 mg/mL	NS[a]	n/a	[h]	12 hr	6 d	7 d	n/a	n/a	n/a	(2)
Bag, Polyvinyl Chloride (PVC)	ZEN	1 mg/mL	NS	n/a	[h]	22 hr	7 d[f]	33 d	n/a	n/a	n/a	(3)(9)
	ZEN	4 mg/mL	NS	n/a	[h]	n/a	7 d	n/a	n/a	n/a	n/a	(7)(9)
	ZEN	10, 20 mg/mL	NS	n/a	[h]	n/a	5 d	n/a	n/a	n/a	n/a	(7)(9)
	ZEN	22 mg/mL	NS	n/a	[h]	17 hr	4 d	11 d	n/a	n/a	n/a	(3)(9)
	UN	10 mg/mL	NS	n/a	[h]	12 hr	n/a	n/a	n/a	n/a	n/a	(18)
	ZEN	1 mg/mL	D5W	n/a	[h]	4 hr	24 hr	24 hr	n/a	n/a	n/a	(3)(9)
	ZEN	1 mg/mL	D5W[b]	n/a	[h]	n/a	18 hr	n/a	n/a	n/a	n/a	(9)
	ZEN	20 mg/mL	D5W[b]	n/a	[h]	n/a	20 hr	n/a	n/a	n/a	n/a	(9)
	ZEN	20 mg/mL	D5W[d]	n/a	[h]	3 hr	18 hr	n/a	n/a	n/a	n/a	(9)
	ZEN	20 mg/mL	D5LR	n/a	[h]	n/a	18 hr	n/a	n/a	n/a	n/a	(9)
	ZEN	22 mg/mL	D5W	n/a	[h]	6 hr	48 hr	7 d	n/a	n/a	n/a	(3)(9)
	ZEN	20 mg/mL	D10W	n/a	[h]	2 hr	8 hr	n/a	n/a	n/a	n/a	(9)
	ZEN	1 mg/mL	D5LR, LR	n/a	[h]	n/a	48 hr	n/a	n/a	n/a	n/a	(9)
	ZEN	20 mg/mL	LR, R	n/a	[h]	8 hr	48 hr	n/a	n/a	n/a	n/a	(9)
	ZEN	1 mg/mL	R	n/a	[h]	10 hr	48 hr	n/a	n/a	n/a	n/a	(9)
	ZEN	20 mg/mL	NMD5W	n/a	[h]	3 hr	24 hr	n/a	n/a	n/a	n/a	(9)
Syringe, Plastic (Unspecified)	HOS	50 mg/mL	SWFI	n/a	[h]	8 hr	44 hr	n/a	n/a	n/a	n/a	(15)
	HOS	50 mg/mL	NS	n/a	[h]	8 hr	40 hr	n/a	n/a	n/a	n/a	(15)
	HOS	50 mg/mL	D5W	n/a	[h]	5 hr	25 hr	n/a	n/a	n/a	n/a	(15)
Syringe, Polypropylene	ASZ, SZ, HOS, FRK	10, 20 mg/mL	NS	n/a	[h]	12 hr	n/a	n/a	n/a	n/a	n/a	(13)
	ASZ, SZ, HOS, FRK	40 mg/mL	NS	n/a	[h]	8 hr	n/a	n/a	n/a	n/a	n/a	(13)
Unspecified	PF	1-20 mg/mL	NS	n/a	[h]	1 hr	15 hr	n/a	n/a	n/a	n/a	(1)(9)
	ASZ	5 mg/mL	NS	n/a	[h]	8 hr	n/a	n/a	n/a	n/a	n/a	(9)

DOI 10.37573/9781585286720.133

Storage Conditions

	Drug Manufacturer	Concentration	Diluents	Osmolality (mOsm/kg)	pH	Temperature Room	Temperature Refrig	Temperature Frozen	Post-thaw Temp Room	Post-thaw Temp Refrig	Body Temp	Refer.
CONTAINER												
Vial, Glass	ZEN	2.5 mg/mL	NS, SWFI	n/a	[h]	24 hr	48 hr	n/a	n/a	n/a	n/a	(6)(9)
	ZEN	2.5 mg/mL	D5W	n/a	[h]	4 hr	24 hr	n/a	n/a	n/a	n/a	(6)(9)
	ZEN	50 mg/mL	NS, SWFI	n/a	[h]	8 hr	48 hr	n/a	n/a	n/a	n/a	(6)(9)
	ZEN	50 mg/mL	D5W	n/a	[h]	3 hr	24 hr	n/a	n/a	n/a	n/a	(6)(9)
	PF	≤ 50 mg/mL	SWFI	n/a	[h]	3 hr	13 hr	n/a	n/a	n/a	n/a	(1)
OTHER INFUSION CONTAINERS												
ADD-Vantage® Flexible Container System (Pfizer)	ZEN	5 mg/mL	½NS	n/a	[h]	22 hr	48 hr	n/a	n/a	n/a	n/a	(9)
	ZEN	20 mg/mL	½NS	n/a	[h]	10 hr	48 hr	n/a	n/a	n/a	n/a	(9)
CADD® Cassette (Smiths Medical)	ZEN	20, 30 mg/mL	NS	n/a	[h]	24 hr[c]	24 hr	n/a	n/a	n/a	n/a	(5)(9)
Dosi-Fuser® (Leventon)	ASZ	5-40 mg/mL	NS	n/a	[h]	24 hr[i]	n/a	n/a	n/a	n/a	n/a	(14)
	ASZ	6 mg/mL	NS	n/a	[h]	24 hr[i]	6 d[i]	n/a	n/a	n/a	n/a	(14)
	FRK	20 mg/mL	NS	n/a	[h]	n/a	4 d	n/a	n/a	n/a	n/a	(14)
Easypump® ST/LT (B. Braun)	UN	5 mg/mL	NS	n/a	[h]	24 hr[i]	10 d[i]	n/a	n/a	n/a	n/a	(11)
	UN	20 mg/mL	NS	n/a	[h]	24 hr[i]	4 d[i]	n/a	n/a	n/a	n/a	(11)
	UN	2.5 mg/mL	NS	n/a	[h]	6 hr[i]	24 hr[i]	n/a	n/a	n/a	n/a	(11)
Homepump Eclipse® / Homepump® (Halyard)	ZEN	4 mg/mL	NS	n/a	[h]	n/a	7 d	n/a	n/a	n/a	n/a	(7)(9)
	UN	5 mg/mL	NS	n/a	[h]	26 hr[i]	4 d[i]	n/a	n/a	n/a	n/a	(8)
	UN	5-10 mg/mL	NS	n/a	[h]	n/a	4 d[i]	n/a	n/a	n/a	n/a	(8)
	UN	10 mg/mL	NS	n/a	[h]	20 hr[i]	4 d[i]	n/a	n/a	n/a	n/a	(8)
	ZEN	10, 20 mg/mL	NS	n/a	[h]	n/a	5 d	n/a	n/a	n/a	n/a	(7)(9)
	UN	20 mg/mL	NS	n/a	[h]	14 hr[i]	72 hr[i]	n/a	n/a	n/a	n/a	(8)
INTERMATE™ (Baxter)[e]	ZEN	5 mg/mL	NS	n/a	[h]	34 hr	4 d[g]	n/a	n/a	n/a	n/a	(9)(16)
	ZEN	5 mg/mL	NS	n/a	[h]	6 hr[j]	72 hr	n/a	n/a	n/a	n/a	(10)
	ASZ	6 mg/mL	NS	n/a	[h]	4 hr	4 d	n/a	n/a	n/a	n/a	(10)
	ZEN	5-40 mg/mL	NS	n/a	[h]	n/a	24 hr	n/a	n/a	n/a	n/a	(10)
	ZEN	10 mg/mL	NS	n/a	[h]	20 hr	4 d[g]	n/a	n/a	n/a	n/a	(9)(16)

Storage Conditions

	Drug Manufacturer	Concentration	Diluents	Osmolality (mOsm/kg)	pH	Temperature: Room	Temperature: Refrig	Temperature: Frozen	Post-thaw Temp: Room	Post-thaw Temp: Refrig	Body Temp	Refer.
OTHER INFUSION CONTAINERS												
INFUSOR™ (Baxter)[e]	RNB	6 mg/mL	NS	n/a	6.5	24 hr[k]	6 d	n/a	n/a	n/a	n/a	(17)
	RNB	12 mg/mL	NS	n/a	6.6	24 hr[l]	72 hr	n/a	n/a	n/a	n/a	(17)
	RNB	20 mg/mL	NS	n/a	6.6	24 hr	72 hr	n/a	n/a	n/a	n/a	(17)
	RNB	25 mg/mL	NS	n/a	6.6	n/a	48 hr	n/a	n/a	n/a	n/a	(17)
SMARTeZ® (Progressive Medical)	UN	5 mg/mL	NS	n/a	[h]	24 hr[i]	10 d[i]	n/a	n/a	n/a	n/a	(12)
	UN	10 mg/mL	NS	n/a	[h]	21 hr[i]	10 d[i]	n/a	n/a	n/a	n/a	(12)
	UN	20 mg/mL	NS	n/a	[h]	24 hr[i]	4 d[i]	n/a	n/a	n/a	n/a	(12)

Flush Compatibility: Sodium chloride 0.9%, heparin.[3,4]

Special Considerations: Due to significant loss of potency, solutions in D5W should be prepared just prior to administration.[1,3]

Notes

[a] Solution contained: tedizolid 0.8 mg/mL.[2]

[b] Solution contained: sodium bicarbonate 0.02%.[9]

[c] Storage in a cold pouch with frozen gel packs replaced every 8 to 12 hours.[5]

[d] Solution contained: potassium chloride 0.15%.[9]

[e] INTERMATE™/INFUSOR™ Portable Elastomeric Infusion System devices are no longer available in the United States.

[f] Study data revealed greater than 90% of initial concentration for 10 days. Study recommends storage for 7 days refrigerated, followed by 6 hours at room temperature prior to administration.[3]

[g] Storage temperature: Refrigerated for 4 days, followed by 6 hours at room temperature.[16]

[h] pH of reconstituted solution is 7.3-8.3.[1,9]

[i] Manufacturer extrapolated data from other source(s).

[j] Following refrigerated storage for 72 hours.[10]

[k] Storage temperature: Refrigerated for 48 hours followed by 24 hours at room temperature.[17]

[l] Storage temperature: Refrigerated for 24 hours followed by 24 hours at room temperature.[17]

REFERENCES

1. Merrem® IV (Meropenem) Injection [package insert]. New York, NY: Pfizer Laboratories Div Pfizer, Inc.; March 2021.
2. Ezquer-Garin C, Ferriols-Lisart R, Martinez-Lopez LM, et al. Stability of tedizolid phosphate-sodium rifampicin and tedizolid phosphate-meropenem admixtures in intravenous infusion bags stored at different temperatures. *Pharmazie*. 2020; 75(5):172-76.
3. Walker S, Varrin S, Yannicelli D, et al. Stability of meropenem in saline and dextrose solutions and compatibility with potassium chloride. *Can J Hosp Pharm*. 2018; 51(4):156-68.

4. Patel PR. Compatibility of meropenem with commonly used injectable drugs. *Am J Health Syst Pharm*. 1996; 53(23):2853-5. Erratum in: *Am J Health Syst Pharm*. 1998; 55(7):735.
5. Grant EM, Zhong MK, Ambrose PG, et al. Stability of meropenem in a portable infusion device in a cold pouch. *Am J Health Syst Pharm*. 2000; 57(10):992-5.
6. Patel PR, Cook SE. Stability of meropenem in intravenous solutions. *Am J Health Syst Pharm*. 1997; 54(4):412-21.
7. Smith DL, Bauer SM, Nicolau DP. Stability of meropenem in polyvinyl chloride bags and an elastomeric infusion device. *Am J Health Syst Pharm*. 2004; 61(16):1682-5.
8. *Stability Data for Drugs Using Homepump Disposable Ambulatory Infusion Systems (MK-00314 rev 3)*, 2015. Alpharetta, GA: Halyard Health; Updated June 2015.
9. ASHP's Interactive Handbook on Injectable Drugs, 2020. Bethesda, MD: American Society of Health-System Pharmacists; Accessed September 2020.
10. Stabforum - Stability Database: Meropenem, Ontario, Canada: Baxter Healthcare; Accessed January 2021.
11. *Drug Stability for Easypump® ST/LT*, 2020. Bethlehem, PA: B. Braun USA; Updated June 2020.
12. *SMARTeZ® - Stability Data for Drugs Using Elastomeric Infusion Pumps*, 2020. Fenton, MO: Progressive Medical, Inc.; Updated May 2020.
13. Carlier M, Stove V, Verstraete AG, et al. Stability of generic brands of meropenem reconstituted in isotonic saline. *Minerva Anestesiol*. 2015; 81(3):283-7.
14. *Drug Stability Table - Dosi-Fuser® Elastomeric Pump (S-CL-00-001v16)*, 2021. Barcelona, Spain: Leventon SAU; Updated May 2021.
15. Fugit KD, Anderson BD. Antibiotic Stability in Freedom 60 Syringe Report by HealthTekTM and the University of Kentucky, Lexington. Chester, NY: RMS Medical Products; 2015.
16. Kramer I. Stability of Meropenem in Elastomeric Portable Infusion Devices. *Eur Hosp Pharm*. 1997; 3(5):168-71.
17. Foy F, Luna G, Martinez J, et al. An investigation of the stability of meropenem in elastomeric infusion devices. *Drug Des Devel Ther*. 2019; 13:2655-65.
18. Venugopalan V, Manigaba K, Borgert SJ, et al. Training a Drug to Do New Tricks: Insights on Stability of Meropenem Administered as a Continuous Infusion. *Microbiol Insights*. 2018; 11:1178636118804549.

Meropenem – Vaborbactam

						Storage Conditions						
						Temperature			Post-thaw Temp			
	Drug Manufacturer	Concentration[a]	Diluents	Osmolality (mOsm/kg)	pH	Room	Refrig	Frozen	Room	Refrig	Body Temp	Refer.
CONTAINER												
Bag, Polyvinyl Chloride (PVC)	MEL	8, 16 mg/mL	NS	n/a	n/a	12 hr	6 d	n/a	n/a	n/a	n/a	(1)
	MEL	4 mg/mL	NS	n/a	n/a	12 hr	5 d	n/a	n/a	n/a	n/a	(1)
OTHER INFUSION CONTAINERS												
Homepump Eclipse® / Homepump® (Halyard)	MEL	11.4 mg/mL	NS	n/a	n/a	12 hr	5 d	n/a	n/a	n/a	n/a	(1)

Flush Compatibility: Sodium chloride 0.9%.[(1)]

Special Considerations: The diluted solution of meropenem-vaborbactam for infusion is administered intravenously over 3 hours. The reconstituted solution is not suitable for direct injection.[(2)]

Notes

[a] Concentration expressed as combination of meropenem and vaborbactam with each component comprising one half the total.

REFERENCES

1. Chen IH, Martin EK, Nicolau DP, et al. Assessment of Meropenem and Vaborbactam Room Temperature and Refrigerated Stability in Polyvinyl Chloride Bags and Elastomeric Devices. *Clin Ther*. 2020; 42(4):606-13.
2. ASHP's Interactive Handbook on Injectable Drugs, 2020. Bethesda, MD: American Society of Health-System Pharmacists; Accessed December 2020.

DOI 10.37573/9781585286720.134

Mesna

Storage Conditions

	Drug Manufacturer	Concentration	Diluents	Osmolality (mOsm/kg)	pH	Temperature: Room	Temperature: Refrig	Temperature: Frozen	Post-thaw Temp: Room	Post-thaw Temp: Refrig	Body Temp	Refer.
CONTAINER												
Bag, Polyethylene	AM	0.54 mg/mL	D5W[k]	n/a	[l]	6 hr	48 hr	n/a	n/a	n/a	n/a	(6)
	AM	3.2 mg/mL	D5W[j]	n/a	[l]	24 hr	48 hr	n/a	n/a	n/a	n/a	(6)
Bag, Polyvinyl Chloride (PVC)	UN	10, 20, 30 mg/mL	NS[b]	n/a	[l]	14 d	n/a	n/a	n/a	n/a	n/a	(4)
Syringe, Polypropylene	UN	40 mg/mL	NS[b]	n/a	[l]	28 d	28 d	n/a	n/a	n/a	n/a	(1)
	AST	100 mg/mL	Undiluted	n/a	[l]	9 d	9 d	n/a	n/a	n/a	9 d[h]	(5)
Vial, Glass	AW	3 mg/mL	D5W[c]	n/a	[l]	48 hr[d]	n/a	n/a	n/a	n/a	n/a	(2)
OTHER INFUSION CONTAINERS												
Dosi-Fuser® (Leventon)	UN	0.4-100 mg/mL	NS[e]	n/a	[l]	n/a	7 d[n]	n/a	n/a	n/a	48 hr[m][n]	(7)
	BA	100 mg/mL	NS[i]	n/a	[l]	10 d	14 d	n/a	n/a	n/a	n/a	(7)
	BA	1 mg/mL	NS[a]	n/a	[l]	10 d	7 d	n/a	n/a	n/a	n/a	(7)
Graseby™ 9000 Cassette (Graseby Medical)	AM	20 mg/mL	SWFI[g]	n/a	[l]	n/a	14 d[f]	n/a	n/a	n/a	7 d[f]	(3)

Flush Compatibility: Sodium chloride 0.9%.[5]

Special Considerations: Multidose vials of mesna may be stored and used for up to 8 d after initial entry.[5]

Notes

[a] Solution contained: ifosfamide 1 mg/mL.[7]

[b] Solution contained: ifosfamide 50 mg/mL.[1,4]

[c] Solution contained: hydrOXYzine hydrochloride 0.5 mg/mL.[2]

[d] Although not specifically stated in this visual compatibility study, room temperature was inferred as the storage temperature.

[e] Solution contained: ifosfamide (AM) 0.8-100 mg/mL.[7]

[f] Protected from light.[3]

[g] Solution contained: ifosfamide (AM) 20 mg/mL.[3]

DOI 10.37573/9781585286720.135

[h] Storage temperature: 35°C.[5]

[i] Solution contained: ifosfamide 100 mg/mL.[7]

[j] Solution contained: cyclophosphamide (AM) 10.8 mg/mL.[6]

[k] Solution contained: cyclophosphamide (AM) 1.8 mg/mL.[6]

[l] pH of undiluted solution is specific to the product, ranging from 6.5-7.3 or 7.5-8.5.[5]

[m] 7 d refrigerated, followed by 48 hr at 33°C.[7]

[n] Manufacturer extrapolated data from other sources.[7]

REFERENCES

1. Adams P, Haines-Nutt R, Bradford E, et al. Pharmaceutical aspects of home infusion therapy for cancer patients. *Pharm J*. 1987; 238:476-78.
2. Marquardt ED. Visual compatibility of hydroxyzine hydrochloride with various antineoplastic agents. *Am J Hosp Pharm*. 1988; 45(10):2127.
3. Priston M, Sewell G. Stability of three cytotoxic drug infusions in the Graseby 9000 ambulatory infusion pump. *J Oncol Pharm Pract*. 1998; 4(3):143-49.
4. Zhang Y, Kawedia JD, Myers AL, et al. Physical and chemical stability of high-dose ifosfamide and mesna for prolonged 14-day continuous infusion. *J Oncol Pharm Pract*. 2014; 20(1):51-7.
5. ASHP's Interactive Handbook on Injectable Drugs, 2020. Bethesda, MD: American Society of Health-System Pharmacists; Accessed July 2020.
6. Menard C, Bourguignon C, Schlatter J, et al. Stability of cyclophosphamide and mesna admixtures in polyethylene infusion bags. *Ann Pharmacother*. 2003; 37(12):1789-92.
7. *Drug Stability Table - Dosi-Fuser® Elastomeric Pump (ES.H.00.73-10)*, 2015. Barcelona, Spain: Leventon SAU; Updated October 2015.

Methadone Hydrochloride

Storage Conditions

						Temperature			Post-thaw Temp			
	Drug Manufacturer	Concentration	Diluents	Osmolality (mOsm/kg)	pH	Room	Refrig	Frozen	Room	Refrig	Body Temp	Refer.
CONTAINER												
Bag, Polyvinyl Chloride (PVC)	LI	1, 2, 5 mg/mL	NS	n/a	[b]	28 d[a]	n/a	n/a	n/a	n/a	n/a	(1)
Vial, Glass	GAL	5 mg/mL	NS	n/a	[b]	180 d	180 d	n/a	n/a	n/a	n/a	(2)

Flush Compatibility: Sodium chloride 0.9%.[1]

Special Considerations: n/a

Notes

[a] Exposed to light.

[b] pH of undiluted solution is 4.5-6.5.[1]

REFERENCES

1. ASHP's Interactive Handbook on Injectable Drugs, 2020. Bethesda, MD: American Society of Health-System Pharmacists; Accessed October 2020.
2. Friciu MM, Alarie H, Beauchemin M, et al. Stability of Methadone Hydrochloride for Injection in Saline Solution. *Can J Hosp Pharm*. 2020; 73(2):141-44.

DOI 10.37573/9781585286720.136

Methotrexate Sodium

Storage Conditions

	Drug Manufacturer	Concentration	Diluents	Osmolality (mOsm/kg)	pH	Temperature Room	Temperature Refrig	Temperature Frozen	Post-thaw Temp Room	Post-thaw Temp Refrig	Body Temp	Refer.
CONTAINER												
Bag, Polyvinyl Chloride (PVC)	UN	0.1, 1, 20 mg/mL	NS	n/a	[g]	n/a	n/a	12 wk[a]	n/a	n/a	n/a	(1)
	UN	0.225, 24 mg/mL	D5W, NS	n/a	[g]	n/a	30 d[b]	n/a	n/a	n/a	n/a	(1)(5)
	LE	0.5 mg/mL	D5W	n/a	[g]	n/a	n/a	30 d[a]	n/a	n/a	n/a	(1)
	UN	1 mg/mL	NS	n/a	[g]	14 d	n/a	n/a	n/a	n/a	n/a	(2)
	FA	1.25, 12.5 mg/mL	NS	n/a	[g]	7 d[b][j]	15 wk[b][j]	n/a	n/a	n/a	n/a	(1)
Bag, Polyethylene	TE	0.2 mg/mL	D5W	n/a	[g]	72 hr[b]	n/a	n/a	n/a	n/a	n/a	(6)
	TE	0.2 mg/mL	NS	n/a	[g]	28 d[b]	n/a	n/a	n/a	n/a	n/a	(6)
	TE	20 mg/mL	D5W, NS	n/a	[g]	28 d[b]	n/a	n/a	n/a	n/a	n/a	(6)
Syringe, Plastic (Unspecified)	LE	2.5 mg/mL	SWFI	n/a	[g]	7 d	7 d	n/a	n/a	n/a	n/a	(1)
	LE	50 mg/mL[c]	Undiluted	[f]	[g]	8 m	n/a	n/a	n/a	n/a	n/a	(1)
	LE	50 mg/mL	Undiluted	[f]	[g]	70 d	n/a	n/a	n/a	n/a	n/a	(1)
Vial, Glass	FA	1.25, 12.5 mg/mL	NS	n/a	[g]	7 d[b][j]	15 wk[b][j]	n/a	n/a	n/a	n/a	(1)
OTHER INFUSION CONTAINERS												
Dosi-Fuser® (Leventon)	BMS	1.25-12.5 mg/mL	NS	n/a	[g]	24 hr[d]	15 wk[d]	n/a	n/a	n/a	n/a	(8)
	TE	2 mg/mL	NS	n/a	[g]	10 d	15 wk	n/a	n/a	n/a	n/a	(8)
Easypump® ST/LT (B. Braun)	UN	0.3, 25 mg/mL	NS	n/a	[g]	7 d	7 d	n/a	n/a	n/a	n/a	(4)
INFUSOR™ (Baxter)[e]	BMS	1.25 mg/mL	NS	n/a	n/a	24 hr[h]	15 wk[h]	n/a	n/a	n/a	n/a	(3)
	BMS	12.5 mg/mL	NS	n/a	n/a	4 d[i]	15 wk[i]	n/a	n/a	n/a	n/a	(3)
SMARTeZ® (Progressive Medical)	UN	0.3, 25 mg/mL	NS	n/a	[g]	7 d	7 d	n/a	n/a	n/a	n/a	(7)

Flush Compatibility: Sodium chloride 0.9%, heparin.[1]

Special Considerations: Protect from light, especially dilute solutions. Preserved isotonic product contains benzyl alcohol; do not use the preserved product for intrathecal or high-dose therapy.

DOI 10.37573/9781585286720.137

Notes

[a] Solution was thawed by microwave irradiation with no loss of potency.[(1)]

[b] Protected from light.

[c] Monoject™ or Plastipak™ syringes.

[d] Manufacturer(s) extrapolated data from other sources.

[e] INTERMATE™/INFUSOR™ Portable Elastomeric Infusion System devices are no longer available in the United States.

[f] Undiluted solution is isotonic.[(1)]

[g] pH of the undiluted solution is approximately 8.5.[(1)]

[h] 15 wk refrigerated, followed by 24 hr at room temperature.

[i] 15 wk refrigerated, followed by 4 d at room temperature.

[j] 15 wk refrigerated, followed by 7 d at room temperature.

REFERENCES

1. ASHP's Interactive Handbook on Injectable Drugs, 2020. Bethesda, MD: American Society of Health-System Pharmacists; Accessed July 2020.
2. Vyas HM, Baptista RJ, Mitrano FP, et al. Drug stability guidelines for a continuous infusion chemotherapy program. *Hosp Pharm*. 1987; 22(7):685-7.
3. Stabforum - Stability Database: Methotrexate, Ontario, Canada: Baxter Healthcare; Accessed August 2020.
4. *Drug Stability for Easypump® ST/LT*, 2020. Bethlehem, PA: B. Braun USA; Updated June 2020.
5. Benaji B, Dine T, Goudaliez F, et al. Compatibility study of methotrexate with PVC bags after repackaging into two types of infusion admixtures. *Int J Pharm*. 1994; 105(1):83-87.
6. Nissen KB, Jorgensen LB, Berg DL, et al. Stability study of methotrexate in 0.9% sodium chloride injection and 5% dextrose injection with limit tests for impurities. *Am J Health Syst Pharm*. 2017; 74(9):e211-e23.
7. *SMARTeZ® - Stability Data for Drugs Using Elastomeric Infusion Pumps*, 2020. Fenton, MO: Progressive Medical, Inc.; Updated May 2020.
8. *Drug Stability Table - Dosi-Fuser® Elastomeric Pump (S-CL-00-001v16)*, 2021. Barcelona, Spain: Leventon SAU; Updated May 2021.

MethylPREDNISolone Sodium Succinate

Storage Conditions

	Drug Manufacturer	Concentration	Diluents	Osmolality (mOsm/kg)	pH[c]	Temperature Room	Temperature Refrig	Temperature Frozen	Post-thaw Temp Room	Post-thaw Temp Refrig	Body Temp	Refer.
CONTAINER												
Bag, Polyvinyl Chloride (PVC)	UP	0.4, 1.25 mg/mL	D5W	[d]	6.92-7.39	24 hr	n/a	n/a	n/a	n/a	n/a	(3)
	UP	4.6 mg/mL	NS	[d]	7.4-7.6	n/a	n/a	12 m[a]	n/a	n/a	n/a	(1)(5)
Syringe, Polypropylene	UP	10 mg/mL	NS	[d]	[c]	4 d	21 d	n/a	n/a	n/a	n/a	(1)(4)
Vial, Glass	UP	4 mg/mL	SWFI	[d]	[c]	24 hr	7 d	n/a	n/a	n/a	n/a	(1)
	UP	62.5 mg/mL	SWFI	[d]	[c]	n/a	n/a	28 d	n/a	n/a	n/a	(1)
OTHER INFUSION CONTAINERS												
Dosi-Fuser® (Leventon)	HOS, UP	10 mg/mL	NS	[d]	[c]	24 hr[b]	7 d[b]	n/a	n/a	n/a	n/a	(6)
Easypump® ST/LT (B. Braun)	UN	10 mg/mL	NS	[d]	[c]	2 hr	7 d	n/a	n/a	n/a	n/a	(8)
Homepump Eclipse® / Homepump® (Halyard)	UN	10 mg/mL	NS	[d]	[c]	24 hr	7 d	n/a	n/a	n/a	n/a	(2)
SMARTeZ® (Progressive Medical)	UN	10 mg/mL	NS	[d]	[c]	2 hr[b]	7 d[b]	n/a	n/a	n/a	n/a	(7)

Flush Compatibility: Sodium chloride 0.9%, heparin.[1]

Special Considerations: The manufacturer states that only Bacteriostatic Water for Injection with Benzyl Alcohol should be used for reconstitution.[9]

Notes

[a] Stored at -20°C.

[b] Manufacturer extrapolated data from other sources.

[c] pH of reconstituted preparation is 7-8.[1]

[d] Calculated osmolality for 5-20 mg/mL in NS ranges from 301-345 mOsm/kg. Calculated osmolality for 5-20 mg/mL in D5W ranges from 275-318 mOsm/kg.[1]

REFERENCES

1. ASHP's Interactive Handbook on Injectable Drugs, 2020. Bethesda, MD: American Society of Health-System Pharmacists; Accessed December 2020.
2. *Stability Data for Drugs Using Homepump Disposable Ambulatory Infusion Systems (MK-00314 rev 3)*, 2015. Alpharetta, GA: Halyard Health; Updated June 2015.

DOI 10.37573/9781585286720.138

3. Strom JG, Jr., Miller SW. Stability and compatibility of methylprednisolone sodium succinate and cimetidine hydrochloride in 5% dextrose injection. *Am J Hosp Pharm*. 1991; 48(6):1237-41.
4. Gupta VD. Chemical stability of methylprednisolone sodium succinate after reconstitution in 0.9% sodium chloride injection and storage in polypropylene syringes. *Int J Pharm Compd*. 2001; 5(2):148-50.
5. Sewell GJ, Palmer AJ. The chemical and physical stability of three intravenous infusions subjected to frozen storage and microwave thawing. *Int J Pharm*. 1991; 72(1):57-63.
6. *Drug Stability Table - Dosi-Fuser® Elastomeric Pump (ES.H.00.73-10)*, 2015. Barcelona, Spain: Leventon SAU; Updated October 2015.
7. *SMARTeZ® - Stability Data for Drugs Using Elastomeric Infusion Pumps*, 2020. Fenton, MO: Progressive Medical, Inc.; Updated May 2020.
8. *Drug Stability for Easypump® ST/LT*, 2020. Bethlehem, PA: B. Braun USA; Updated June 2020.
9. Methylprednisolone Sodium Succinate Injection [package insert]. Lake Zurich, IL: Fresenius Kabi USA, LLC; December 2019.

Metoclopramide Hydrochloride

Storage Conditions

	Drug Manufacturer	Concentration	Diluents	Osmolality (mOsm/kg)	pH	Temperature: Room	Temperature: Refrig	Temperature: Frozen	Post-thaw Temp: Room	Post-thaw Temp: Refrig	Body Temp	Refer.
CONTAINER												
Bag, Polyvinyl Chloride (PVC)	RB	0.2 mg/mL	D5W	n/a	[c]	24 hr	n/a	14 d[f]	24 hr[f]	n/a	n/a	(1)
	RB	0.2, 3.2 mg/mL	NS	n/a	[c]	24 hr	n/a	28 d	24 hr	n/a	n/a	(1)
	SKB	0.5 mg/mL	NS[a]	n/a	[c]	5 wk	26 wk[b]	n/a	n/a	n/a	7 d[b]	(1)
Syringe, Polypropylene	BA	0.5 mg/mL	NS	n/a	[c]	21 d	n/a	n/a	n/a	n/a	n/a	(2)
	AST	0.74 mg/mL	[d]	n/a	[c]	n/a	n/a	n/a	n/a	n/a	10 d[e][g]	(5)
	SO	2.5 mg/mL	NS	n/a	[c]	24 hr	24 hr	n/a	n/a	n/a	n/a	(1)
OTHER INFUSION CONTAINERS												
CADD® Cassette (Smiths Medical)[i]	UN	1 mg/mL	unspec.[h]	n/a	[c]	7 d	n/a	n/a	n/a	n/a	n/a	(4)
Easypunp® ST/LT (B. Braun)	UN	5 mg/mL[j]	NS[j]	n/a	n/a	48 hr	48 hr	n/a	n/a	n/a	n/a	(6)
MiniMed™ Syringe (Medtronic)	RB	5 mg/mL	Undiluted	280	4.5-6.5	60 d	90 d	n/a	n/a	n/a	7 d[g]	(1)
SMARTeZ® (Progressive Medical)	UN	5 mg/mL[j]	NS[j]	n/a	n/a	48 hr	48 hr	n/a	n/a	n/a	n/a	(3)

Flush Compatibility: Sodium chloride 0.9%, heparin.[1]

Special Considerations: Do not freeze undiluted (5 mg/mL) product.[1]

Notes

[a] Solution contained: morphine sulfate 1 mg/mL (EV).[1]

[b] 26 weeks refrigerated, followed by 7 d at 32°C.[1]

[c] pH of undiluted solution is 4.5-6.5.[1]

[d] Solution contained: fentaNYL 0.037 mg/mL (DB) and midazolam 0.55 mg/mL (RC).[5]

[e] Protected from light.[5]

[f] 14 days at -20°C, followed by 24 hr at room temperature.[1]

[g] Storage temperature: 32°C.[5]

[h] Solution contained: morphine 15 mg/mL.[4]

[i] Container information: Tested in PVC (CADD®) cassettes manufactured by Pharmacia Deltec, Inc.; CADD® Cassette is now a registered trademark of Smiths Medical.

[j] Published materials note a concentration of 5 mg/mL with a diluent of NS despite the concentration of the undiluted product being 5 mg/mL.[3,6]

DOI 10.37573/9781585286720.139

REFERENCES

1. ASHP's Interactive Handbook on Injectable Drugs, 2020. Bethesda, MD: American Society of Health-System Pharmacists; Accessed October 2020.
2. Gupta VD. Chemical stability of metoclopramide hydrochloride injection diluted with 0.9% sodium chloride injection in polypropylene syringes at room temperature. *Int J Pharm Compd*. 2005; 9(1):72-4.
3. *SMARTeZ® - Stability Data for Drugs Using Elastomeric Infusion Pumps*, 2020. Fenton, MO: Progressive Medical, Inc.; Updated May 2020.
4. Swanson G, Smith J, Bulich R, et al. Patient-controlled analgesia for chronic cancer pain in the ambulatory setting: a report of 117 patients. *J Clin Oncol*. 1989; 7(12):1903-8.
5. Peterson GM, Miller KA, Galloway JG, et al. Compatibility and stability of fentanyl admixtures in polypropylene syringes. *J Clin Pharm Ther*. 1998; 23(1):67-72.
6. *Drug Stability for Easypump® ST/LT*, 2020. Bethlehem, PA: B. Braun USA; Updated June 2020.

MetroNIDAZOLE

Storage Conditions

	Drug Manufacturer	Concentration	Diluents	Osmolality (mOsm/kg)	pH	Temperature			Post-thaw Temp			
						Room	Refrig	Frozen	Room	Refrig	Body Temp	Refer.
CONTAINER												
Bag, Polyvinyl Chloride (PVC)	AB	5 mg/mL	RTU[c]	n/a	n/a	14 d	14 d[a]	n/a	n/a	n/a	n/a	(1)
OTHER INFUSION CONTAINERS												
Dosi-Fuser® (Leventon)	UN	5 mg/mL	RTU	n/a	n/a	24 hr[b]	10 d[a][b]	n/a	n/a	n/a	n/a	(5)
EasyPump® ST/LT (B. Braun)	UN	5 mg/mL	RTU	n/a	n/a	24 hr	10 d[a][d]	n/a	n/a	n/a	n/a	(3)
Homepump Eclipse® / Homepump® (Halyard)	UN	5 mg/mL	RTU	n/a	n/a	24 hr	10 d[a]	n/a	n/a	n/a	n/a	(2)
SMARTeZ® (Progressive Medical)	UN	5 mg/mL	NS	n/a	n/a	24 hr	10 d[a]	n/a	n/a	n/a	n/a	(4)

Flush Compatibility: Sodium chloride 0.9%, heparin.[1]

Special Considerations: Short-term exposure to normal room light does not adversely affect stability. Direct sunlight should be avoided.[1]

Notes

[a] MetroNIDAZOLE solution is susceptible to crystallization when refrigerated. The crystals redissolve on warming to room temperature.[1]

[b] Manufacturer(s) extrapolated data from other sources.[5]

[c] Solution contained: cefepime (ELN) 3.3, 6.6, 10, 20 mg/mL.[1]

[d] Storage for 10 days refrigerated followed by 24 hours at room temperature.[3]

REFERENCES

1. ASHP's Interactive Handbook on Injectable Drugs, 2020. Bethesda, MD: American Society of Health-System Pharmacists; Accessed May 2020.
2. *Stability Data for Drugs Using Homepump Disposable Ambulatory Infusion Systems (MK-00314 rev 3)*, 2015. Alpharetta, GA: Halyard Health; Updated June 2015.
3. *Drug Stability for Easypump® ST/LT*, 2020. Bethlehem, PA: B. Braun USA; Updated June 2020.
4. *SMARTeZ® - Stability Data for Drugs Using Elastomeric Infusion Pumps*, 2020. Fenton, MO: Progressive Medical, Inc.; Updated May 2020.
5. *Drug Stability Table - Dosi-Fuser® Elastomeric Pump (ES.H.00.73-10)*, 2015. Barcelona, Spain: Leventon SAU; Updated October 2015.

DOI 10.37573/9781585286720.140

Micafungin Sodium

Storage Conditions

	Drug Manufacturer	Concentration	Diluents	Osmolality (mOsm/kg)	pH	Temperature			Post-thaw Temp			
						Room	Refrig	Frozen	Room	Refrig	Body Temp	Refer.
CONTAINER												
Bag, Polyethylene	ASP	0.25, 3 mg/mL	D5W, NS	n/a	[c]	72 hr[b]	72 hr[b]	n/a	n/a	n/a	n/a	(1)
	ASP	4 mg/mL	D5W, NS	n/a	[c]	4 d[b]	n/a	n/a	n/a	n/a	n/a	(1)
	ASP	1 mg/mL	D5¼NS, LR	n/a	[c]	7 d	n/a	n/a	n/a	n/a	n/a	(1)
Syringe, Polypropylene	ASP	0.5, 1 mg/mL	NS	n/a	[c]	15 d[b]	n/a	n/a	n/a	n/a	n/a	(4)
Vial, Glass	ASP	0.25, 3, 5 mg/mL	D5W, NS	n/a	[c]	48 hr[b]	n/a	n/a	n/a	n/a	n/a	(1)
OTHER INFUSION CONTAINERS												
Easypump® ST/LT (B. Braun)	UN	0.5, 2 mg/mL	NS	n/a	[c]	24 hr	4 d[a]	n/a	n/a	n/a	n/a	(3)
Homepump® Eclipse / Homepump® (Halyard)	ASP	0.2, 1 mg/mL	D5W, NS	n/a	[c]	n/a	10 d	n/a	n/a	n/a	n/a	(1)
SMARTeZ® (Progressive Medical)	UN	0.5, 2 mg/mL	NS	n/a	[c]	24 hr	4 d	n/a	n/a	n/a	n/a	(5)

Flush Compatibility: Sodium chloride 0.9%.[2]

Special Considerations: Reconstitute only with NS or D5W; do not vigorously shake vial. Original vial is coated with light protective film. Dilute to final concentration between 0.5 and 4 mg/mL prior to administration. Protect diluted solution from light. It is not necessary to cover the IV tubing or the infusion drip chamber.[2]

Notes

[a] Stored for 4 d refrigerated followed by 1 d at room temperature.[3]

[b] Protected from light.

[c] pH of reconstituted solution in NS is 5-7.[2]

REFERENCES

1. Micafungin for Injection: Stability Medication Information Letter (Ref#: 00070821) [personal communication]. Northbrook, IL: Astellas Pharma Global Development, Inc.; 2021:5.
2. Mycamine® (Micafungin) Injection [package insert]. Northbrook, IL: Astellas Pharma US, Inc.; July 2020.
3. *Drug Stability for Easypump® ST/LT*, 2020. Bethlehem, PA: B. Braun USA; Updated June 2020.
4. Briot T, Vrignaud S, Lagarce F. Stability of micafungin sodium solutions at different concentrations in glass bottles and syringes. *Int J Pharm*. 2015; 492(1-2):137-40.
5. *SMARTeZ® - Stability Data for Drugs Using Elastomeric Infusion Pumps*, 2020. Fenton, MO: Progressive Medical, Inc.; Updated May 2020.

DOI 10.37573/9781585286720.141

Midazolam Hydrochloride

Storage Conditions

	Drug Manufacturer	Concentration	Diluents	Osmolality (mOsm/kg)	pH	Temperature: Room	Temperature: Refrig	Temperature: Frozen	Post-thaw Temp: Room	Post-thaw Temp: Refrig	Body Temp	Refer.
CONTAINER												
Bag, Polyethylene	RC	0.035 mg/mL	D5W, NS	[k]	[i]	24 hr	24 hr	n/a	n/a	n/a	n/a	(2)
	NL	0.12-0.8 mg/mL	D5W, NS[a]	n/a	3.3-3.6	4 d	7 d	n/a	n/a	n/a	n/a	(3)
Bag, Polyolefin	RC	0.5 mg/mL	D5W, NS	[k]	[i]	30 d[b]	30 d[b]	n/a	n/a	n/a	n/a	(2)
	HOS	1 mg/mL	D5W	n/a	3.2-3.4	27 d[b][c]	27 d[b]	n/a	n/a	n/a	n/a	(4)
Bag, Polyvinyl Chloride (PVC)	RC	0.03 mg/mL	D5W, NS	[k]	[i]	72 hr	n/a	n/a	n/a	n/a	n/a	(2)
	RC	1 mg/mL	NS	[k]	[i]	7 wk[b][c]	7 wk[c]	n/a	n/a	n/a	n/a	(2)
	HOS	1 mg/mL	D5W	n/a	3.2-3.4	27 d[b][c]	27 d	n/a	n/a	n/a	n/a	(4)
	RC	1 mg/mL	NS[j]	[k]	[i]	10 d[b][c]	n/a	n/a	n/a	n/a	n/a	(2)
Syringe, Polypropylene	RC	1 mg/mL	Undiluted	n/a	[i]	28 d[b]	n/a	n/a	n/a	n/a	n/a	(2)
	RC	2 mg/mL	NS	[k]	[i]	10 d	10 d	n/a	n/a	n/a	n/a	(2)
	RC	3 mg/mL	NS	[k]	[i]	13 d[g]	n/a	n/a	n/a	n/a	13 d[g]	(2)
	RC	5 mg/mL	Undiluted	n/a	[i]	36 d[b]	n/a	n/a	n/a	n/a	n/a	(2)
	MYL	1 mg/mL	NS	n/a	3.4	90 d	365 d	365 d	n/a	n/a	n/a	(1)
Unspecified	RC	0.1, 0.5 mg/mL	D5W, NS[h]	[k]	[i]	23 d	23 d	n/a	n/a	n/a	n/a	(2)
Vial, Cyclic Olefin Copolymer (COC)	MYL	1 mg/mL	NS	n/a	3.4	180 d	365 d	365 d	n/a	n/a	n/a	(1)
Vial, Glass	RC	0.03 mg/mL	D5W, NS	[k]	[i]	72 hr	n/a	n/a	n/a	n/a	n/a	(2)
	RC	0.5 mg/mL	D5W, NS	[k]	[i]	36 d[b]	36 d[b]	n/a	n/a	n/a	36 d[b][d]	(2)
	RC	3 mg/mL	NS	[k]	[i]	n/a	n/a	n/a	n/a	n/a	13 d[f]	(2)
OTHER INFUSION CONTAINERS												
INFUSOR™ / INTERMATE™ (Baxter)[l]	RC	0.5, 1.5 mg/mL	NS[e]	n/a	n/a	7 d[b]	n/a	n/a	n/a	n/a	n/a	(2)

Flush Compatibility: Sodium chloride 0.9%, heparin.[2]

Special Considerations: Store product at controlled room temperature and protect from light. Admixtures do not require protection from light for short term storage and administration.[2]

DOI 10.37573/9781585286720.142

Notes

[a] Solution contained: haloperidol 0.04-0.08 mg/mL.[3]

[b] Protected from light.

[c] Exposed to fluorescent light.

[d] Storage temperature: 40°C.[2]

[e] Solution contained: traMADol hydrochloride 11.18 and 33.3 mg/mL, respectively.[2]

[f] Storage temperature: 32°C.[2]

[g] Storage temperature: 20°C and 32°C.[2]

[h] Solution contained: HYDROmorphone HCl 2 mg/mL and 20 mg/mL.[2]

[i] pH of undiluted injection is 2.9-3.7.[2]

[j] Benzyl alcohol added to a concentration of 1%.[2]

[k] Diluted in NS to 0.625, 1.25, and 1.67 mg/mL, osmolality is 274, 262, and 259 mOsm/kg.[2]

[l] INTERMATE™/INFUSOR™ Portable Elastomeric Infusion System devices are no longer available in the United States.

REFERENCES

1. Gilliot S, Masse M, Feutry F, et al. Long-term stability of ready-to-use 1-mg/mL midazolam solution. *Am J Health Syst Pharm*. 2020; 77(9):681-89.
2. ASHP's Interactive Handbook on Injectable Drugs, 2020. Bethesda, MD: American Society of Health-System Pharmacists; Accessed August 2020.
3. Estan-Cerezo G, Rodríguez-Lucena FJ, Chirivella CM, et al. Midazolam and haloperidol for palliative sedation: physicochemical stability and compatibility of parenteral admixtures. *Braz J Pharm Sci*. 2019; 55:e17351.
4. Karlage K, Earhart Z, Green-Boesen K, et al. Stability of midazolam hydrochloride injection 1-mg/mL solutions in polyvinyl chloride and polyolefin bags. *Am J Health Syst Pharm*. 2011; 68(16):1537-40.

Milrinone Lactate

Storage Conditions

	Drug Manufacturer	Concentration	Diluents	Osmolality (mOsm/kg)	pH	Temperature Room	Temperature Refrig	Temperature Frozen	Post-thaw Temp Room	Post-thaw Temp Refrig	Body Temp	Refer.
CONTAINER												
Bag, Polyolefin	SW	400, 600, 800 mcg/mL	NS	n/a	[a]	14 d	14 d	n/a	n/a	n/a	n/a	(1)(4)
Bag, Polyvinyl Chloride (PVC)	SW	200 mcg/mL	NS, D5W	n/a	[a]	14 d	14 d	n/a	n/a	n/a	n/a	(1)(2)
	SW	400 mcg/mL	D5W, LR, NS, ½NS	n/a	[a]	7 d	n/a	n/a	n/a	n/a	n/a	(1)(3)
	SW	400, 600, 800 mcg/mL	D5W	n/a	[a]	14 d	14 d	n/a	n/a	n/a	n/a	(1)(4)
Vial, Glass	WI	200 mcg/mL	D5W, NS, ½NS	n/a	[a]	72 hr	n/a	n/a	n/a	n/a	n/a	(1)
COMMERCIAL PREPARATIONS (RTU)												
Flexible Plastic Container (Hospira)	HOS	200 mcg/mL	D5W	n/a	[a]	[b]	n/a	n/a	n/a	n/a	n/a	(6)
IntraVia® Plastic Container (Baxter)	BA	200 mcg/mL	D5W	n/a	3.5	[b]	n/a	n/a	n/a	n/a	n/a	(5)

Flush Compatibility: Sodium chloride 0.9%, heparin.[1,3]

Special Considerations: Avoid freezing, avoid excessive heat.[5–7]

Notes

[a] pH ranges from 3.2-4.[5–7]

[b] Expiration date per manufacturer's label when stored in the protective overwrap under labeled storage conditions.

REFERENCES

1. ASHP's Interactive Handbook on Injectable Drugs, 2020. Bethesda, MD: American Society of Health-System Pharmacists; Accessed July 2020.
2. Wong F, Gill MA. Stability of Milrinone Lactate 200 micrograms/mL in 5% Dextrose Injection and 0.9% Sodium Chloride Injection. *Int J Pharm Compd*. 1998; 2(2):168169.
3. Akkerman SR, Zhang H, Mullins RE, et al. Stability of milrinone lactate in the presence of 29 critical care drugs and 4 i.v. solutions. *Am J Health Syst Pharm*. 1999; 56(1):63-8.
4. Nguyen D, Gill MA, Wong F. Stability of Milrinone Lactate in 5% Dextrose Injection and 0.9% Sodium Chloride Injection at Concentrations of 400, 600, and 800 micrograms/mL. *Int J Pharm Compd*. 1998; 2(3):246-8.
5. Milrinone Lactate in Dextrose Injection [package insert]. Deerfield, IL: Baxter Healthcare Corporation; May 2018.
6. Milrinone Lactate in 5% Dextrose Injection [package insert]. Lake Forest, IL: Hospira, Inc.; June 2020.
7. Milrinone Lactate Injection [package insert]. Lake Forest, IL: Hospira, Inc.; November 2019.

DOI 10.37573/9781585286720.143

MitoMYcin

Storage Conditions

CONTAINER	Drug Manufacturer	Concentration	Diluents	Osmolality (mOsm/kg)	pH	Temperature: Room	Temperature: Refrig	Temperature: Frozen	Post-thaw Temp: Room	Post-thaw Temp: Refrig	Body Temp	Refer.
Bag, Polyvinyl Chloride (PVC)	BR	0.4 mg/mL	NS	n/a	[d]	24 hr	n/a	n/a	n/a	n/a	n/a	(5)
	BR	0.5 mg/mL	BWFI	n/a	[d]	14 d	n/a	n/a	n/a	n/a	n/a	(1)
	KY	0.6 mg/mL	NS	n/a	[d]	n/a	4 d[c]	n/a	n/a	n/a	n/a	(5)
	BR	0.6 mg/mL	NS	n/a	[d]	n/a	n/a	8 wk[a]	n/a	n/a	n/a	(2)(5)
	KY	0.6 mg/mL	½NS	n/a	[d]	n/a	7 d[c]	n/a	n/a	n/a	n/a	(5)
	KY	0.4 mg/mL	[e]	n/a	[d]	n/a	7 d[c]	n/a	n/a	n/a	n/a	(5)
	BR	0.02 mg/mL	LR	n/a	[d]	5 d	n/a	n/a	n/a	n/a	n/a	(4)(5)
	BR	0.04 mg/mL	LR	n/a	[d]	n/a	15 d	n/a	n/a	n/a	n/a	(4)(5)
	BR	0.04 mg/mL	NS	n/a	[d]	n/a	5 d	n/a	n/a	n/a	n/a	(4)(5)
	CH	0.05 mg/mL	D5W	n/a	[b]	15 d[b]	120 d[b]	n/a	n/a	n/a	n/a	(3)
Syringe, Polypropylene	BMS	0.5 mg/mL	SWFI	n/a	[d]	11 d[c]	6 wk[c]	n/a	n/a	n/a	n/a	(5)
Unspecified	BR	0.05 mg/mL	NS	n/a	[d]	5 d	n/a	n/a	n/a	n/a	n/a	(5)
	BR	0.05 mg/mL	LR	n/a	[d]	43 hr	n/a	n/a	n/a	n/a	n/a	(5)
	UN	0.02, 0.04 mg/mL	[f]	n/a	[d]	24 hr	n/a	n/a	n/a	n/a	n/a	(5)
	UN	0.02, 0.04 mg/mL	NS	n/a	[d]	12 hr	n/a	n/a	n/a	n/a	n/a	(5)
Vial, Glass	BR	0.4 mg/mL	NS	n/a	[d]	24 hr	n/a	n/a	n/a	n/a	n/a	(5)
	KY	0.6 mg/mL	½NS	n/a	[d]	n/a	7 d[c]	n/a	n/a	n/a	n/a	(5)
	KY	0.6 mg/mL	NS	n/a	[d]	n/a	4 d[c]	n/a	n/a	n/a	n/a	(5)
	BR	0.02 mg/mL	LR	n/a	[d]	6 d	n/a	n/a	n/a	n/a	n/a	(4)(5)
	BR	0.04 mg/mL	LR	n/a	[d]	n/a	20 d	n/a	n/a	n/a	n/a	(4)(5)
	BR	0.04 mg/mL	NS	n/a	[d]	n/a	5 d	n/a	n/a	n/a	n/a	(4)(5)
	BR	0.04 mg/mL	D5W	n/a	[d]	n/a	24 hr	n/a	n/a	n/a	n/a	(5)
	ACD	0.5 mg/mL	SWFI	n/a	[d]	7 d[c]	14 d[c]	n/a	n/a	n/a	n/a	(6)

DOI 10.37573/9781585286720.144

Flush Compatibility: Sodium chloride 0.9%, heparin.[5,6]

Special Considerations: Protect reconstituted solution from light. Unless buffered to a pH of approximately 7.8, avoid long-term storage in dextrose-containing solutions.[3,4,6]

Notes

[a] Buffered and unbuffered solutions were frozen at -30°C for 28 days, then thawed. The unbuffered solutions were refrozen for another 28 days. Freezing at -20°C resulted in a precipitate forming in the solution.

[b] Solutions buffered to achieve a pH of approximately 7.8.

[c] Protected from light.

[d] pH of reconstituted product is 6-8.[5]

[e] Diluent: Sodium chloride 0.6%.[5]

[f] Diluent: Sodium lactate (1/6) M.[5]

REFERENCES

1. Vyas HM, Baptista RJ, Mitrano FP, et al. Drug stability guidelines for a continuous infusion chemotherapy program. *Hosp Pharm*. 1987; 22(7):685-7.
2. Stolk LM, Fruijtier A, Umans R. Stability after freezing and thawing of solutions of mitomycin C in plastic minibags for intravesical use. *Pharm Weekbl Sci*. 1986; 8(6):286-8.
3. Quebbeman EJ, Hoffman NE, Ausman RK, et al. Stability of mitomycin admixtures. *Am J Hosp Pharm*. 1985; 42(8):1750-4.
4. Dorr R, Liddil JD. Stability of mitomycin C in different infusion fluids: Compatibility with heparin and glucocorticosteroids. *J Oncol Pharm Pract*. 1995; 1:19-24.
5. ASHP's Interactive Handbook on Injectable Drugs, 2020. Bethesda, MD: American Society of Health-System Pharmacists; Accessed July 2020.
6. Mitomycin Injection, Lyophilized [package insert]. Durham, NC: Accord Healthcare, Inc.; September 2020.

MitoXANTRONE Hydrochloride

Storage Conditions

						Temperature			Post-thaw Temp			
	Drug Manufacturer	Concentration	Diluents	Osmolality (mOsm/kg)	pH	Room	Refrig	Frozen	Room	Refrig	Body Temp	Refer.
CONTAINER												
Bag, Polyvinyl Chloride (PVC)	LE	0.02-0.5 mg/mL	D5W, NS	n/a	[a]	7 d	7 d	n/a	n/a	n/a	n/a	(1)
Syringe, Plastic (Unspecified)	LE	2 mg/mL	Undiluted	n/a	3.43-3.65	6 wk	6 wk	n/a	n/a	n/a	n/a	(1)(3)
Syringe, Polypropylene	UN	0.2 mg/mL	NS	n/a	[a]	28 d	28 d	n/a	n/a	n/a	n/a	(1)
	UN	0.2 mg/mL	SWFI	n/a	[a]	14 d	14 d	n/a	n/a	n/a	24 hr	(1)
Vial, Glass	LE	0.02-0.5 mg/mL	NS	n/a	[a]	48 hr	n/a	n/a	n/a	n/a	n/a	(1)
	APP	2 mg/mL	Undiluted	n/a	[a]	7 d	14 d	n/a	n/a	n/a	n/a	(1)(2)
OTHER INFUSION CONTAINERS												
Dosi-Fuser® (Leventon)	SZ	2 mg/mL	NS	n/a	[a]	7 d	7 d	n/a	n/a	n/a	n/a	(4)

Flush Compatibility: Sodium chloride 0.9%. Heparin may cause precipitation.[1,2]

Special Considerations: Do not freeze. Refrigeration of the concentrate may cause a precipitate, which redissolves upon warming to room temperature.[1]

Notes

[a] pH of undiluted solution is 3-4.5. pH of maximum stability is 2-4.5. Solution is unstable at pH 7.4[1]

REFERENCES

1. ASHP's Interactive Handbook on Injectable Drugs, 2020. Bethesda, MD: American Society of Health-System Pharmacists; Accessed June 2020.
2. Mitoxantrone Injection [package insert]. Lake Forest, IL: Hospira, Inc.; May 2018.
3. Walker S, Lau DWC, Deangelis C, et al. Mitoxantrone Stability in Syringes and Glass Vials and Evaluation of Chemical Contamination. *Can J Hosp Pharm*. 1991; 44(3):143-51.
4. *Drug Stability Table - Dosi-Fuser® Elastomeric Pump (S-CL-00-001v16)*, 2021. Barcelona, Spain: Leventon SAU; Updated May 2021.

DOI 10.37573/9781585286720.145

Morphine Sulfate

Storage Conditions

	Drug Manufacturer	Concentration	Diluents	Osmolality (mOsm/kg)	pH	Temperature			Post-thaw Temp			
						Room	Refrig	Frozen	Room	Refrig	Body Temp	Refer.
CONTAINER												
Bag, Polypropylene	AST	0.02 mg/mL	NS[o]	5.4-5.73	[p]	30 d[a]	n/a	n/a	n/a	n/a	n/a	(1)(7)
	AST	0.02, 0.1 mg/mL	NS[m]	5.4-5.65	[p]	30 d[a]	n/a	n/a	n/a	n/a	n/a	(1)(7)
Bag, Polyvinyl Chloride (PVC)	AB, AH	0.04, 0.4 mg/mL	D5W, NS	[e]	[p]	7 d	7 d	n/a	n/a	n/a	n/a	(1)
	LI	1, 2 mg/mL	D5W, NS	[e]	[p]	n/a	n/a	14 wk	n/a	n/a	n/a	(1)
	UN	2, 15 mg/mL	SWFI	[e]	[p]	15 d	15 d	n/a	n/a	n/a	n/a	(1)
	AH	5 mg/mL	D5W, NS	[e]	[p]	30 d	n/a	n/a	n/a	n/a	n/a	(1)
	AH	10 mg/mL	Undiluted	[e]	[p]	30 d	n/a	n/a	n/a	n/a	n/a	(1)
Syringe, Polypropylene	LI	1, 5 mg/mL	D5W, NS[b]	[e]	[p]	6 wk[a]	6 wk[a]	6 wk[a]	n/a	n/a	n/a	(1)(3)
	UN	5 mg/mL	NS	[e]	[p]	60 d	60 d	n/a	n/a	n/a	48 hr	(4)
	UN	50 mg/mL	NS, SWFI	[e]	[p]	60 d	n/a	n/a	n/a	n/a	48 hr	(4)
	UN	2 mg/mL	NS	[e]	[p]	6 wk[a]	n/a	n/a	n/a	n/a	n/a	(1)
	UN	5 mg/mL	NS	[e]	[p]	60 d	60 d[a]	n/a	n/a	n/a	48 hr	(1)
	UN	50 mg/mL	NS, SWFI	[e]	[p]	60 d[c]	n/a	n/a	n/a	n/a	48 hr	(1)
OTHER INFUSION CONTAINERS												
CADD® Cassette (Smiths Medical)	ES	1, 5 mg/mL	NS	[e]	[p]	14 d	30 d	n/a	n/a	n/a	n/a	(1)
	UN	1, 5 mg/mL	NS	[e]	[p]	30 d	30 d	n/a	n/a	n/a	14 d[d]	(6)
	UN	1, 10 mg/mL	NS	[e]	[p]	n/a	n/a	n/a	n/a	n/a	16 d[i][a]	(1)
	SAB	10 mg/mL	D5W, NS[k]	[e]	[w]	31 d	31 d	n/a	n/a	n/a	n/a	(1)(10)
	AGT	1, 40 mg/mL	NS	[e]	[p]	30 d[a]	n/a	n/a	n/a	n/a	n/a	(1)
	UN	15, 25 mg/mL	Undiluted	[e]	[p]	30 d	30 d	n/a	n/a	n/a	14 d[d]	(6)
	SAB	25, 50 mg/mL[n]	Undiluted	[e]	[p]	31 d	31 d	n/a	n/a	n/a	n/a	(1)(10)
Cormed™ III Bag (Kalex)	UN	0.5, 15, 30 mg/mL	NS	[e]	[p]	n/a	14 d	n/a	n/a	n/a	5 d[r]	(1)
	UN	60 mg/mL	NS	[e]	[p]	n/a	n/a	n/a	n/a	n/a	5 d[r]	(1)
Easypump® ST/LT (B. Braun)	UN	1, 20 mg/mL	NS	[e]	[p]	7d	n/a	n/a	n/a	n/a	n/a	(8)

DOI 10.37573/9781585286720.146

Storage Conditions

	Drug Manufacturer	Concentration	Diluents	Osmolality (mOsm/kg)	pH	Temperature Room	Temperature Refrig	Temperature Frozen	Post-thaw Temp Room	Post-thaw Temp Refrig	Body Temp	Refer.
OTHER INFUSION CONTAINERS												
Homepump Eclipse® / Homepump® (Halyard)	UN	20 mg/mL	NS	[e]	[p]	7 d	n/a	n/a	n/a	n/a	n/a	(5)
Infusaid® Model 400 Implantable Pump (Infusaid)	CI	15 mg/mL	NS[s]	154.6	4.75-4.95	n/a	n/a	n/a	n/a	n/a	30 d	(11)
INFUSOR™ (Baxter)[u]	STE	0.025 mg/mL	NS[t]	[e]	[p]	n/a	120 d[l]	n/a	n/a	n/a	7 d [l]	(2)
	BA	1-15 mg/mL	D5W	[e]	[p]	13 wk	102 d	n/a	n/a	n/a	n/a	(2)
	BA	1-15 mg/mL	NS	[e]	[p]	4 d[q]	14 d[q]	n/a	n/a	n/a	n/a	(2)
	UN	2, 15 mg/mL	SWFI	[e]	[p]	12 d	12 d	n/a	n/a	n/a	12 d[j]	(1)
INTERMATE™ (Baxter)[u]	UN	2, 15 mg/mL	SWFI	[e]	[p]	15 d	15 d	n/a	n/a	n/a	15 d[j]	(1)
MEDI-FLO™ Elastomeric Pump (Wolf Medical)	UN	1, 20 mg/mL	NS	[e]	[p]	7 d	n/a	n/a	n/a	n/a	n/a	(13)
PVC/Kalex Cassette (Pharmacia Deltec)	CNF	0.5, 1.5, 2.5 mg/mL	NS	[e]	[p]	n/a	n/a	n/a	n/a	n/a	60 d[i]	(1)
SMARTeZ® (Progressive Medical)	UN	1, 20 mg/mL	NS	[e]	[p]	7 d[v]	n/a	n/a	n/a	n/a	n/a	(9)
SynchroMed® EL Implantable Pump (Medtronic)	UN	2 mg/mL	unspec.[g]	[e]	[p]	n/a	n/a	n/a	n/a	n/a	12 wk	(1)
	WW	20 mg/mL	unspec.[h]	[e]	[p]	n/a	n/a	n/a	n/a	n/a	12 wk	(1)
SynchroMed® II Implantable Pump (Medtronic)	WW	25 mg/mL	Undiluted	n/a	[p]	n/a	n/a	n/a	n/a	n/a	180 d	(12)
	UN	50 mg/mL	SWFI[f]	[e]	[p]	n/a	n/a	n/a	n/a	n/a	90 d	(1)
VIP 30 Implantable Pump (Fresenius)	UN	10 mg/mL	Undiluted	[e]	[p]	n/a	n/a	n/a	n/a	n/a	8 wk	(1)

Flush Compatibility: Sodium chloride 0.9%, heparin.[1]

Special Considerations: Morphine sulfate darkens with age and upon prolonged exposure to light and solutions should not be used if darker than pale yellow. Solutions have demonstrated formation of precipitate at refrigerated temperatures. Use only preservative-free diluents and drug products for intraspinal administration.[1]

Notes

[a] Protected from light.[1,3,7]

[b] Solution contained: meperidine 5-10 mg/mL.[1,3]

[c] Visual inspection reported yellow discoloration after 30 days.[1]

[d] Storage temperature: 35°C.[6]

[e] Osmolality of 7.5 mg/mL in NS is 236 mOsm/kg.[(1)]
[f] Solution contained: bupivacaine HCl 25 mg/mL and cloNIDine HCl 2 mg/mL.[(1)]
[g] Solution contained: cloNIDine HCl 1.84 mg/mL.[(1)]
[h] Solution contained: cloNIDine HCl (BI) 50 mcg/mL.[(1)]
[i] Storage temperature: 32°C.[(1)]
[j] Storage temperature: 31°C.[(1)]
[k] Solution compounded using preservative-free and preserved morphine sulfate 50 mg/mL.[(1,10)]
[l] 120 d refrigerated, followed by 7 d at 33°C.[(2)]
[m] Solution contained: ropivacaine HCl (ASZ) 2 mg/mL.[(1,7)]
[n] Solution compounded using preservative-free and preserved morphine sulfate 25 mg/mL and 50 mg/mL.[(1,10)]
[o] Solution contained: ropivacaine HCl (ASZ) 1 mg/mL.[(1,7)]
[p] pH of undiluted solutions range from 2.5-6.5.[(1)]
[q] 14 d refrigerated, followed by 4 d at room temperature.[(2)]
[r] Visual inspection reported light brown color change after 5 days at 37°C.[(1)]
[s] Solution contained: baclofen 1 mg/mL.[(11)]
[t] Solution contained: ropivacaine 2 mg/mL (ASZ).[(2)]
[u] INTERMATE™/INFUSOR™ Portable Elastomeric Infusion System devices are no longer available in the United States.
[v] Manufacturer extrapolated data from other sources.[(9)]
[w] pH of solution ranged from 2.9-3.4.[(1,10)]

REFERENCES

1. ASHP's Interactive Handbook on Injectable Drugs, 2020. Bethesda, MD: American Society of Health-System Pharmacists; Accessed December 2020.
2. Stabforum - Stability Database: Morphine; Morphine+Ropivacaine, Ontario, Canada: Baxter Healthcare; Accessed February 2021.
3. Strong ML, Schaaf LJ, Pankaskie MC, et al. Shelf-lives and factors affecting the stability of morphine sulphate and meperidine (pethidine) hydrochloride in plastic syringes for use in patient-controlled analgesic devices. *J Clin Pharm Ther*. 1994; 19(6):361-9.
4. Trissel LA, Xu QA, Pham L. Physical and Chemical Stability of Morphine Sulfate 5mg/mL and 50mg/mL Packaged in Plastic Syringes. *Int J Pharm Compd*. 2002; 6(1):62-5.
5. *Stability Data for Drugs Using Homepump Disposable Ambulatory Infusion Systems (MK-00314 rev 3)*, 2015. Alpharetta, GA: Halyard Health; Updated June 2015.
6. *Pharmaceutical report on chemical and physical stability of drugs commonly used with CADD® infusion pumps (IN193109GB-122019)*, 2019. Minneapolis, MN: Smiths Medical ASD, Inc.; Updated December 2019.
7. Oster Svedberg K, McKenzie J, Larrivee-Elkins C. Compatibility of ropivacaine with morphine, sufentanil, fentanyl, or clonidine. *J Clin Pharm Ther*. 2002; 27(1):39-45.
8. *Drug Stability for Easypump® ST/LT*, 2020. Bethlehem, PA: B. Braun USA; Updated June 2020.
9. *SMARTeZ® - Stability Data for Drugs Using Elastomeric Infusion Pumps*, 2020. Fenton, MO: Progressive Medical, Inc.; Updated May 20.
10. Walker SE, Iazzetta J, Lau DWC. Stability of Sulfite Free High Potency Morphine Sulfate Solutions in Portable Infusion Pump Cassettes. *Can J Hosp Pharm*. 1989; 42(5):195-200.
11. Sitaram BR, Tsui M, Rawicki HB, et al. Stability and compatibility of intrathecal admixtures containing baclofen and high concentrations of morphine. *Int J Pharm*. 1997; 153(1):13-24.
12. *Indications, drug stability, and emergency procedures - SynchroMed® and IsoMed® implantable infusion systems (M961293A001 Rev E)*, 2017. Minneapolis, MN: Medtronic, Inc.; Updated December 2017.
13. *MEDI-FLO™ - Drug Stability Guide: Antibiotics, Chemotherapy and Pain Management Infusions (REV01)*, 2019. Sunrise, FL: Wolf Medical Supply; Updated September 2019.

Mycophenolate Mofetil

Storage Conditions

						Temperature			Post-thaw Temp			
	Drug Manufacturer	Concentration	Diluents	Osmolality (mOsm/kg)	pH	Room	Refrig	Frozen	Room	Refrig	Body Temp	Refer.
CONTAINER												
Bag, Polypropylene	RC, ACD	1, 4, 10 mg/mL	D5W	n/a	[a]	n/a	n/a	5 wk[b]	n/a	n/a	n/a	(4)
	RC, ACD	1, 4 mg/mL	D5W	n/a	[a]	14 d[c]	5 wk[c]	n/a	n/a	n/a	n/a	(4)
	RC	10 mg/mL	D5W	n/a	[a]	14 d[c]	5 wk[c]	n/a	n/a	n/a	n/a	(4)
	ACD	10 mg/mL	D5W	n/a	[a]	21 d[c]	5 wk[c]	n/a	n/a	n/a	n/a	(4)
Bag, Polyvinyl Chloride (PVC)	RC	1, 5, 10 mg/mL	D5W	n/a	[a]	7 d[d]	7 d[d]	n/a	n/a	n/a	n/a	(5)

Flush Compatibility: D5W.[1]

Special Considerations: Mycophenolate mofetil is a white to off-white lyophilized powder that forms slightly yellow solution upon reconstitution and dilution.[2,3]

Notes

[a] pH of injectable solution is 2.4-4.1 (AKN) or 2.7-4.1 (ZYD).[2,3]

[b] Storage temperature: –15 to –25°C.[4]

[c] Protected from light. Loss due to chemical sorption when compounded using Equashield® closed-system transfer device negligible.[4]

[d] Progressive discoloration occurred after 72 hours in bags exposed to light and stored at room temperature. No discoloration occurred in bags indirectly protected from light stored under refrigeration.[5]

REFERENCES

1. ASHP's Interactive Handbook on Injectable Drugs, 2020. Bethesda, MD: American Society of Health-System Pharmacists; Accessed August 2020.
2. Mycophenolate Mofetil Injection [package insert]. Lake Forest, IL: Akorn, Inc.; January 2020.
3. Mycophenolate Mofetil Injection [package insert]. Pennington, NJ: Zydus Pharmaceuticals (USA), Inc.; January 2020.
4. Ezquer-Garin C, Ferriols-Lisart R, Alos-Alminana M. Stability of mycophenolate mofetil in polypropylene 5% dextrose infusion bags and chemical compatibility associated with the use of the Equashield® closed-system transfer device. *Biomed Chromatogr*. 2019; 33(7):e4529.
5. Certain E, Beteta F, Goudou-Sinha C, et al. Stability of i.v. mycophenolate mofetil in 5% dextrose injection in polyvinyl chloride infusion bags. *Am J Health Syst Pharm*. 2002; 59(24):2434-9.

DOI 10.37573/9781585286720.147

Nafcillin Sodium

Storage Conditions

	Drug Manufacturer	Concentration	Diluents	Osmolality (mOsm/kg)	pH	Temperature Room	Temperature Refrig	Temperature Frozen	Post-thaw Temp Room	Post-thaw Temp Refrig	Body Temp	Refer.
CONTAINER												
Bag, Polyvinyl Chloride (PVC)	WY	20 mg/mL	NS	361	[e]	72 hr	24 d	n/a	n/a	n/a	n/a	(1)
	WY	20 mg/mL	D5W	334	[e]	7 d	15 d	30 d	24 hr	n/a	n/a	(1)
Syringe, Glass	WY	250 mg/mL	unspec.	n/a	[e]	n/a	n/a	9 m	n/a	n/a	n/a	(1)
Syringe, Polypropylene	APC	10 mg/mL	NS	n/a	[e]	7 d	44 d	n/a	n/a	n/a	n/a	(1)
Unspecified	AUR	10-200 mg/mL	SWFI, NS	n/a	[e]	24 hr	7 d	n/a	n/a	n/a	n/a	(3)
	AUR	2-30 mg/mL	D5W, D5½NS	n/a	[e]	24 hr	n/a	n/a	n/a	n/a	n/a	(3)
	AUR	10-30 mg/mL	LR	n/a	[e]	24 hr	n/a	n/a	n/a	n/a	n/a	(3)
	AUR	10-30 mg/mL	D5W, D5½NS, LR	n/a	[e]	n/a	7 d	n/a	n/a	n/a	n/a	(3)
	AUR	250 mg/mL	SWFI, NS	n/a	[e]	n/a	n/a	90 d	n/a	n/a	n/a	(3)
	AUR	10-250 mg/mL	D5W, D5½NS, LR	n/a	[e]	n/a	n/a	90 d	n/a	n/a	n/a	(3)
Vial, Glass	AUR	250 mg/mL	BWFI, SWFI, NS	n/a	[e]	72 hr	7 d	90 d	n/a	n/a	n/a	(3)
OTHER INFUSION CONTAINERS												
CADD® Cassette (Smiths Medical)	MAR	20, 120 mg/mL	SWFI	n/a	[e]	72 hr	14 d	n/a	n/a	n/a	n/a	(1)
	WY	80 mg/mL	NS	n/a	[e]	48 hr[g]	24 hr[g]	n/a	n/a	n/a	n/a	(1)
Dosi-Fuser® (Leventon)	SI	5 mg/mL	NS	n/a	[e]	72 hr	14 d	30 d	24 hr	n/a	n/a	(6)
	BR	5-40 mg/mL	D5W, NS	n/a	[e]	n/a	10 d[c]	30 d[c]	n/a	n/a	n/a	(6)
	BR	10-40 mg/mL	D5W	n/a	[e]	24 hr[c]	14 d[c]	30 d	n/a	n/a	n/a	(8)
Easypump® ST/LT (B. Braun)	UN	5, 50 mg/mL	NS	n/a	[e]	30 hr	14 d	n/a	n/a	n/a	n/a	(9)
Homepump Eclipse® / Homepump® (Halyard)	UN	10 mg/mL	NS	n/a	[e]	24 hr	72 hr	n/a	n/a	n/a	n/a	(4)
INFUSOR™ (Baxter)[d]	BR	10 mg/mL	D5W	n/a	[e]	72 hr[f]	14 d[f]	n/a	n/a	n/a	n/a	(2)
	BR	10-40 mg/mL	D5W	n/a	[e]	24 hr[a]	14 d[a]	n/a	n/a	n/a	n/a	(2)
INTERMATE™ (Baxter)[d]	BR	5 mg/mL	D5W	n/a	[e]	24 hr	10 d	30 d	n/a	n/a	n/a	(2)
	BR	5-40 mg/mL	D5W, NS	n/a	[e]	n/a	10 d	30 d	n/a	n/a	n/a	(2)
SMARTeZ® (Progressive Medical)	UN	50 mg/mL	NS	n/a	[e]	48 hr[c]	14 d[c]	n/a	n/a	n/a	n/a	(6)

DOI 10.37573/9781585286720.148

Storage Conditions

	Drug Manufacturer	Concentration	Diluents	Osmolality (mOsm/kg)	pH	Temperature Room	Temperature Refrig	Temperature Frozen	Post-thaw Temp Room	Post-thaw Temp Refrig	Body Temp	Refer.
COMMERCIAL PREPARATIONS (RTU)												
GALAXY™ Plastic Container (Baxter)	SKB	20 mg/mL	D5W	iso	6-8.5	n/a	n/a	n/a	72 hr[b]	21 d[b]	n/a	(1)(5)

Flush Compatibility: Sodium chloride 0.9%, heparin.[1]

Special Considerations: Precipitation was observed after 48 hours in a solution incubated at 34° to 36°C, at concentrations ≥ 40 mg/mL in NS.[7]

Notes

[a] 14 days refrigerated, followed by 24 hours at room temperature.[2]

[b] Expiration date per manufacturer's label. Do not extrapolate commercial premix stability data to extemporaneously compounded solutions.

[c] Manufacturer extrapolated data from other sources.

[d] INTERMATE™/INFUSOR™ Portable Elastomeric Infusion System devices are no longer available in the United States.

[e] pH of reconstituted preparation is 6-8.5.[1]

[f] 14 days refrigerated, followed by 72 hours at room temperature.[2]

[g] Followed by 48 hours of simulated administration at 30°C.[1]

REFERENCES

1. ASHP's Interactive Handbook on Injectable Drugs, 2020. Bethesda, MD: American Society of Health-System Pharmacists; Accessed September 2020.
2. Stabforum - Stability Database: Nafcillin, Ontario, Canada: Baxter Healthcare; Accessed February 2021.
3. Nafcillin Sodium Injection [package insert]. E. Windsor, NJ: AuroMedics Pharma, LLC.; January 2021.
4. *Stability Data for Drugs Using Homepump Disposable Ambulatory Infusion Systems (MK-00314 rev 3)*, 2015. Alpharetta, GA: Halyard Health; Updated June 2015.
5. Nafcillin Injection in GALAXY™ Container (PL 2040 Plastic) [package insert]. Deerfield, IL: Baxter Healthcare Corporation; September 2018.
6. *Drug Stability Table - Dosi-Fuser® Elastomeric Pump (S-CL-00-001v16)*, 2021. Barcelona, Spain: Leventon SAU; Updated May 2021.
7. Chan V. Influence of temperature and drug concentration on nafcillin precipitation. *Am J Health Syst Pharm*. 2005; 62(13):1347-8.
8. *SMARTeZ® - Stability Data for Drugs Using Elastomeric Infusion Pumps*, 2020. Fenton, MO: Progressive Medical, Inc.; Updated May 2020.
9. *Drug Stability for Easypump® ST/LT*, 2020. Bethlehem, PA: B. Braun USA; Updated June 2020.

NORepinephrine

Storage Conditions

						Temperature			Post-thaw Temp			
	Drug Manufacturer	Concentration	Diluents	Osmolality (mOsm/kg)	pH	Room	Refrig	Frozen	Room	Refrig	Body Temp	Refer.
CONTAINER												
Bag, Polyvinyl Chloride (PVC)	WI	0.016 mg/mL	D5W	n/a	[a]	n/a	47 d[b]	n/a	n/a	n/a	n/a	(1)
	WI	0.04 mg/mL	D5W	n/a	[a]	n/a	87 d[b]	n/a	n/a	n/a	n/a	(1)
	SX	0.004, 0.016 mg/mL	D5W	n/a	[a]	7 d	n/a	n/a	n/a	n/a	n/a	(1)
	SZ	0.0645 mg/mL	D5W, NS	n/a	[a]	61 d[b]	61 d[b]	n/a	n/a	n/a	n/a	(1)
	SAB	0.004, 0.016 mg/mL	D5W, NS	n/a	[a]	7 d[d]	n/a	n/a	n/a	n/a	n/a	(3)
Syringe, Polypropylene	AGT	0.24 mg/mL	NS	n/a	[a]	n/a	30 d[b]	n/a	n/a	n/a	n/a	(1)
	UN	0.5, 1.16 mg/mL	D5W	n/a	[a]	48 hr[c]	n/a	n/a	n/a	n/a	n/a	(1)
	MYL	0.2 mg/mL	NS	n/a	3.3-3.6	180 d	365 d	365 d	n/a	n/a	n/a	(2)
	MYL	0.5 mg/mL	NS	n/a	3.3-3.6	n/a	365 d	365 d	n/a	n/a	n/a	(2)
	AGT	0.12, 0.24 mg/mL[e]	NS	n/a	[a]	48 hr	n/a	n/a	n/a	n/a	n/a	(1)
Vial, Plastic (Unspecified)	MYL	0.2 mg/mL	NS	n/a	3.3-3.6	330 d	365 d	365 d	n/a	n/a	n/a	(2)
	MYL	0.5 mg/mL	NS	n/a	3.3-3.6	365 d	365d	365 d	n/a	n/a	n/a	(2)

Flush Compatibility: Sodium chloride 0.9%.[1]

Special Considerations: Caution should be employed in mixing additives that may result in a final pH above 6 since NORepinephrine bitartrate is alkali labile.[1] Do not use the solution if its color is pinkish or darker than slightly yellow or if it contains a precipitate. Protect from light.[4]

Notes

[a] pH from 3 to 4.5. NORepinephrine bitartrate is stable at pH 3.6 to 6 in dextrose 5%.[1]

[b] Protected from light.

[c] Stored with and without light protection.

[d] Exposed to light.

[e] Tartrate salt.

DOI 10.37573/9781585286720.149

REFERENCES

1. ASHP's Interactive Handbook on Injectable Drugs, 2020. Bethesda, MD: American Society of Health-System Pharmacists; Accessed August 2020.
2. Gilliot S, Masse M, Genay S, et al. Long-term stability of ready-to-use norepinephrine solution at 0.2 and 0.5 mg/mL. *Eur J Hosp Pharm*. 2020; 27 e1:e93-e98.
3. Tremblay M, Lessard MR, Trepanier CA, et al. Stability of norepinephrine infusions prepared in dextrose and normal saline solutions. *Can J Anaesth*. 2008; 55(3):163-7.
4. Levophed® (Norepinephrine Bitartrate) Injection [package insert]. Lake Forest, IL: Hospira, Inc.; November 2020.

Octreotide Acetate

Storage Conditions

						Temperature			Post-thaw Temp			
CONTAINER	Drug Manufacturer	Concentration	Diluents	Osmolality (mOsm/kg)	pH	Room	Refrig	Frozen	Room	Refrig	Body Temp	Refer.
Bag, Polyvinyl Chloride (PVC)	SZ	1.5 mcg/mL	NS	n/a	[c]	48 hr[a]	n/a	n/a	n/a	n/a	n/a	(1)
Syringe, Polypropylene	SZ	200 mcg/mL	Undiluted	n/a	[c]	7 d[d]	29 d[d]	n/a	n/a	n/a	n/a	(3)
	SZ	200 mcg/mL	Undiluted	n/a	[c]	7 d[a]	22 d[a]	n/a	n/a	n/a	n/a	(1)
	SZ	200 mcg/mL	Undiluted	n/a	[c]	n/a	60 d[b]	60 d[b]	n/a	n/a	n/a	(4)

Flush Compatibility: Sodium chloride 0.9%.[1]

Special Considerations: Store preservative-free single dose vials and preserved multi-dose vials refrigerated and protected from light.[2] Do not confuse octreotide acetate injection with the injectable depot suspension product, which must not be administered IV or SC.[1]

Notes

[a] Exposed to light.
[b] Light conditions unspecified.
[c] pH of undiluted solution is 3.9-4.5.[2]
[d] Protected from light.

REFERENCES

1. ASHP's Interactive Handbook on Injectable Drugs, 2020. Bethesda, MD: American Society of Health-System Pharmacists; Accessed December 2020.
2. Octreotide Acetate Injection [package insert]. Schaumburg, IL: Sagent Pharmaceuticals, Inc.; June 2019.
3. Stiles ML, Allen LV, Jr., Resztak KE, et al. Stability of octreotide acetate in polypropylene syringes. *Am J Hosp Pharm*. 1993; 50(11):2356-8.
4. Ripley RG, Ritchie DJ, Holstad SG. Stability of octreotide acetate in polypropylene syringes at 5 and -20 degrees C. *Am J Health Syst Pharm*. 1995; 52(17):1910-1.

DOI 10.37573/9781585286720.150

Omadacycline

Storage Conditions

						Temperature			Post-thaw Temp			
	Drug Manufacturer	Concentration	Diluents	Osmolality (mOsm/kg)	pH	Room	Refrig	Frozen	Room	Refrig	Body Temp	Refer.
CONTAINER												
Bag, Unspecified	PRK	1, 2 mg/mL	NS, D5W	n/a	n/a	24 hr[b]	7 d[a]	n/a	n/a	n/a	n/a	(1)(3)
SMARTeZ® (Progressive Medical)	PRK	1, 2 mg/mL	NS, D5W	n/a	n/a	n/a	9 d[a]	n/a	n/a	n/a	n/a	(3)(4)

Flush Compatibility: Sodium chloride 0.9%.[2]

Special Considerations: Omadacycline must not be administered through the same intravenous line with any solution containing multivalent cations (e.g., calcium, magnesium). The manufacturer states that diluted solutions of omadacycline should not be frozen. If the diluted solution has been stored under refrigeration, it should be removed from refrigerator, and kept at room temperature in an upright position for 1 hour prior to use.[2]

Notes

[a] Storage temperature: 2-8°C.

[b] Storage temperature: 25°C.

REFERENCES

1. Nuzyra® (Omadacycline) Injection, Lyophilized [package insert]. Boston, MA: Paratek Pharmaceuticals, Inc.; November 2020.
2. ASHP's Interactive Handbook on Injectable Drugs, 2020. Bethesda, MD: American Society of Health-System Pharmacists; Accessed August 2020.
3. Nuzyra® Stability Medication Information Letter (Ref#: US-OMC-SRL-0022) [personal communication]. King of Prussia, PA: Paratek Pharmaceuticals, Inc.; 2020:4.
4. *SMARTeZ® - Stability Data for Drugs Using Elastomeric Infusion Pumps*, 2020. Fenton, MO: Progressive Medical, Inc.; Updated May 2020.

DOI 10.37573/9781585286720.151

Ondansetron Hydrochloride

Storage Conditions

						Temperature			Post-thaw Temp			
	Drug Manufacturer	Concentration	Diluents	Osmolality (mOsm/kg)	pH	Room	Refrig	Frozen	Room	Refrig	Body Temp	Refer.
CONTAINER												
Bag, Polyolefin	GSK	0.08 mg/mL	NS[m]	n/a	[k]	n/a	30 d	n/a	n/a	n/a	n/a	(2)
Bag, Polyvinyl Chloride (PVC)	GL	0.016, 0.08 mg/mL	D5W, NS	n/a	[k]	7 d[a]	7 d	n/a	n/a	n/a	n/a	(1)
	GL	0.03, 0.3 mg/mL	D5W, NS	n/a	[k]	48 hr	14 d	12 wk	n/a	n/a	n/a	(1)
	GL	0.024, 0.096 mg/mL	D5W, LR, NS	n/a	[k]	14 d	14 d[l]	n/a	n/a	n/a	n/a	(1)(9)
	GL	0.08 mg/mL	NS	n/a	[k]	n/a	120 d	120 d	n/a	n/a	n/a	(1)
	GL	0.1, 1 mg/mL	NS[q]	n/a	[k]	31 d	31 d	n/a	n/a	n/a	7 d[e]	(1)
	CER	0.1, 0.2, 0.4, 0.64 mg/mL	NS	n/a	[k]	48 hr[c]	30 d[c]	n/a	n/a	n/a	n/a	(1)
	CER	0.1, 0.2, 0.4, 0.64 mg/mL	NS[b]	n/a	[k]	48 hr[c]	30 d[c]	n/a	n/a	n/a	n/a	(1)(4)
	GL	0.15 mg/mL	NS[g]	n/a	[k]	28 d	28 d	n/a	n/a	n/a	n/a	(1)(6)
	GL	0.15 mg/mL	D5W[g]	n/a	[k]	72 hr	28 d	n/a	n/a	n/a	n/a	(1)
	GL	0.75 mg/mL	D5W[n]	n/a	[k]	72 hr	72 hr	n/a	n/a	n/a	n/a	(1)
	GL	0.75 mg/mL	NS[n]	n/a	[k]	7 d	28 d	n/a	n/a	n/a	n/a	(1)
Syringe, Polypropylene	UN	0.25, 0.5, 1 mg/mL	D5W, NS	n/a	[k]	48 hr	14 d	90 d	48 hr[o]	14 d[o]	n/a	(7)(13)
	GL	2 mg/mL	Undiluted	n/a	[k]	48 hr	14 d	90 d	48 hr[o]	14 d[o]	n/a	(7)
Unspecified	GL	0.1, 1 mg/mL	NS[d]	n/a	[k]	31 d	31 d	n/a	n/a	n/a	7 d[e]	(1)
OTHER INFUSION CONTAINERS												
CADD® Cassette (Smiths Medical)	GL	0.24 mg/mL	NS	n/a	[k]	24 hr [f][h]	30 d[f]	n/a	n/a	n/a	n/a	(11)(14)
	GL	2 mg/mL	Undiluted	n/a	[k]	7 d [f][h]	30 d[f]	n/a	n/a	n/a	n/a	(11)(14)
Dosi-Fuser® (Leventon)	GSK	0.1-0.7 mg/mL	D5W, NS	n/a	[k]	24 hr[j]	10 d[j]	n/a	n/a	n/a	12 hr[j]	(10)
Easypump® ST/LT (B. Braun)	UN	0.03 mg/mL	D5W, NS	n/a	[k]	7 d	21 d	n/a	n/a	n/a	n/a	(12)
	UN	0.7 mg/mL	D5W, NS	n/a	[k]	4 d	10 d	n/a	n/a	n/a	n/a	(12)

DOI 10.37573/9781585286720.152

Storage Conditions

	Drug Manufacturer	Concentration	Diluents	Osmolality (mOsm/kg)	pH	Temperature Room	Temperature Refrig	Frozen	Post-thaw Temp Room	Post-thaw Temp Refrig	Body Temp	Refer.
OTHER INFUSION CONTAINERS												
Homepump Eclipse® / Homepump® (Halyard)	GL	0.03, 0.3 mg/mL	D5W, NS	n/a	[k]	n/a	14 d[a]	n/a	n/a	n/a	n/a	(1)(5)
INTERMATE™ (Baxter)[p]	GL	0.1-0.7 mg/mL	D5W, NS	n/a	[k]	24 hr[i]	10 d[i]	n/a	n/a	n/a	12 hr[i]	(3)
Polyester Container (CR3)	CER	0.64 mg/mL	D5W[b]	n/a	[k]	48 hr[c]	30 d[c]	n/a	n/a	n/a	n/a	(1)(4)
SMARTeZ® (Progressive Medical)	UN	0.03-0.3 mg/mL	D5W, NS	n/a	[k]	7 d[j]	21 d[j]	n/a	n/a	n/a	n/a	(8)
		0.7 mg/mL	D5W, NS	n/a	[k]	4 d[j]	10 d[j]	n/a	n/a	n/a	n/a	(8)

Flush Compatibility: Sodium chloride 0.9%, heparin.[1]

Special Considerations: n/a

Notes

a Exposed to light.[1]

b Solution contained: dexAMETHasone 0.2 and 0.4 mg/mL (ES).[1,4]

c 30 d refrigerated followed by 48 hr at room temperature.[1,4]

d Solution contained: morphine sulfate (AST) 1 mg/mL or HYDROmorphone HCl (ES) 0.5 mg/mL.[1]

e Storage temperature: 32°C.[1]

f 30 d refrigerated, followed by 24 hr at 30°C.[11,14]

g Solution contained: dexAMETHasone sodium phosphate (MSD) 0.4 mg/mL.[1,6]

h Storage temperature: 30°C.[11]

i 10 d refrigerated, followed by 24 hr at room temperature, followed by 12 hr at 33°C.[3]

j Manufacturer(s) extrapolated data from other sources.[10]

k pH of undiluted solutions is 3.3-4.[1]

l 14 d refrigerated, followed by 48 hr at room temperature.[1,9]

m Solution contained: dexAMETHasone sodium phosphate (ASN) 0.1 mg/mL.[2]

n Solution contained: dexAMETHasone sodium phosphate (MSD) 0.23 mg/mL.[1]

o 90 d at -20°C, followed by 14 d at 4°C, then 48 hr at 24°C.[7,13]

p INTERMATE™/INFUSOR™ Portable Elastomeric Infusion System devices are no longer available in the United States.

q Solution contained: meperidine HCl (WY) 4 mg/mL.[1]

REFERENCES

1. ASHP's Interactive Handbook on Injectable Drugs, 2020. Bethesda, MD: American Society of Health-System Pharmacists; Accessed October 2020.
2. Simar J, Godet M, Hecq JD, et al. Long-term stability of dexamethasone and alizapride or ondansetron in sodium chloride 0.9% polyolefin bag at 5+/-3 degrees C. *Ann Pharm Fr*. 2017; 75(1):30-39.
3. Stabforum - Stability Database: Ondansetron, Ontario, Canada: Baxter Healthcare; Accessed January 2021.
4. Hagan RL, Mallett MS, Fox JL. Stability of ondansetron hydrochloride and dexamethasone sodium phosphate in infusion bags and syringes for 32 days. *Am J Health Syst Pharm*. 1996; 53(12):1431-5. Erratum in: *Am J Health Syst Pharm*. 1997; 54(9):1110.
5. *Stability Data for Drugs Using Homepump Disposable Ambulatory Infusion Systems (MK-00314 rev 3)*, 2015. Alpharetta, GA: Halyard Health; Updated June 2015.
6. Evrard B, Ceccato A, Gaspard O, et al. Stability of ondansetron hydrochloride and dexamethasone sodium phosphate in 0.9% sodium chloride injection and in 5% dextrose injection. *Am J Health Syst Pharm*. 1997; 54(9):1065-8.
7. Casto DT. Stability of ondansetron stored in polypropylene syringes. *Ann Pharmacother*. 1994; 28(6):712-4.
8. *SMARTeZ® - Stability Data for Drugs Using Elastomeric Infusion Pumps*, 2020. Fenton, MO: Progressive Medical, Inc.; Updated May 2020.
9. Graham CL, Dukes GE, Kao CF, et al. Stability of ondansetron in large-volume parenteral solutions. *Ann Pharmacother*. 1992; 26(6):768-71.
10. *Drug Stability Table - Dosi-Fuser® Elastomeric Pump (S-CL-00-001v16)*, 2021. Barcelona, Spain: Leventon SAU; Updated May 2021.
11. Stiles ML, Allen LV, Jr., Fox JL. Stability of ondansetron hydrochloride in portable infusion-pump reservoirs. *Am J Hosp Pharm*. 1992; 49(6):1471-3.
12. *Drug Stability for Easypump® ST/LT*, 2020. Bethlehem, PA: B. Braun USA; Updated June 2020.
13. Estan-Cerezo G, Jimenez-Pulido I, Rodriguez Lucena FJ, et al. Chemical stability of ondansetron hydrochloride with other drugs in admixtures via parenteral; a review. *Farm Hosp*. 2017; 41(5):625-29.
14. *Pharmaceutical report on chemical and physical stability of drugs commonly used with CADD® infusion pumps (IN193109GB-122019)*, 2019. Minneapolis, MN: Smiths Medical ASD, Inc.; Updated December 2019.

Oritavancin Diphosphate

Storage Conditions

						Temperature			Post-thaw Temp			
	Drug Manufacturer	Concentration	Diluents	Osmolality (mOsm/kg)	pH	Room	Refrig	Frozen	Room	Refrig	Body Temp	Refer.
CONTAINER												
Bag, Polyvinyl Chloride (PVC)	TMC	1.2 mg/mL	D5W	n/a	[(a)]	6 hr[(b)]	12 hr[(b)]	n/a	n/a	n/a	n/a	(1)(2)

Flush Compatibility: D5W. Incompatible with sodium chloride 0.9% and heparin.[(1)] Intravenous unfractionated heparin sodium is contraindicated for 120 hours (5 days) after drug administration.[(2)]

Special Considerations: Reconstitute three - 400 mg vials with 40 mL SWFI per vial to provide a 10 mg/mL solution. To avoid foaming, gently swirl vials. Withdraw and discard 120 mL D5W from a 1,000 mL bag, then add 120 mL (1,200 mg) of drug to the D5W bag for a final concentration of 1.2 mg/mL. Use only D5W for dilution.[(2)]

Notes

[a] pH range is 3.1-4.3.[(1)]

[b] Combined reconstituted and diluted storage time, including the 3 hr infusion time, should not exceed 6 hr at room temperature or 12 hr if refrigerated.[(2)]

REFERENCES

1. ASHP's Interactive Handbook on Injectable Drugs, 2020. Bethesda, MD: American Society of Health-System Pharmacists; Accessed August 2020.
2. Orbactiv® (Oritavancin) Injection [package insert]. Parsippany, NJ: The Medicines Company; February 2020.

DOI 10.37573/9781585286720.153

Oxacillin Sodium

Storage Conditions

						Temperature			Post-thaw Temp			
	Drug Manufacturer	Concentration	Diluents	Osmolality (mOsm/kg)	pH	Room	Refrig	Frozen	Room	Refrig	Body Temp	Refer.
CONTAINER												
Bag, Polyvinyl Chloride (PVC)	BR	1 mg/mL	[f]	n/a	[e]	n/a	24 hr	n/a	n/a	n/a	n/a	(1)
	BR	10 mg/mL	D5W	295	[e]	24 hr	n/a	30 d	24 hr	n/a	n/a	(1)
Syringe, Plastic (Unspecified)	BR	200 mg/mL	SWFI	[b]	[e]	n/a	n/a	12 wk	n/a	n/a	n/a	(1)
Syringe, Polypropylene	AUR	100 mg/mL	NS	[b]	[e]	92 hr	14 d	n/a	n/a	n/a	n/a	(5)
	AUR	200 mg/mL	SWFI	[b]	[e]	84 hr	n/a	n/a	n/a	n/a	n/a	(5)
	AUR	200 mg/mL	D5W	[b]	[e]	42 hr	n/a	n/a	n/a	n/a	n/a	(5)
Unspecified	BR	1, 10, 50 mg/mL	D5W, NS	[b]	[e]	24 hr	n/a	n/a	n/a	n/a	n/a	(1)
	UN	10-30 mg/mL	D5W, LR	[b]	[e]	n/a	4 d	30 d	n/a	n/a	n/a	(1)
	UN	10-100 mg/mL	NS	[b]	[e]	4 d	7 d	30 d	n/a	n/a	n/a	(1)
	UN	10-30 mg/mL	D5½NS	[b]	[e]	24 hr	4 d	30 d	n/a	n/a	n/a	(1)
Vial, Glass	BR	1 mg/mL	[f]	[b]	[e]	n/a	24 hr	n/a	n/a	n/a	n/a	(1)
	BR	200 mg/mL	SWFI	[b]	[e]	n/a	n/a	12 wk	n/a	n/a	n/a	(1)
OTHER INFUSION CONTAINERS												
Accufuser® (Vygon)	FLU	5 mg/mL	NS	[b]	5.3-5.6	7 d	6 wk	n/a	n/a	n/a	n/a	(6)
	FLU	5 mg/mL	D5W	[b]	3.6-5.6	48 hr	6 wk	n/a	n/a	n/a	n/a	(6)
AutoDose™ (Tandem Medical)	UN	10 mg/mL	NS	[b]	[e]	7 d	30 d	n/a	n/a	n/a	n/a	(7)
CADD® Cassette (Smiths Medical)	MAR	120 mg/mL	SWFI	[b]	[e]	72 hr	14 d	n/a	n/a	n/a	n/a	(1)
Dosi-Fuser® (Leventon)	BR	10-80 mg/mL	D5W, NS	[b]	[e]	24 hr[a]	10 d[a]	30 d[a]	24 hr[a]	n/a	n/a	(4)
	BMS	10-100 mg/mL	NS	[b]	[e]	4 d	14 d	30 d	24 hr	n/a	n/a	(4)
	BR	40 mg/mL	SWFI	[b]	[e]	n/a	10 d[a]	n/a	n/a	n/a	n/a	(4)
Easypump® ST/LT (B. Braun)	UN	10,100 mg/mL	NS	[b]	n/a	4 d[a]	8 d[a]	n/a	n/a	n/a	n/a	(9)

DOI 10.37573/9781585286720.154

Storage Conditions

	Drug Manufacturer	Concentration	Diluents	Osmolality (mOsm/kg)	pH	Temperature Room	Temperature Refrig	Temperature Frozen	Post-thaw Temp Room	Post-thaw Temp Refrig	Body Temp	Refer.
OTHER INFUSION CONTAINERS												
Homepump Eclipse® / Homepump® (Halyard)	UN	10-30 mg/mL	D5W	[b]	[e]	n/a	4 d[a]	n/a	n/a	n/a	n/a	(8)
	UN	10-100 mg/mL	NS	[b]	[e]	4 d[a]	7 d[a]	n/a	n/a	n/a	n/a	(8)
	UN	10-100 mg/mL	D5W	[b]	[e]	n/a	n/a	30 d[a]	n/a	n/a	n/a	(8)
INTERMATE™ (Baxter)[d]	BR	10-80 mg/mL	D5W, NS	[b]	[e]	24 hr	10 d	30 d	24 hr	n/a	n/a	(2)
	BR	40 mg/mL	SWFI	[b]	n/a	n/a	10 d	n/a	n/a	n/a	n/a	(2)
SMARTeZ® (Progressive Medical)	UN	10, 100 mg/mL	NS	[b]	n/a	4 d[a]	8 d[a]	n/a	n/a	n/a	n/a	(10)
COMMERICAL PREPARATIONS (RTU)												
GALAXY™ Plastic Container (Baxter)	BA	20, 40 mg/mL	D	iso	6-8.5	n/a	n/a	[c]	48 hr[c]	21 d[c]	n/a	(1)(3)

Flush Compatibility: Sodium chloride 0.9%, heparin.[1]

Special Considerations: Oxacillin sodium at higher concentrations is a venous irritant.

Notes

[a] Manufacturer(s) extrapolated data from other sources.

[b] 166 mg/mL (BR) in SWFI is 596 mOsm/kg by freezing-point depression and 657 mOsm/kg by vapor pressure. 50 mg/mL (BE) is 381 mOsm/kg in D5W and 396 mOsm/kg in NS.[1]

[c] Frozen expiration date per manufacturer's label. Do not extrapolate commercial premix stability data to extemporaneously compounded solutions. Store in a freezer capable of maintaining -20°C or colder. Do not refreeze after thawing.[3]

[d] INTERMATE™/INFUSOR™ Portable Elastomeric Infusion System devices are no longer available in the United States.

[e] pH of 10 mg/mL is 7.4-7.94 in D5W and 7.73 in NS.[1]

[f] Diluents: D5W, D5LR, D5NS, LR, NS.[1]

REFERENCES

1. ASHP's Interactive Handbook on Injectable Drugs, 2020. Bethesda, MD: American Society of Health-System Pharmacists; Accessed October 2020.
2. Stabforum - Stability Database: Oxacillin, Ontario, Canada: Baxter Healthcare; Accessed February 2021.
3. Oxacillin Injection, USP in GALAXY™ Plastic Container (PL 2040) [package insert]. Deerfield, IL: Baxter Healthcare Corporation; September 2018.

4. *Drug Stability Table - Dosi-Fuser® Elastomeric Pump (S-CL-00-001v16)*, 2021. Barcelona, Spain: Leventon SAU; Updated May 2021.
5. Fugit KD, Anderson BD. Antibiotic Stability in Freedom 60 Syringe Report by HealthTek™ and the University of Kentucky, Lexington. Chester, NY: RMS Medical Products; 2015.
6. Kim MJ, Lee GY, Park YS, et al. Intravenous Suitability Studies of Commonly Used Oxacillin Sodium Solutions in the Accufuser® Infusion Device. *Pharmacology & Pharmacy*. 2011; 2(3):189-93.
7. Zhang Y, Trissel LA. Stability of Ampicillin Sodium, Nafcillin Sodium, And Oxacillin Sodium in AutoDose Infusion System Bags. *Int J Pharm Compd*. 2002; 6(3):226-9.
8. *Stability Data for Drugs Using Homepump Disposable Ambulatory Infusion Systems (MK-00314 rev 3)*, 2015. Alpharetta, GA: Halyard Health; Updated June 2015.
9. *Drug Stability for Easypump® ST/LT*, 2020. Bethlehem, PA: B. Braun USA; Updated June 2020.
10. *SMARTeZ® - Stability Data for Drugs Using Elastomeric Infusion Pumps*, 2020. Fenton, MO: Progressive Medical, Inc.; Updated May 2020.

Oxaliplatin

Storage Conditions

	Drug Manufacturer	Concentration	Diluents	Osmolality (mOsm/kg)	pH	Temperature			Post-thaw Temp			
						Room	Refrig	Frozen	Room	Refrig	Body Temp	Refer.
CONTAINER												
Bag, Polyethylene	SAA	0.2, 1.3 mg/mL	D5W	n/a	n/a	14 d	14 d	n/a	n/a	n/a	n/a	(5)
Bag, Polyolefin	AVE	0.25 mg/mL	D5W	n/a	n/a	90 d	90 d	n/a	n/a	n/a	n/a	(4)
	SAA	0.7 mg/mL	D5W	n/a	n/a	30 d	30 d	n/a	n/a	n/a	n/a	(1)
Bag, Polypropylene	SAA	0.2, 1.3 mg/mL	D5W	n/a	n/a	14 d	14 d	n/a	n/a	n/a	n/a	(5)
Bag, Polyvinyl Chloride (PVC)	SAA	0.2, 1.3 mg/mL	D5W	n/a	n/a	14 d	14 d	n/a	n/a	n/a	n/a	(5)
OTHER INFUSION CONTAINERS												
Dosi-Fuser® (Leventon)	SW	0.1-1 mg/mL	D5W	n/a	n/a	28 d[c]	28 d[c]	n/a	n/a	n/a	n/a	(7)
INTERMATE (Baxter)[a]	SAA	0.1-1 mg/mL	D5W	n/a	n/a	28 d	n/a	n/a	n/a	n/a	n/a	(6)
	SAA	0.1-1 mg/mL	D5W	n/a	n/a	9 d	28 d[b]	n/a	n/a	n/a	n/a	(6)

Flush Compatibility: D5W. Incompatible with sodium chloride 0.9%, heparin flush, alkaline drugs, and chloride-containing solutions.[2,3]

Special Considerations: Do not freeze. Do not use needles or sets containing aluminum.[2]

Notes

[a] INTERMATE™/INFUSOR™ Portable Elastomeric Infusion System devices are no longer available in the United States.

[b] Stored for 28 days refrigerated, followed by 9 days at 25°C.[6]

[c] Manufacturer extrapolated data from other sources.

REFERENCES

1. Andre P, Cisternino S, Roy AL, et al. Stability of oxaliplatin in infusion bags containing 5% dextrose injection. *Am J Health Syst Pharm*. 2007; 64(18):1950-4.
2. ASHP's Interactive Handbook on Injectable Drugs, 2020. Bethesda, MD: American Society of Health-System Pharmacists; Accessed July 2020.
3. Oxaliplatin Injection [package insert]. Weston, FL: Apotex Corp.; November 2020.
4. Junker A, Roy S, Desroches MC, et al. Stability of oxaliplatin solution. *Ann Pharmacother*. 2009; 43(2):390-1.
5. Eiden C, Philibert L, Bekhtari K, et al. Physicochemical stability of oxaliplatin in 5% dextrose injection stored in polyvinyl chloride, polyethylene, and polypropylene infusion bags. *Am J Health Syst Pharm*. 2009; 66(21):1929-33.
6. Stabforum - Stability Database: Oxaliplatin, Ontario, Canada: Baxter Healthcare; Accessed January 2021.
7. *Drug Stability Table - Dosi-Fuser® Elastomeric Pump (S-CL-00-001v16)*, 2021. Barcelona, Spain: Leventon SAU; Updated May 2021.

DOI 10.37573/9781585286720.155

Oxytocin

Storage Conditions

	Drug Manufacturer	Concentration	Diluents	Osmolality (mOsm/kg)	pH	Temperature Room	Temperature Refrig	Temperature Frozen	Post-thaw Temp Room	Post-thaw Temp Refrig	Body Temp	Refer.
CONTAINER												
Bag, Polyvinyl Chloride (PVC)	APP	0.08 units/mL	NS, D5W	n/a	[a]	90 d[b]	n/a	n/a	n/a	n/a	n/a	(1)(2)
	APP	0.08 units/mL	LR	n/a	[a]	28 d[b]	n/a	n/a	n/a	n/a	n/a	(1)(2)
	APP	0.02, 0.06 units/mL	LR	n/a	[a]	31 d	31 d	n/a	n/a	n/a	n/a	(3)

Flush Compatibility: Sodium chloride 0.9%, heparin.[1]

Special Considerations: Protect from freezing.[1]

Notes

[a] pH of undiluted product is 3-5.[1]

[b] Protected from light.

REFERENCES

1. ASHP's Interactive Handbook on Injectable Drugs, 2020. Bethesda, MD: American Society of Health-System Pharmacists; Accessed July 2020.
2. Trissel LA, Zhang Y, Douglas K, et al. Extended stability of oxytocin in common infusion solutions. *Int J Pharm Compd*. 2006; 10(2):156-8.
3. Boothby L, Madabushi R, Kumar V, et al. Extended Stability of Oxytocin in Ringer's Lactate Solution at 4° and 25°C. *Hospital Pharmacy*. 2006; 41:437-41.

DOI 10.37573/9781585286720.156

PACLitaxel

Storage Conditions

	Drug Manufacturer	Concentration	Diluents	Osmolality (mOsm/kg)	pH	Temperature: Room	Temperature: Refrig	Temperature: Frozen	Post-thaw Temp: Room	Post-thaw Temp: Refrig	Body Temp	Refer.
CONTAINER												
Bag, Ethylene Vinyl Acetate (EVA)	FAU	0.3, 1.2 mg/mL	D5W, NS	n/a	[a]	24 hr[i]	n/a	n/a	n/a	n/a	24 hr[b][i]	(1)
Bag, Polyethylene	TE	0.3 mg/mL	NS	n/a	[f]	72 hr[e]	16 d[e]	n/a	n/a	n/a	n/a	(6)
	TE	0.3 mg/mL	D5W	n/a	[f]	72 hr[e]	18 d[e]	n/a	n/a	n/a	n/a	(6)
	BMS	0.4, 1.2 mg/mL	D5W	n/a	[a]	5 d[e]	5 d[e]	n/a	n/a	n/a	n/a	(1)
	TE	1.2 mg/mL	D5W, NS	n/a	[f]	72 hr[e]	12 d[e]	n/a	n/a	n/a	n/a	(6)
Bag, Polyolefin	TE	0.3 mg/mL	D5W, NS	n/a	[f]	72 hr[g]	13 d[g]	n/a	n/a	n/a	n/a	(6)
	BMS	0.3, 1.2 mg/mL	D5W, NS	n/a	[a]	n/a	n/a	n/a	n/a	n/a	72 hr[g][h]	(1)
	TE	1.2 mg/mL	NS	n/a	[f]	72 hr[g]	9 d[g]	n/a	n/a	n/a	n/a	(6)
	TE	1.2 mg/mL	D5W	n/a	[f]	72 hr[g]	10 d[g]	n/a	n/a	n/a	n/a	(6)
	BR	0.1, 1 mg/mL	D5W, NS	n/a	[a]	72 hr	72 hr	n/a	n/a	n/a	72 hr[b]	(1)
	MJ	1 mg/mL	D5W[c]	n/a	[a]	7 d[d]	7 d[d]	n/a	n/a	n/a	7 d[b]	(2)
	MAY	0.3 mg/mL	D5W	n/a	3.5-4.1	8 d[j]	28 d[j]	n/a	n/a	n/a	n/a	(11)
	MAY	0.3 mg/mL	NS	n/a	3.4-4	6 d[j]	28 d[j]	n/a	n/a	n/a	n/a	(11)
	MAY	0.75 mg/mL	D5W	n/a	3.6-3.9	4 d[j]	20 d[j]	n/a	n/a	n/a	n/a	(11)
	MAY	0.75 mg/mL	NS	n/a	3.5-3.9	6 d[j]	20 d[j]	n/a	n/a	n/a	n/a	(11)
	MAY	1.2 mg/mL	D5W, NS	n/a	3.5-4	4 d[j]	12 d[j]	n/a	n/a	n/a	n/a	(11)
Vial, Glass	TE	0.3 mg/mL	NS	n/a	[f]	72 hr	13 d	n/a	n/a	n/a	n/a	(6)
	TE	0.3 mg/mL	D5W	n/a	[f]	7 d	20 d	n/a	n/a	n/a	n/a	(6)
	TE	1.2 mg/mL	NS	n/a	[f]	5 d	8 d	n/a	n/a	n/a	n/a	(6)
	TE	1.2 mg/mL	D5W	n/a	[f]	7 d	10 d	n/a	n/a	n/a	n/a	(6)
OTHER INFUSION CONTAINER												
Easypump® ST/LT (B. Braun)	UN	0.3, 1.2 mg/mL	D5W, NS	n/a	[a]	24 hr	7 d	n/a	n/a	n/a	n/a	(8)
SMARTeZ® (Progressive Medical)	UN	0.3, 1.2 mg/mL	D5W, NS	n/a	[a]	24 hr[k]	7 d[k]	n/a	n/a	n/a	n/a	(9)

DOI 10.37573/9781585286720.157

Flush Compatibility: Sodium chloride 0.9%, heparin.[1]

Special Considerations: Precipitation may be exacerbated by the use of peristaltic pumps. Volumetric pumps may reduce this problem.[3-5] Since the mechanism of this irregular precipitation has not been identified, care and vigilance are required throughout the infusion. Precipitation is sporadic and unpredictable and may occur within recommended concentration range of 0.3-1.2mg/mL.[1] Containers and administration sets should not contain DEHP plasticizer. Administer through a 0.22-micron filter.[1] Precipitants, which may form during refrigeration of vials, should dissolve upon warming to room temperature.

Do not confuse PAClitaxel injection, USP, with PAClitaxel protein-bound particles for injectable suspension (Abraxane®). These have different physicochemical properties, dosing, preparation, administration procedures, and clinical applications.

Neither freezing nor refrigeration adversely affects the stability of the product.[10]

Notes

[a] pH of 0.6, 1.2 mg/mL in D5W, NS or D5LR is 4.4-5.6.[1]

[b] Storage temperature: 32°C.[1]

[c] Solution contained: 20 or 25% ethanol.[2]

[d] Author recommends maximum 7 d stability due to unpredictability of precipitation. Studies showed stability up to 14 d.[2]

[e] Container information: Ecoflac® low-density polyethylene bag (BRN).

[f] pH range of tested solutions was 3.5-4.2 (approx.).[6]

[g] Container information: Viaflo® polyolefin bag (BA).[6]

[h] Protected from light.[1]

[i] Although physically compatible and stable for 72 hr, unknown material leached from EVA container by 24 hr.[1]

[j] Container information: Freeflex® polyolefin with polypropylene film layer (FRK).[7]

[k] Manufacturer extrapolated data from other sources.[9]

REFERENCES

1. ASHP's Interactive Handbook on Injectable Drugs, 2020. Bethesda, MD: American Society of Health-System Pharmacists; Accessed August 2020.
2. Trissel LA, Xu Q, Martinez JF. Compounding an extended-stability admixture of Paclitaxel for long-term infusion. *Int J Pharm Compd*. 1997; 1(1):49-53.
3. Woloschuk DM. Drug precipitation and peristaltic pumps. *Am J Hosp Pharm*. 1994; 51(11):1473.
4. Pfeifer RW, Hale KN, Cronquist SE, et al. Precipitation of paclitaxel during infusion by pump. *Am J Hosp Pharm*. 1993; 50(12):2518, 21.
5. Trissel LA. Pharmaceutical properties of paclitaxel and their effects on preparation and administration. *Pharmacotherapy*. 1997; 17(5 Pt 2):133S-39S.
6. Donyai P, Sewell GJ. Physical and chemical stability of paclitaxel infusions in different container types. *J Oncol Pharm Pract*. 2006; 12(4):211-22.
7. 0.9% Sodium Chloride Injection, USP [package insert]. Lake Zurich, IL: Fresenius Kabi USA, Inc.; August 2016.
8. *Drug Stability for Easypump® ST/LT*, 2020. Bethlehem, PA: B. Braun USA; Updated June 2020.
9. *SMARTeZ® - Stability Data for Drugs Using Elastomeric Infusion Pumps*, 2020. Fenton, MO: Progressive Medical, Inc.; Updated May 2020.
10. Paclitaxel Injection [package insert]. Lake Forest, IL: Hospira, Inc.; May 2020.
11. Kattige A. Long-term physical and chemical stability of a generic paclitaxel infusion under simulated storage and clinical-use conditions. *Eur J Hosp Pharm*. 2006; 12(6):129-34.

Palonosetron Hydrochloride

Storage Conditions

	Drug Manufacturer	Concentration	Diluents	Osmolality (mOsm/kg)	pH	Temperature		Post-thaw Temp			Body Temp	Refer.
						Room	Refrig	Frozen	Room	Refrig		
CONTAINER												
Bag, Polyvinyl Chloride (PVC)	MGI	5, 30 mcg/mL	D5W, NS, D5LR, D5½NS	n/a	[a]	48 hr	14 d	n/a	n/a	n/a	n/a	(1)
	MGI	5 mcg/mL[b]	D5W, NS	n/a	[a]	48 hr	14 d[d]	n/a	n/a	n/a	n/a	(3)
Syringe, Polypropylene	MGI	25 mcg/mL[c]	D5W, NS	n/a	[a]	48 hr	14 d[d]	n/a	n/a	n/a	n/a	(3)

Flush Compatibility: Sodium chloride 0.9%, heparin.[1]

Special Considerations: Protect from light. Do not freeze.[2]

Notes

[a] pH of undiluted solution is 4.5-5.5.[2]

[b] Solution contained dexAMETHasone sodium phosphate (AMR) 0.2 mg/mL and 0.4 mg/mL.[3]

[c] Solution contained dexAMETHasone sodium phosphate (AMR) 0.33 mg/mL.[3]

[d] Protected from light.[3]

REFERENCES

1. ASHP's Interactive Handbook on Injectable Drugs, 2020. Bethesda, MD: American Society of Health-System Pharmacists; Accessed December 2020.
2. Palonosetron Hydrochloride Injection [package insert]. Lake Forest, IL: Hospira, Inc.; June 2020.
3. Trissel LA, Zhang Y. Compatibility and stability of Aloxi (palonosetron hydrochloride) admixed with dexamethasone sodium phosphate. *Int J Pharm Compd*. 2004; 8(5):398-403.

DOI 10.37573/9781585286720.158

Pantoprazole Sodium

Storage Conditions

						Temperature			Post-thaw Temp			
	Drug Manufacturer	Concentration	Diluents	Osmolality (mOsm/kg)	pH	Room	Refrig	Frozen	Room	Refrig	Body Temp	Refer.
CONTAINER												
Bag, Polyvinyl Chloride (PVC)	ALT[a]	0.16-0.8 mg/mL	NS	n/a	[h]	6 hr[e]	20 d[e]	n/a	n/a	n/a	n/a	(2)
	ALT[a]	0.16 mg/mL	NS	n/a	[h]	48 hr	21 d	n/a	n/a	n/a	n/a	(2)(3)
	ALT[a]	0.16-0.8 mg/mL	D5W	n/a	[h]	8 hr[f]	11 d[f]	n/a	n/a	n/a	n/a	(2)
	ALT[a]	0.16 mg/mL	D5W	n/a	[h]	24 hr	14 d	n/a	n/a	n/a	n/a	(2)(3)
	SZ[b]	0.4 mg/mL	D5W	n/a	[c]	48 hr[d]	14 d[d]	n/a	n/a	n/a	n/a	(4)
	SZ[b]	0.4, 0.8 mg/mL	NS	n/a	[c]	72 hr[d]	28 d[d]	n/a	n/a	n/a	n/a	(4)
	SZ[b]	0.8 mg/mL	D5W	n/a	[c]	72 hr[d]	28 d[d]	n/a	n/a	n/a	n/a	(4)
	ALT[a]	0.8 mg/mL	NS	n/a	[h]	28 hr[g]	10 d[g]	n/a	n/a	n/a	n/a	(2)
	ALT[a]	0.8 mg/mL	NS	n/a	[h]	7 d	21 d	n/a	n/a	n/a	n/a	(2)(3)
	ALT[a]	0.8 mg/mL	D5W	n/a	[h]	24 hr	7 d	n/a	n/a	n/a	n/a	(2)
Syringe, Polypropylene	SZ[b]	4 mg/mL	NS	n/a	[c]	n/a	28 d[d]	n/a	n/a	n/a	n/a	(4)
	WY[a]	4 mg/mL	NS	n/a	[c]	4 d	4 d	n/a	n/a	n/a	n/a	(3)(7)
Unspecified	PH[b]	0.4 mg/mL	NS	n/a	[c]	48 hr	n/a	n/a	n/a	n/a	n/a	(6)
	PH[b]	0.4 mg/mL	D5W	n/a	[c]	48 hr	n/a	n/a	n/a	n/a	n/a	(6)

Flush Compatibility: Sodium chloride 0.9%. [1,3]

Special Considerations: Do not freeze reconstituted product.[1,5] Some formulations of pantoprazole sodium injection contain edetate disodium, the salt form of EDTA. Edetate disodium may chelate metal ions (e.g., zinc), and therefore some formulations of pantoprazole sodium injection may not be compatible with products that contain zinc. Admixtures of pantoprazole sodium may undergo a slight yellow discoloration when stored at room temperature or when exposed to light. This discoloration does not appear to be associated with decomposition of the drug.[3]

Notes

[a] Formulated with EDTA.[3]

[b] Formulated with*out* EDTA.[3]

[c] pH of reconstituted Protonix® I.V.[a] in NS is 9-10.5.[1]

[d] Protected from light.[4]

[e] Stored at 4°C for 20 d, followed by 6 hr at 23°C.[2]

[f] Stored at 4°C for 11 d, followed by 8 hr at 23°C.[2]

[g] Stored at 4°C for 10 d, followed by 28 hr at 23°C.[2]

[h] pH of 1% aqueous Panto® IV[a] Solution is 10.05; pH of 10% aqueous solution is 10.85.[5]

DOI 10.37573/9781585286720.159

REFERENCES

1. Protonix® I.V. (Pantoprazole Sodium) Injection [package insert]. Philadelphia, PA: Wyeth Pharmaceuticals LLC; November 2020.
2. Walker S, Iazzetta J, Law S. Extended stability of pantoprazole for injection in 0.9% sodium chloride or 5% dextrose at 4 degrees c and 23 degrees c. *Can J Hosp Pharm*. 2009; 62(2):135-41.
3. ASHP's Interactive Handbook on Injectable Drugs, 2020. Bethesda, MD: American Society of Health-System Pharmacists; Accessed July 2020.
4. Donnelly RF. Stability of pantoprazole sodium in glass vials, polyvinyl chloride minibags, and polypropylene syringes. *Can J Hosp Pharm*. 2011; 64(3):192-8.
5. Panto® IV (Pantoprazole Sodium) Injection [product monograph]. Oakville, Ontario: Takeda Canada Inc; August 2017.
6. Carpenter JF, McNulty MA, Dusci LJ, et al. Stability of Omeprazole Sodium and Pantoprazole Sodium Diluted for Intravenous Infusion. *J Pharm Technol*. 2006; 22(2):95-98.
7. Johnson CE. Stability of pantoprazole in 0.9% sodium chloride injection in polypropylene syringes. *Am J Health Syst Pharm*. 2005; 62(22):2410-2.

PEMEtrexed Disodium

Storage Conditions

						Temperature			Post-thaw Temp			
	Drug Manufacturer	Concentration	Diluents	Osmolality (mOsm/kg)	pH	Room	Refrig	Frozen	Room	Refrig	Body Temp	Refer.
CONTAINER												
Bag, Polyvinyl Chloride (PVC)	LI	2, 10, 20 mg/mL	NS, D5W[d]	n/a	[b]	48 hr	24 hr[a][c]	[e]	n/a	n/a	n/a	(1)(3)
Syringe, Polypropylene	LI	25 mg/mL	NS	n/a	[b]	48 hr	31 d[c]	n/a	n/a	n/a	n/a	(2)(3)

Flush Compatibility: Sodium chloride 0.9%, heparin.[3]

Special Considerations: Incompatible with calcium-containing solutions (e.g., LR).[3]

Notes

[a] Although no drug loss occurred in 31 d, unidentified microparticulates developed during refrigerated storage exceeding 24 hr in PVC bags.[1]

[b] The pH of reconstituted product is 6.6-7.8.[3]

[c] Protected from light.

[d] Manufacturer recommends reconstitution and dilution only with NS.[3]

[e] Due to development of substantial microparticulates, avoid freezing in PVC bags.[4]

REFERENCES

1. Zhang Y, Trissel LA. Physical and chemical stability of pemetrexed in infusion solutions. *Ann Pharmacother*. 2006; 40(6):1082-5.
2. Zhang Y, Trissel LA. Physical and chemical stability of pemetrexed solutions in plastic syringes. *Ann Pharmacother*. 2005; 39(12):2026-8.
3. ASHP's Interactive Handbook on Injectable Drugs, 2020. Bethesda, MD: American Society of Health-System Pharmacists; Accessed September 2020.
4. Zhang Y, Trissel LA. Physical instability of frozen pemetrexed solutions in PVC bags. *Ann Pharmacother*. 2006; 40(7-8):1289-92.

DOI 10.37573/9781585286720.160

Penicillin G Potassium

Storage Conditions

	Drug Manufacturer	Concentration	Diluents	Osmolality (mOsm/kg)	pH	Temperature: Room	Temperature: Refrig	Temperature: Frozen	Post-thaw Temp: Room	Post-thaw Temp: Refrig	Body Temp	Refer.
CONTAINER												
Bag, Polyvinyl Chloride (PVC)	SQ	10,000 units/mL	NS	n/a	[c]	n/a	24 hr	n/a	n/a	n/a	n/a	(1)
	SQ	10,000 units/mL	D5W	n/a	[c]	24 hr	24 hr	30 d	24 hr	n/a	n/a	(1)
	PD	20,000 units/mL	NS	n/a	[c]	24 hr	4 d[d]	25 d[e]	n/a	n/a	n/a	(1)
	UN	40,000 units/mL	D5W, NS	n/a	[c]	24 hr	24 hr	n/a	n/a	n/a	n/a	(1)
Unspecified	UN	5,000 units/mL	NS, D5NS	n/a	[c]	n/a	48 hr	n/a	n/a	n/a	n/a	(1)
	UN	100,000 units/mL	D5W	501	[c]	48 hr	48 hr	n/a	n/a	n/a	n/a	(1)
	UN	100,000 units/mL	NS	527	[c]	n/a	48 hr	n/a	n/a	n/a	n/a	(1)
OTHER INFUSION CONTAINERS												
CADD® Cassette (Smiths Medical)	MAR	100,000 units/mL	SWFI	n/a	[c]	72 hr	n/a	n/a	n/a	n/a	n/a	(1)(4)
	MAR	200,000 units/mL	SWFI	n/a	[c]	72 hr	14 d	n/a	n/a	n/a	n/a	(1)(4)
Dosi-Fuser® (Leventon)	UN	20,000-100,000 units/mL	NS	n/a	n/a	48 hr	10 d	30 d	24 hr	n/a	n/a	(2)
Easypump® ST/LT (B. Braun)	UN	20,000 units/mL	NS	n/a	[c]	24 hr	4 d	n/a	n/a	n/a	n/a	(6)
Homepump Eclipse® / Homepump® (Halyard)	UN	10,000 units/mL	D5W	n/a	[c]	24 hr[a]	24 hr[a]	30 d[a]	n/a	n/a	n/a	(5)
	UN	20,000 units/mL	NS	n/a	[c]	24 hr[a]	4 d[a]	n/a	n/a	n/a	n/a	(5)
SMARTeZ® (Progressive Medical)	UN	20,000 units/mL	NS	n/a	[c]	24 hr[a]	14 d[a]	n/a	n/a	n/a	n/a	(7)
	UN	100,000 units/mL	NS	n/a	[c]	24 hr	14 d	n/a	n/a	n/a	n/a	(7)
COMMERCIAL PREPARATIONS (RTU)												
GALAXY™ Plastic Container (Baxter)	BA	20,000, 40,000, 60,000 units/mL	D	300	5.5-8	n/a	n/a	[b]	24 hr[b]	14 d[b]	n/a	(1)(3)

Flush Compatibility: Sodium chloride 0.9%, heparin.[1]

Special Considerations: n/a

DOI 10.37573/9781585286720.161

Notes

[a] Manufacturer extrapolated data from other sources.

[b] Frozen expiration date per manufacturer's label. Do not extrapolate commercial premix stability data to extemporaneously compounded solutions.

[c] pH of reconstituted powder for injection is 6-8.5.[1]

[d] Storage temperature: 4°C.[1]

[e] Storage temperature: -7°C.[1]

REFERENCES

1. ASHP's Interactive Handbook on Injectable Drugs, 2020. Bethesda, MD: American Society of Health-System Pharmacists; Accessed August 2020.
2. *Drug Stability Table - Dosi-Fuser® Elastomeric Pump (S-CL-00-001v16)*, 2021. Barcelona, Spain: Leventon SAU; Updated May 2021.
3. Penicillin G Potassium Injection in GALAXY™ Container (PL 2040 Plastic) [package insert]. Deerfield, IL: Baxter Healthcare Corporation; July 2018.
4. Stiles ML, Allen LV, Jr. Stability of nafcillin sodium, oxacillin sodium, penicillin G potassium, penicillin G sodium, and tobramycin sulfate in polyvinyl chloride drug reservoirs. *Am J Health Syst Pharm*. 1997; 54(9):1068-70.
5. *Stability Data for Drugs Using Homepump Disposable Ambulatory Infusion Systems (MK-00314 rev 3)*, 2015. Alpharetta, GA: Halyard Health; Updated June 2015.
6. *Drug Stability for Easypump® ST/LT*, 2020. Bethlehem, PA: B. Braun USA; Updated June 2020.
7. *SMARTeZ® - Stability Data for Drugs Using Elastomeric Infusion Pumps*, 2020. Fenton, MO: Progressive Medical, Inc.; Updated May 2020.

Penicillin G Sodium

Storage Conditions

	Drug Manufacturer	Concentration	Diluents	Osmolality (mOsm/kg)	pH	Temperature: Room	Temperature: Refrig	Frozen	Post-thaw Temp: Room	Post-thaw Temp: Refrig	Body Temp	Refer.
CONTAINER												
Bag, Polyvinyl Chloride (PVC)	GL	20,000 units/mL[a]	NS	n/a	[c]	n/a	8 wk	n/a	n/a	n/a	n/a	(1)
	GL	20,000, 80,000 units/mL	NS	n/a	[c]	n/a	48 hr	n/a	n/a	n/a	n/a	(1)
	AY	50,000 units/mL	D5W	394	[c]	n/a	n/a	39 d	n/a	31 d	n/a	(1)
	UN	180,000 units/mL	SWFI	n/a	[c]	n/a	n/a	30 d[b]	n/a	12 hr[b]	12 hr[b]	(4)
	TE	2,500, 50,000 units/mL	D5W, NS	n/a	[c]	n/a	21 d	n/a	n/a	n/a	n/a	(1)(2)
Vial, Glass	UN	unspec.	unspec.	n/a	[c]	24 hr[d]	3-7 d[e]	n/a	n/a	n/a	n/a	(1)
OTHER INFUSION CONTAINERS												
CADD® Cassette (Smiths Medical)	UN	100,000, 200,000 units/mL	SWFI	n/a	[c]	72 hr	n/a	n/a	n/a	n/a	n/a	(1)
Dosi-Fuser® (Leventon)	UN	10,000 units/mL	D5W	n/a	[c]	24 hr[g]	7 d[g]	4 wk[g]	n/a	n/a	n/a	(3)
Easypump® ST/LT (B. Braun)	UN	2,000 units/mL	NS	n/a	[c]	2 hr	72 hr	n/a	n/a	n/a	n/a	(5)
	UN	100,000 units/mL	NS	n/a	[c]	2 hr[h]	24 hr	n/a	n/a	n/a	n/a	(5)
INTERMATE™ (Baxter)[f]	TE	2,500 units/mL	NS	n/a	[c]	n/a	21 d	n/a	n/a	n/a	n/a	(2)
	TE	2,500 units/mL	D5W	n/a	[c]	n/a	28 d	n/a	n/a	n/a	n/a	(2)
	TE	50,000 units/mL	D5W, NS	n/a	[c]	n/a	28 d	n/a	n/a	n/a	n/a	(2)

Flush Compatibility: Sodium chloride 0.9%, heparin.[1]

Special Considerations: The calculated osmolality of 100,000 units/mL is 502 mOsm/kg in D5W and 529 mOsm/kg in NS. The osmolality of 50,000 units/mL is 394 mOsm/kg in D5W and 421 in NS.[1]

Notes

[a] Reconstituted with citrate buffer (pH 6.5-7.5). Reconstituting with citrate buffers having pH values of 6.5, 7, and 7.5 increases stability.[1]

[b] Little loss after 30 d at -20°C; 12-16% penicillin loss after 30 d frozen when followed by 4 d refrigerated, then 24 hr at 37°C. Penicillin G sodium should not be administered for more than 12 hr after a cycle of freezing and thawing.[4]

[c] pH of solutions range from 5-7.5.[1]

[d] Diluted in infusion solutions.

[e] After reconstitution.

[f] INTERMATE™/INFUSOR™ Portable Elastomeric Infusion System devices are no longer available in the United States.

[g] Manufacturer extrapolated data from other sources.

[h] When combined storage conditions of refrigerated and room temperature, the beyond use date is 2 hours. When stored only at room temperature, the beyond use date is 6 hours.[5]

DOI 10.37573/9781585286720.162

REFERENCES

1. ASHP's Interactive Handbook on Injectable Drugs, 2020. Bethesda, MD: American Society of Health-System Pharmacists; Accessed July 2020.
2. Hossain MA, Friciu M, Aubin S, et al. Stability of penicillin G sodium diluted with 0.9% sodium chloride injection or 5% dextrose injection and stored in polyvinyl chloride bag containers and elastomeric pump containers. *Am J Health Syst Pharm*. 2014; 71(8):669-73.
3. *Drug Stability Table - Dosi-Fuser® Elastomeric Pump (ES.H.00.73-10)*, 2015. Barcelona, Spain: Leventon SAU; Updated October 2015.
4. Stiles ML, Tu YH, Allen LV, Jr. Stability of cefazolin sodium, cefoxitin sodium, ceftazidime, and penicillin G sodium in portable pump reservoirs. *Am J Hosp Pharm*. 1989; 46(7):1408-12.
5. *Drug Stability for Easypump® ST/LT*, 2020. Bethlehem, PA: B. Braun USA; Updated June 2020.

Pentamidine Isethionate

Storage Conditions

						Temperature			Post-thaw Temp			
	Drug Manufacturer	Concentration	Diluents	Osmolality (mOsm/kg)	pH	Room	Refrig	Frozen	Room	Refrig	Body Temp	Refer.
CONTAINER												
Bag, Polyvinyl Chloride (PVC)	APP	0.8-29.54 mg/mL	D5W	n/a	n/a	n/a	30 d	90 d[a]	n/a	n/a	n/a	(3)
	FRK	0.8-98 mg/mL	D5W, SWFI	[c]	[b]	n/a	30 d	n/a	n/a	n/a	n/a	(1)
	FRK	0.8-2.5 mg/mL	D5W	[c]	[b]	n/a	n/a	120 d	n/a	n/a	n/a	(1)
	APP	0.842, 29.74 mg/mL	SWFI	n/a	n/a	n/a	n/a	90 d	n/a	n/a	n/a	(3)
	APP	0.86, 29.14 mg/mL	NS	n/a	n/a	n/a	n/a	90 d	n/a	n/a	n/a	(3)
	LY	1, 2 mg/mL	D5W, NS	n/a	n/a	48 hr	n/a	n/a	n/a	n/a	n/a	(1)
	FRK	1-30 mg/mL	D5W, SWFI	[c]	[b]	n/a	n/a	90 d	n/a	n/a	n/a	(1)
Syringe, Plastic (Unspecified)	APP	0.8-96.65 mg/mL	D5W	[c]	[b]	n/a	30 d	120 d	n/a	n/a	n/a	(3)
	APP	0.933-91 mg/mL	SWFI	[c]	[b]	n/a	30 d	120 d	n/a	n/a	n/a	(3)
Unspecified	APP	60-100 mg/mL	SWFI	[c]	5.4	48 hr[e]	n/a	n/a	n/a	n/a	n/a	(4)
Vial, Glass	APP	0.7-30.7 mg/mL	NS	n/a	n/a	n/a	n/a	90 d	n/a	n/a	n/a	(3)
	FRK	0.8-98 mg/mL	D5W, SWFI	[c]	[b]	n/a	30 d	n/a	n/a	n/a	n/a	(1)
	APP	0.93, 2.9, 93.4 mg/mL	SWFI	[c]	[b]	n/a	30 d	90 d	n/a	n/a	n/a	(3)
	APP	50 mg/mL	SWFI	n/a	n/a	48 hr	90 d	90 d	n/a	n/a	n/a	(3)
	APP	91.9, 97.96 mg/mL	D5W	[c]	[b]	n/a	30 d	90 d	n/a	n/a	n/a	(3)
OTHER INFUSION CONTAINERS												
Dosi-Fuser® (Leventon)	LI	2 mg/mL	NS	[c]	[b]	24 hr[f]	n/a	n/a	n/a	n/a	n/a	(6)
	LI	2-6 mg/mL	D5W	[c]	[b]	24 hr[f]	10 d[f]	30 d[f]	n/a	n/a	n/a	(6)
INTERMATE™ (Baxter)[d]	LY	2 mg/mL	NS	n/a	n/a	24 hr	n/a	n/a	n/a	n/a	n/a	(2)
	LY	2 mg/mL	D5W	n/a	n/a	n/a	n/a	30 d	n/a	n/a	n/a	(2)
	LY	6 mg/mL	D5W	n/a	n/a	24 hr	10 d	n/a	n/a	n/a	n/a	(2)

Flush Compatibility: Sodium chloride 0.9%.[1]

Special Considerations: Do not use sodium chloride 0.9% to reconstitute as precipitation will occur.[1] Reconstituted solution should be protected from light. Keep at room temperature (22°C to 30°C) to avoid crystallization.[4]

DOI 10.37573/9781585286720.163

Notes

[a] Frozen stability was 89.5% of initial concentration after 120 d at 0.8965 mg/mL, 90% or greater of initial concentration at 120 d at 2.444 mg/mL.

[b] pH of reconstituted solutions at 60-100 mg/mL is 5.4 in SWFI.[(5)]

[c] Osmolality of 100 mg/mL is 160 mOsm/kg in SWFI and 455 mOsm/kg in D5W.[(1)]

[d] INTERMATE™/INFUSOR™ Portable Elastomeric Infusion System devices are no longer available in the United States.

[e] Protected from light.

[f] Manufacturer extrapolated data from other sources.

REFERENCES

1. ASHP's Interactive Handbook on Injectable Drugs, 2020. Bethesda, MD: American Society of Health-System Pharmacists; Accessed December 2020.
2. Stabforum - Stability Database: Pentamidine, Ontario, Canada: Baxter Healthcare; Accessed December 2020.
3. Pentam® 300 Stability Medication Information Letter (Ref#: N/A) [personal communication]. Melrose Park, IL: American Pharmaceutical Partners, Inc.; 2002:3.
4. Pentam® 300 (Pentamidine Isethionate) Injection [package insert]. Lake Zurich, IL: Fresenius Kabi USA, LLC; September 2019.
5. Miller RF, Godfrey-Faussett P, Semple SJ. Nebulised pentamidine as treatment for Pneumocystis carinii pneumonia in the acquired immunodeficiency syndrome. *Thorax*. 1989; 44(7):565-9.
6. *Drug Stability Table - Dosi-Fuser® Elastomeric Pump (S-CL-00-001v16)*, 2021. Barcelona, Spain: Leventon SAU; Updated May 2021.

Pertuzumab

Storage Conditions

						Temperature			Post-thaw Temp			
	Drug Manufacturer	Concentration	Diluents	Osmolality (mOsm/kg)	pH	Room	Refrig	Frozen	Room	Refrig	Body Temp	Refer.
CONTAINER												
Bag, Polyolefin	GEN	Various[a]	NS	n/a	[b]	n/a	24 hr	n/a	n/a	n/a	n/a	(1)
	GEN	1.5 mg/mL[h]	NS	n/a	[b]	24 hr[d]	n/a	n/a	n/a	n/a	n/a	(2)
	GEN	1.5 mg/mL[h]	NS[e]	n/a	[b]	24 hr[d]	n/a	n/a	n/a	n/a	n/a	(2)
	GEN	2.7 mg/mL[h]	NS[c]	n/a	[b]	24 hr	24 hr	n/a	n/a	n/a	n/a	(2)
	GEN	3 mg/mL[h]	NS	n/a	[b]	24 hr	24 hr	n/a	n/a	n/a	n/a	(2)
Bag, Polyvinyl Chloride (PVC)	GEN	Various[a]	NS	n/a	[b]	n/a	24 hr	n/a	n/a	n/a	n/a	(1)
	GEN	2.7 mg/mL[h]	NS[c]	n/a	[b]	24 hr	24 hr	n/a	n/a	n/a	n/a	(2)
	GEN	3 mg/mL[h]	NS	n/a	[b]	24 hr	24 hr	n/a	n/a	n/a	n/a	(2)
OTHER INFUSION CONTAINERS												
INFUSOR™ (Baxter)[f]	GEN	1.5, 3.5 mg/mL	NS	n/a	n/a	48 hr[g]	60 d[g]	n/a	n/a	n/a	n/a	(3)

Flush Compatibility: Sodium chloride 0.9%.[1]

Special Considerations: Do not mix with dextrose 5% solution. Do not freeze or shake.[1]

Notes

[a] Dose diluted in 250 mL sodium chloride 0.9%.[1]

[b] pH of product at 30 mg/mL is 6.0.[2]

[c] Solution contained: trastuzumab 2.3 mg/mL (approx.).[2]

[d] Storage temperature: 30°C, protected from light.[2]

[e] Solution contained: trastuzumab 1.5 mg/mL (approx.).[2]

[f] INTERMATE™/INFUSOR™ Portable Elastomeric Infusion System devices are no longer available in the United States.

[g] 60 days at refrigerated temperature, followed by 48 hours at room temperature.[3]

[h] Approximate concentration based on diluent volume and volume of admixed medication(s).

DOI 10.37573/9781585286720.164

REFERENCES

1. Perjeta® (Pertuzumab) Injection [package insert]. South San Francisco, CA: Genentech, Inc.; October 2020.
2. Glover ZW, Gennaro L, Yadav S, et al. Compatibility and stability of pertuzumab and trastuzumab admixtures in i.v. infusion bags for coadministration. *J Pharm Sci*. 2013; 102(3):794-812.
3. Stabforum - Stability Database: Pertuzumab, Ontario, Canada: Baxter Healthcare; Accessed February 2021.

Phenylephrine Hydrochloride

Storage Conditions

						Temperature			Post-thaw Temp			
CONTAINER	Drug Manufacturer	Concentration	Diluents	Osmolality (mOsm/kg)	pH	Room	Refrig	Frozen	Room	Refrig	Body Temp	Refer.
Bag, Plastic (Unspecified)	HIK, AVD	20, 100 mcg/mL	D5W, NS	n/a	[a]	4 hr	24 hr	n/a	n/a	n/a	n/a	(2)(3)
	WI	2,500 mcg/mL	NS	n/a	[a]	24 hr	n/a	n/a	n/a	n/a	n/a	(1)
	UN	2,500 mcg/mL	SWFI	n/a	[a]	n/a	n/a	n/a	n/a	n/a	12 wk[f]	(1)
Bag, Polyvinyl Chloride (PVC)	BA	100, 200 mcg/mL	NS	n/a	[a]	14 d	n/a	n/a	n/a	n/a	n/a	(7)
	SZ	200, 400 mcg/mL	NS	n/a	[a]	60 d[c]	n/a	n/a	n/a	n/a	n/a	(6)
Syringe, Polypropylene	GNS	100 mcg/mL	NS	n/a	[a]	30 d[c]	30 d[d]	30 d[b][d]	n/a	n/a	n/a	(4)
Syringe, Plastic (Unspecified)	UN	2,500 mcg/mL	unspec.[i]	n/a	5.8-6.0	66 d	n/a	n/a	n/a	n/a	n/a	(5)
Unspecified	WI	2,500 mcg/mL	D5W, NS[e]	n/a	[a]	24 hr	n/a	n/a	n/a	n/a	n/a	(1)
	WI	2,500 mcg/mL	D5W[g]	n/a	[a]	24 hr	n/a	n/a	n/a	n/a	n/a	(1)
	WI	20 mcg/mL	unspec.[h]	n/a	n/a	24 hr	n/a	n/a	n/a	n/a	n/a	(1)

Flush Compatibility: Sodium chloride 0.9%, D5W.[2,3]

Special Considerations: Phenylephrine hydrochloride is available as a 1% solution. Each mL of solution contains phenylephrine hydrochloride 10 mg with sodium citrate dihydrate 4 mg, citric acid monohydrate 1 mg, sodium chloride 3.5 mg, and sodium metabisulfite 2 mg in water for injection.[2,3]

Notes

[a] The 10% solution of phenylephrine (HIK) has a pH ranging from 3.0-6.5.[2] The 10% solution of phenylephrine (AVD) has a pH ranging from 3.5-5.5.[3]

[b] Storage temperature: -20° C.[4]

[c] Exposed to fluorescent light.[4]

[d] Protected from light.

[e] Solution contained: chloramphenicol sodium succinate (PD) 0.5 mg/mL with and without sodium bicarbonate 7.5 gm/L.[1]

[f] Storage temperature: 60° C.[1]

[g] Solution contained: potassium chloride (AB) 0.04 mEq/mL.[1]

[h] Solution contained: sodium bicarbonate 5%.[1]

[i] Solution contained: lidocaine hydrochloride 2%.[1]

DOI 10.37573/9781585286720.165

REFERENCES

1. ASHP's Interactive Handbook on Injectable Drugs, 2020. Bethesda, MD: American Society of Health-System Pharmacists; Accessed August 2020.
2. Phenylephrine Hydrochloride Injection [package insert]. Eatontown, NJ: Hikma Pharmaceuticals USA Inc.; March 2020.
3. Vazculep® (Phenylephrine Hydrochloride) Injection [package insert]. Chesterfield, MO: Avadel Legacy Pharmaceuticals, LLC; April 2020.
4. Kiser TH, Oldland AR, Fish DN. Stability of phenylephrine hydrochloride injection in polypropylene syringes. *Am J Health Syst Pharm*. 2007; 64(10):1092-5.
5. Das Gupta V, Stewart KR. Chemical stabilities of lignocaine hydrochloride and phenylephrine hydrochloride in aqueous solution. *J Clin Hosp Pharm*. 1986; 11(6):449-52.
6. Jansen JJ, Oldland AR, Kiser TH. Evaluation of phenylephrine stability in polyvinyl chloride bags. *Hosp Pharm*. 2014; 49(5):455-7.
7. Gupta VD. Chemical stability of phenylephrine hydrochloride after reconstitution in 0.9% sodium chloride injection for infusion. *Int J Pharm Compd*. 2004; 8(2):153-5.

Piperacillin Sodium – Tazobactam Sodium

Storage Conditions

	Drug Manufacturer	Concentration[c]	Diluents	Osmolality (mOsm/kg)	pH	Temperature Room	Temperature Refrig	Temperature Frozen	Post-thaw Temp Room	Post-thaw Temp Refrig	Body Temp	Refer.
CONTAINER												
Bag, Plastic (Unspecified)	HOS[f], WY[d]	unspec.[g]	D5W, NS, SWFI	n/a	[e]	24 hr[b]	7 d[b]	n/a	n/a	n/a	n/a	(3)(8)
Bag, Polyolefin	WY[f]	40 mg/mL	NS	n/a	4.5-5.3	67 hr[a]	17 d	n/a	n/a	n/a	n/a	(10)
	WY[f]	40 mg/mL	[j]	n/a	5.2-6.6	7 d[a] 10 d	58 d	n/a	n/a	n/a	n/a	(10)
Bag, Polyvinyl Chloride (PVC)	UN[f]	10 mg/mL	D5W, NS	n/a	n/a	48 hr	28 d	71 d	n/a	n/a	n/a	(10)
	WY[d]	20, 80 mg/mL	D5W, NS	n/a	[e]	72 hr[a]	28 d	n/a	n/a	n/a	n/a	(1)
	WY[f]	40 mg/mL	NS	n/a	4.5-5.3	72 hr[a] 4 d	5 d	n/a	n/a	n/a	n/a	(10)
	UN[f]	60 mg/mL	D5W, NS	n/a	n/a	48 hr	28 d	n/a	n/a	n/a	n/a	(10)
	UN[f]	80 mg/mL	D5W, NS	n/a	n/a	n/a	n/a	30 d	n/a	n/a	n/a	(1)
Syringe, Polypropylene	UN[f]	150, 200 mg/mL	D5W, NS	n/a	n/a	24 hr	7 d	30 d	n/a	7 d	n/a	(1)
Vial, Glass	WY[d]	unspec.[g]	D5W, NS, SWFI	n/a	[e]	24 hr	48 hr	n/a	n/a	n/a	n/a	(3)
OTHER INFUSION CONTAINERS												
ADD-Vantage® Flexible Container System (Pfizer)	HOS	unspec.	D5W, NS	n/a	n/a	24 hr	n/a	n/a	n/a	n/a	n/a	(1)
Dosi-Fuser® (Leventon)	LE	10-80 mg/mL	D5W, NS	n/a	n/a	24 hr[h]	7 d[h]	5 wk[h]	24 hr[h]	n/a	n/a	(6)
	UN	40 mg/mL	NS	n/a	n/a	n/a	22 d	n/a	n/a	n/a	n/a	(6)
Easypump® ST/LT (B. Braun)	UN	10, 80 mg/mL	NS	n/a	n/a	48 hr	28 d	n/a	n/a	n/a	n/a	(9)
Homepump Eclipse® / Homepump® (Halyard)	UN	10-80 mg/mL	NS	n/a	n/a	24 hr	28 d	n/a	n/a	n/a	n/a	(4)
	UN	18 mg/mL	D5W	n/a	n/a	7 d	n/a	n/a	n/a	n/a	n/a	(4)
INTERMATE™ (Baxter)[i]	LE	10-80 mg/mL	D5W, NS	n/a	n/a	24 hr	7 d	5 wk	24 hr	n/a	n/a	(2)
SMARTeZ® (Progressive Medical)	UN	10-80 mg/mL	NS	n/a	n/a	24 hr[h]	28 d[h]	n/a	n/a	n/a	n/a	(5)

DOI 10.37573/9781585286720.166

Storage Conditions

						Temperature			Post-thaw Temp			
	Drug Manufacturer	Concentration[c]	Diluents	Osmolality (mOsm/kg)	pH	Room	Refrig	Frozen	Room	Refrig	Body Temp	Refer.
COMMERCIAL PREPARATIONS (RTU)												
GALAXY™ Plastic Container (Baxter)	WY[d]	40, 60 mg/mL	D	iso	[e]	n/a	n/a	[k]	24 hr[k]	14 d[k]	n/a	(3)

Flush Compatibility: Sodium chloride 0.9%, heparin.[1]

Special Considerations: Zosyn® (WY) brand was formulated to include EDTA (a metal-chelating agent) and sodium citrate (a buffer) to provide for consistent potency and minimal particulate development in commercially available diluents; this also improved the EDTA-containing formulation compatibility with calcium-containing diluents and certain aminoglycosides.[7] The compatibility profile of generic formulations is not equivalent to Zosyn® (WY) brand. Generic formulations do not contain EDTA. Compatibility tests conducted prior to 2007 evaluated the non-EDTA formulation.[1] Non-EDTA formulations are incompatible with Lactated Ringer's Solutions.[8]

Notes

[a] Exposed to light.[1,10]

[b] Chemically stable for up to 24 hr at room temperature and 7 d refrigerated in IV bags (unspecified).[3,8]

[c] Stated concentrations expressed as piperacillin sodium content. Concentration, as displayed on manufacturer packaging, is a ratio of 8 parts piperacillin sodium and 1 part tazobactam sodium (e.g., 4.5 gm is 4 gm piperacillin sodium and 0.5 gm tazobactam sodium). Stability data applies to both components.[1,3,8]

[d] EDTA formulation.

[e] pH of WY products is 5.5-6.8.[1]

[f] Non-EDTA formulation.

[g] Reconstituted per manufacturer labeling; dose diluted in 50-150 mL NS, D5W, or up to 50 mL SWFI.[3,8]

[h] Manufacturer extrapolated data from other sources.

[i] INTERMATE™/INFUSOR™ Portable Elastomeric Infusion System devices are no longer available in the United States.

[j] Buffered sodium chloride solution was an isotonic mixture of a citrate buffer and 0.72% sodium chloride with a nominal pH of 7.0.[10]

[k] Frozen expiration date per manufacturer's label. Do not extrapolate commercial premix stability data to extemporaneously compounded solutions. Thawed solutions should not be refrozen.[1]

REFERENCES

1. ASHP's Interactive Handbook on Injectable Drugs, 2020. Bethesda, MD: American Society of Health-System Pharmacists; Accessed August 2020.
2. Stabforum - Stability Database: Piperacillin + Tazobactam, Ontario, Canada: Baxter Healthcare; Accessed January 2021.
3. Zosyn® (Piperacillin and Tazobactam) Injection in GALAXY™ Containers [package insert]. Philadelphia, PA: Wyeth Pharmaceuticals LLC; August 2020.
4. *Stability Data for Drugs Using Homepump Disposable Ambulatory Infusion Systems (MK-00314 rev 3)*, 2015. Alpharetta, GA: Halyard Health; Updated June 2015.

5. *SMARTeZ® - Stability Data for Drugs Using Elastomeric Infusion Pumps*, 2020. Fenton, MO: Progressive Medical, Inc.; Updated May 2020.
6. *Drug Stability Table - Dosi-Fuser® Elastomeric Pump (S-CL-00-001v16)*, 2021. Barcelona, Spain: Leventon SAU; Updated May 2021.
7. Desai NR, Shah SM, Cohen J, et al. Zosyn (piperacillin/tazobactam) reformulation: Expanded compatibility and coadministration with lactated Ringer's solutions and selected aminoglycosides. *Ther Clin Risk Manag*. 2008; 4(2):303-14.
8. Piperacillin and Tazobactam Injection, lyophilized [package insert]. Lake Forest, IL: Hospira, Inc.; June 2020.
9. *Drug Stability for Easypump® ST/LT*, 2020. Bethlehem, PA: B. Braun USA; Updated June 2020.
10. Rigge DC, Jones MF. Shelf lives of aseptically prepared medicines: stability of piperacillin/tazobactam in PVC and non-PVC bags. *J Pharm Biomed Anal*. 2005; 39(1-2):339-43.

Plazomicin

Storage Conditions

						Temperature			Post-thaw Temp			
	Drug Manufacturer	Concentration	Diluents	Osmolality (mOsm/kg)	pH	Room	Refrig	Frozen	Room	Refrig	Body Temp	Refer.
CONTAINER												
Bag, Polyvinyl Chloride (PVC)	CIP	2.5, 45 mg/mL	NS, LR	n/a	[a]	24 hr	7 d	n/a	n/a	n/a	n/a	(1)(3)
Bag, Polyolefin	ACH	2.5, 40 mg/mL	NS	n/a	[a]	24 hr	n/a	n/a	n/a	n/a	n/a	(3)
Syringe, Polypropylene	ACH	2.5, 40 mg/mL	NS	n/a	[a]	24 hr	n/a	n/a	n/a	n/a	n/a	(3)
Vial, Glass	ACH	2.5, 40 mg/mL	NS	n/a	[a]	24 hr	n/a	n/a	n/a	n/a	n/a	(3)
OTHER INFUSION CONTAINERS												
Homepump Eclipse® / Homepump® (Halyard)	ACH	2.5, 40 mg/mL	NS, LR	n/a	[a]	n/a	7 d	n/a	n/a	n/a	n/a	(3)

Flush Compatibility: Sodium chloride 0.9%. Incompatible with heparin.[2]

Special Considerations: n/a

Notes

[a] Undiluted solution (50 mg/mL) is adjusted to pH of 6.5 with sodium hydroxide.[1,2]

REFERENCES

1. Zemdri® (Plazomicin) Injection [package insert]. Warren, NJ: Cipla USA, Inc.; July 2020.
2. ASHP's Interactive Handbook on Injectable Drugs, 2020. Bethesda, MD: American Society of Health-System Pharmacists; Accessed August 2020.
3. Zemdri® Stability Medication Information Letter (Ref#: MRC_0090_R_1018) [personal communication]. San Francisco, CA: Achaogen, Inc.; 2018:4.

DOI 10.37573/9781585286720.167

Quinupristin – Dalfopristin

Storage Conditions

						Temperature			Post-thaw Temp			
	Drug Manufacturer	Concentration	Diluents	Osmolality (mOsm/kg)	pH	Room	Refrig	Frozen	Room	Refrig	Body Temp	Refer.
CONTAINER												
Unspecified	PF	Various[a]	D5W	n/a	n/a	5 hr	54 hr	n/a	n/a	n/a	n/a	(1)(2)
OTHER INFUSION CONTAINERS												
Homepump Eclipse® / Homepump® (Haylard)	UN	2 mg/mL	D5W	n/a	n/a	5 hr[b]	54 hr[b]	n/a	n/a	n/a	n/a	(3)

Flush Compatibility: Flush with D5W before and after administration. Not compatible with sodium chloride 0.9% or heparin.[1]

Special Considerations: Incompatible with sodium chloride-containing solutions. Reconstituted solution may foam; allow foam to dissipate to a clear solution prior to further dilution. Do not freeze. Dilute in 250 mL D5W; 100 mL may be used for central line infusions. If moderate to severe venous irritation occurs following peripheral administration, consider increasing infusion volume to 500-750 mL, changing the infusion site, or infusion by a central line.[1]

Notes

[a] Concentration of combined agents in 100 mL to 750 mL of diluent.[1]

[b] Manufacturer extrapolated data from other sources.

REFERENCES

1. Synercid® IV (Quinupristin and Dalfopristin) Injection [package insert]. New York, NY: Pfizer Inc; August 2019.
2. ASHP's Interactive Handbook on Injectable Drugs, 2020. Bethesda, MD: American Society of Health-System Pharmacists; Accessed December 2020.
3. *Stability Data for Drugs Using Homepump Disposable Ambulatory Infusion Systems (MK-00314 rev 3)*, 2015. Alpharetta, GA: Halyard Health; Updated June 2015.

DOI 10.37573/9781585286720.168

RifAMPin

Storage Conditions

						Temperature			Post-thaw Temp			
	Drug Manufacturer	Concentration	Diluents	Osmolality (mOsm/kg)	pH	Room	Refrig	Frozen	Room	Refrig	Body Temp	Refer.
CONTAINER												
Bag, Polypropylene	MMD	2.4 mg/mL	NS[b]	n/a	n/a	7 hr[a]	6 d[a]	28 d[a]	n/a	n/a	n/a	(1)
OTHER INFUSION CONTAINERS												
Easypump® ST/LT (B. Braun)	UN	0.5, 3 mg/mL	NS	n/a	n/a	24 hr	6 d	n/a	n/a	n/a	n/a	(2)
Homepump Eclipse® / Homepump® (Halyard)	UN	0.75 mg/mL	D5W	n/a	n/a	7 d	n/a	n/a	n/a	n/a	n/a	(3)
SMARTeZ® (Progressive Medical)	UN	0.5, 3 mg/mL	NS	n/a	n/a	24 hr	6 d	n/a	n/a	n/a	n/a	(4)

Flush Compatibility: Sodium chloride 0.9%.

Special Considerations: n/a

Notes

[a] Protected from light.[1]

[b] Solution contained tedizolid phosphate 0.8 mg/mL.[1]

REFERENCES

1. Ezquer-Garin C, Ferriols-Lisart R, Martinez-Lopez LM, et al. Stability of tedizolid phosphate-sodium rifampicin and tedizolid phosphate-meropenem admixtures in intravenous infusion bags stored at different temperatures. *Pharmazie*. 2020; 75(5):172-76.
2. *Drug Stability for Easypump® ST/LT*, 2020. Bethlehem, PA: B. Braun USA; Updated June 2020.
3. *Stability Data for Drugs Using Homepump Disposable Ambulatory Infusion Systems (MK-00314 rev 3)*, 2015. Alpharetta, GA: Halyard Health; Updated June 2015.
4. *SMARTeZ® - Stability Data for Drugs Using Elastomeric Infusion Pumps*, 2020. Fenton, MO: Progressive Medical, Inc.; Updated May 2020.

DOI 10.37573/9781585286720.169

RiTUXimab

Storage Conditions

						Temperature			Post-thaw Temp			
	Drug Manufacturer	Concentration	Diluents	Osmolality (mOsm/kg)	pH	Room	Refrig	Frozen	Room	Refrig	Body Temp	Refer.
CONTAINER												
Bag, Polyethylene	BGD, GEN	1-4 mg/mL	NS, D5W	n/a	[b]	24 hr	24 hr	n/a	n/a	n/a	n/a	(1)
	SZ	1 mg/mL	NS	n/a	[b]	24 hr[a]	30 d[a]	n/a	n/a	n/a	n/a	(4)
Bag, Polyolefin	RC	1 mg/mL	NS	n/a	[b]	n/a	180 d[d]	n/a	n/a	n/a	n/a	(3)
	TE	1, 4 mg/mL	NS	300-321	6.4-6.6	24 hr[d][e]	6 wk[d]	n/a	n/a	n/a	n/a	(5)
Bag, Polypropylene	SZ	1 mg/mL	NS	n/a	[b]	24 hr[a]	30 d[a]	n/a	n/a	n/a	n/a	(4)
Bag, Polyvinyl Chloride (PVC)	BGD, GEN	1-4 mg/mL	NS, D5W	n/a	[b]	24 hr	24 hr	n/a	n/a	n/a	n/a	(1)
	TE	1, 4 mg/mL	NS	289-313	6.4-6.6	24 hr[d][e]	6 wk[d]	n/a	n/a	n/a	n/a	(5)
	GEN	1.5 mg/mL	NS	n/a	[b]	n/a	14 d[c]	n/a	n/a	n/a	n/a	(2)
Vial, Glass	GEN	10 mg/mL	Undiluted	n/a	[b]	n/a	14 d[c]	n/a	n/a	n/a	n/a	(2)

Flush Compatibility: Sodium chloride 0.9%, heparin.[1]

Special Considerations: Do not freeze or shake. Protect vials from direct sunlight. Keep vials refrigerated.[1]

Notes

[a] Storage temperature: 2-8°C for 30 days, followed by 24 hours at room temperature.[4]

[b] The pH of undiluted product is 6.5.[1]

[c] Stability was defined as average retention of at least 85% of initial activity.[2]

[d] Protected from light.[3,5]

[e] Storage temperature: 2-8°C for 6 weeks, followed by 24 hours at room temperature.[5]

REFERENCES

1. Rituxan® (Rituximab) Injection [package insert]. South San Francisco, CA: Genentech, Inc.; August 2020.
2. Zhang Y, Vermeulen LC, Kolesar JM. Stability of stock and diluted rituximab. *Am J Health Syst Pharm*. 2013; 70(5):436-8.
3. ASHP's Interactive Handbook on Injectable Drugs, 2020. Bethesda, MD: American Society of Health-System Pharmacists; Accessed May 2020.
4. Lamanna WC, Heller K, Schneider D, et al. The in-use stability of the rituximab biosimilar Rixathon®/Riximyo® upon preparation for intravenous infusion. *J Oncol Pharm Pract*. 2019; 25(2):269-78.
5. Kim SJ, Kim KW, Shin YK, et al. In-Use Stability of the Rituximab Biosimilar CT-P10 (Truxima®) Following Preparation for Intravenous Infusion and Storage. *BioDrugs*. 2019; 33(2):221-28.

DOI 10.37573/9781585286720.170

Ropivacaine Hydrochloride

Storage Conditions

	Drug Manufacturer	Concentration	Diluents	Osmolality (mOsm/kg)	pH	Temperature: Room	Temperature: Refrig	Temperature: Frozen	Post-thaw Temp: Room	Post-thaw Temp: Refrig	Body Temp	Refer.
CONTAINER												
Bag, Ethylene Vinyl Acetate (EVA)	ASZ	1.5 mg/mL	NS[e]	[f]	[d]	51 d	51 d	n/a	n/a	n/a	n/a	(1)
Bag, Polyolefin	QI	1-2 mg/mL	NS[h]	[f]	4.9-5.1	15 d	15 d	n/a	n/a	n/a	n/a	(6)
Bag, Polypropylene	ASZ	1, 2 mg/mL	NS[b]	[f]	[d]	n/a	n/a	n/a	n/a	n/a	30 d[c]	(1)
Bag, Polyvinyl Chloride (PVC)	ASZ	1.5 mg/mL	NS[e]	[f]	[d]	7 d	7 d	n/a	n/a	n/a	n/a	(1)
Syringe, Polypropylene	AST	1.2 mg/mL	[a]	[f]	[d]	30 d	30 d	n/a	n/a	n/a	n/a	(1)
Vial, Glass	ASZ	1.5 mg/mL	NS[e]	[f]	[d]	51 d	51 d	n/a	n/a	n/a	n/a	(1)
OTHER INFUSION CONTAINERS												
Dosi-Fuser® (Leventon)	ASZ	1-10 mg/mL	NS	n/a	n/a	7 d	120 d	n/a	n/a	n/a	n/a	(3)
Easypump® ST/LT (B. Braun)	UN	0.2, 5 mg/mL	NS	n/a	n/a	24 hr	14 d	n/a	n/a	n/a	n/a	(7)
	UN	1, 7.5 mg/mL	NS	n/a	n/a	30 d	n/a	n/a	n/a	n/a	n/a	(7)
INFUSOR™ (Baxter)[i]	AST	1-10 mg/mL	NS	n/a	n/a	7 d	120 d[g]	n/a	n/a	n/a	n/a	(2)
SynchroMed™ II Implantable Pump (Medtronic)	ASZ	7.5 mg/mL	NS[j]	1030	3.46	n/a	n/a	n/a	n/a	n/a	5 wk	(4)

Flush Compatibility: Sodium chloride 0.9%.[5]

Special Considerations: Ropivacaine hydrochloride solubility is reduced above pH of 6.[1]

Ropivacaine vials, ampules, bottles, and bags are preservative free and are intended for single use only. Commercially available continuous (epidural) infusion preparations should not be left in place for more than 24 hours. Ropivacaine is indicated for epidural injection or infusion, for local infiltration, and major nerve block. Unintended intravenous injection or infusion may result in cardiac arrhythmia or arrest.[5]

DOI 10.37573/9781585286720.171

Notes

[a] Solution prepared with 3 mL ropivacaine hydrochloride 2 mg/mL and 2 mL methylPREDNISolone acetate (PHU) 40 mg/mL, for a final concentration of 1.2 mg/mL ropivacaine hydrochloride and 16 mg/mL methylPREDNISolone acetate.

[b] Solutions of ropivacaine hydrochloride 1 mg/mL tested with: morphine sulfate (AST) 20 mcg/mL; SUFentanil citrate (JN) 0.4 mcg/mL; fentaNYL citrate (JN) 1 mcg/mL; and cloNIDine hydrochloride (BI) 5 and 50 mcg/mL in Mark II Polybags. Solutions of ropivacaine hydrochloride 2 mg/mL tested with: morphine sulfate (AST) 20 and 100 mcg/mL; SUFentanil citrate (JN) 0.4 and 4 mcg/mL; fentaNYL citrate (JN) 1 and 10 mcg/mL; and cloNIDine hydrochloride (BI) 5 mcg/mL in Mark II Polybags.

[c] Storage temperature: 30°C, Protected from light.

[d] pH of the undiluted solution is 4-6.5.[1]

[e] Solution contained: fentaNYL citrate (CUR) 3 mcg/mL, tested at 20°C and 4°C.

[f] Commercially available solutions of ropivacaine hydrochloride are isotonic.[1,5]

[g] Storage temperature: 120 days refrigerated, followed by 7 d at 33°C.

[h] Solution contained: butorphanol 50 mcg/mL (HE).

[i] INTERMATE™/INFUSOR™ Portable Elastomeric Infusion System devices are no longer available in the United States.

[j] Tested in vitro combined with morphine sulfate (LAV) 7.5 mg/mL, cloNIDine hydrochloride (BI) 15 mcg/mL, and ziconotide (EI) 0.1, 0.25, 0.5, and 0.75 mcg/mL. While ziconotide concentration decreased to 53.4% after 5 weeks, ropivacaine, morphine, and cloNIDine remained stable.

REFERENCES

1. ASHP's Interactive Handbook on Injectable Drugs, 2020. Bethesda, MD: American Society of Health-System Pharmacists; Accessed August 2020.
2. Stabforum - Stability Database: Ropivacaine, Ontario, Canada: Baxter Healthcare; Accessed December 2020.
3. *Drug Stability Table - Dosi-Fuser® Elastomeric Pump (S-CL-00-001v16)*, 2021. Barcelona, Spain: Leventon SAU; Updated May 2021.
4. Dupoiron D, Richard H, Chabert-Desnot V, et al. In vitro stability of low-concentration ziconotide alone or in admixtures in intrathecal pumps. *Neuromodulation*. 2014; 17(5):472-82; discussion 82.
5. Naropin® (Ropivacaine Hydrochloride) Injection [package insert]. Lake Zurich, IL: Fresenius Kabi; February 2020.
6. Chen F, Li P, Zhou B, et al. Stability of an epidural analgesic admixture containing butorphanol tartrate and ropivacaine hydrochloride. *Eur J of Hosp Pharm*. 2015; 22(1):7-11.
7. *Drug Stability for Easypump® ST/LT*, 2020. Bethlehem, PA: B. Braun USA; Updated June 2020.

Sargramostim

Storage Conditions

	Drug Manufacturer	Concentration	Diluents	Osmolality (mOsm/kg)	pH	Temperature Room	Temperature Refrig	Temperature Frozen	Post-thaw Temp Room	Post-thaw Temp Refrig	Body Temp	Refer.
CONTAINER												
Syringe, Plastic (Unspecified)	SAA	250, 500 mcg/mL[(a)(c)]	BWFI	n/a	[(b)]	n/a	21 d	n/a	n/a	n/a	n/a	(1)
Vial, Glass	SAA	250 mcg/mL[(c)]	SWFI	n/a	[(b)]	n/a	14 d	n/a	n/a	n/a	n/a	(1)
	SAA	250 mcg/mL[(c)]	BWFI	n/a	[(b)]	n/a	30 d	n/a	n/a	n/a	n/a	(1)
	SAA	500 mcg/mL[(a)]	Undiluted	n/a	[(b)]	n/a	20 d	n/a	n/a	n/a	n/a	(1)(3)

Flush Compatibility: Sodium chloride 0.9%, heparin.[(2)]

Special Considerations: Store liquid, reconstituted, and lyophilized product at 2°C to 8°C. Do not freeze. Dilute for intravenous infusions only with NS. Concentrations below 10 mcg/mL require the addition of albumin 1 mg per 1 mL of solution prior to the addition of sargramostim to prevent adsorption. Do not infuse through an inline membrane filter because of possible absorption.[(3)]

Notes

[a] Liquid formulation (500 mcg/mL), preserved with 1.1% benzyl alcohol.[(3)]

[b] pH of liquid product is 6.7-7.7. pH of reconstituted lyophilized product is 7.1-7.7.[(3)]

[c] Lyophilized formulation (250 mcg), contains no preservatives.[(3)]

REFERENCES

1. Leukine® Medication Information Letter (Ref#: 1-818723726) [personal communication]. Bridgewater, NJ: Sanofi-Aventis U.S., LLC; 2016:7.
2. ASHP's Interactive Handbook on Injectable Drugs, 2020. Bethesda, MD: American Society of Health-System Pharmacists; Accessed December 2020.
3. Leukine® (Sargramostim) Injection [package insert]. Bridgewater, NJ: Sanofi-Aventis U.S., LLC; June 2018.

DOI 10.37573/9781585286720.172

Sodium Bicarbonate

Storage Conditions

CONTAINER	Drug Manufacturer	Concentration	Diluents	Osmolality (mOsm/kg)	pH	Temperature: Room	Temperature: Refrig	Temperature: Frozen	Post-thaw Temp: Room	Post-thaw Temp: Refrig	Body Temp	Refer.
Bag, Ethylene Vinyl Acetate (EVA)	POL	0.2 mEq/mL	D5W	[a]	[b]	n/a	7 d	n/a	n/a	n/a	n/a	(2)
Bag, Polyolefin	HOS	0.05 mEq/mL	D5W, SWFI	[a]	8.2-8.5	5 d	7 d	n/a	n/a	n/a	n/a	(4)
	HOS	0.1, 0.15 mEq/mL	D5W, SWFI	[a]	8.0-8.5	7 d	7 d	n/a	n/a	n/a	n/a	(4)
	HOS	0.1 mEq/mL	D5W	[a]	8.1-8.5	7 d	21 d	21 d	n/a	n/a	n/a	(5)
	HOS	0.15 mEq/mL	D5W	[a]	8.2-8.5	15 d	21 d	30 d	n/a	n/a	n/a	(5)
	PHE	0.4 mEq/mL	NS	[a]	8.1-8.3	48 hr	n/a	n/a	n/a	n/a	n/a	(6)
Bag, Polyvinyl Chloride (PVC)	AB	0.048 mEq/mL	NS, D5W, D5NS	[a]	[b]	n/a	24 hr	n/a	n/a	n/a	n/a	(3)
Syringe, Glass[h]	HOS	1 mEq/mL	Undiluted	[a]	7.9-8.1	n/a	5 wk	n/a	n/a	n/a	n/a	(8)
Syringe, Polypropylene	AB	0.89 mEq/mL	Undiluted	[a]	7.8-8.0	7 d	60 d[c]	n/a	n/a	n/a	n/a	(3)(7)
	UN	0.89 mEq/mL	[g]	[a]	7.49-8.12	45 d[e][f]	90 d[d][f]	n/a	n/a	n/a	n/a	(3)(9)
Vial, Glass	AB	0.048 mEq/mL	NS, D5W, D5NS	[a]	[b]	n/a	24 hr	n/a	n/a	n/a	n/a	(3)

Flush Compatibility: Sodium chloride 0.9%, heparin.[3]

Special Considerations: Sodium Bicarbonate 7.5% (75 mg/mL) equates to 0.89 mEq/mL bicarbonate and sodium concentrations. Sodium Bicarbonate 8.4% (84 mg/mL) equates to 1 mEq/mL bicarbonate and sodium concentrations. pH is used to determine stability of the drug, using the range 7.0-8.5 defined by USP.[4,5] Sodium bicarbonate may raise the pH of an admixture above 6 and cause significant decomposition of alkali-labile drugs.[3]

Notes

[a] Osmolality of sodium bicarbonate 7.5% solution is 1467.3 mOsm/kg.[1]

[b] pH of undiluted solution is 7-8.5.[3]

[c] Storage temperature: 5-10°C.

[d] Storage temperature: 12-14°C.[9]

[e] Storage temperature: 23°C.[9]

[f] Terminal expiration of 90 days after packaging in syringes stored at 12-14°C or 30 days after syringes are removed from refrigeration.[9]

[g] Sodium bicarbonate 7.5% (0.89 mEq/mL) solution prepared with 750 gm of analytical reagent grade sodium bicarbonate diluted in 10 L of cooled water.[9]

[h] Hospira Glass LifeShield™ syringe; 50 mL pre-filled syringe.[8]

DOI 10.37573/9781585286720.173

REFERENCES

1. Mostert JW. The pH and osmolality of intravenously used drugs. *JAMA*. 1971; 216(9):1483.
2. Stawny M, Gostynska A, Gorecka A, et al. Stability studies of two compounded solutions potentially used in tumor lysis syndrome. *J Oncol Pharm Pract*. 2019; 25(6):1434-38.
3. ASHP's Interactive Handbook on Injectable Drugs, 2020. Bethesda, MD: American Society of Health-System Pharmacists; Accessed August 2020.
4. Wear J, McPherson TB, Kolling WM. Stability of sodium bicarbonate solutions in polyolefin bags. *Am J Health Syst Pharm*. 2010; 67(12):1026-9. Erratum in: *Am J Health Syst Pharm*. 2010; 67(19):1586.
5. Sayre BE, Prettyman T, Kaushal G. Extended Stability of Sodium Bicarbonate Infusions Prepared in Polyolefin Bags. *Hosp Pharm*. 2012; 47(7):538-43.
6. Naorungroj T, Neto AS, Fujii T, et al. Stability of bicarbonate in normal saline: a technical report. *Crit Care Resusc*. 2020; 22(1):83-85.
7. DeLuca PP, Kowalsky RJ. Problems arising from the transfer of sodium bicarbonate injection from ampuls to plastic disposable syringes. *Am J Hosp Pharm*. 1972; 29(3):217-22.
8. Seki JT, Wang TQ, Yip PM, et al. Stability of sodium bicarbonate injection 8.4% in syringes over a six-week period in refrigerated temperature. *J Oncol Pharm Pract*. 2018; 24(3):198-200.
9. Hicks CI, Gallardo JP, Guillory JK. Stability of sodium bicarbonate injection stored in polypropylene syringes. *Am J Hosp Pharm*. 1972; 29(3):210-6.

Succinylcholine Chloride

Storage Conditions

CONTAINER	Drug Manufacturer	Concentration	Diluents	Osmolality (mOsm/kg)	pH	Temperature: Room	Temperature: Refrig	Temperature: Frozen	Post-thaw Temp: Room	Post-thaw Temp: Refrig	Body Temp	Refer.
Bag, Polyvinyl Chloride (PVC)	TR	1 mg/mL	NS, LR, D5W, D5NS, D5LR	n/a	n/a	n/a	24 hr	n/a	n/a	n/a	n/a	(3)
Syringe, Polypropylene	AB	20 mg/mL[a]	Undiluted	n/a	3.50-3.55	45 d[b][d]	90 d[b]	n/a	n/a	n/a	n/a	(1)
	BW	20 mg/mL	NS, D5W	n/a	n/a	90 d[c]	107 d[c]	n/a	n/a	n/a	n/a	(2)
	UN	10 mg/mL	NS	n/a	n/a	7 d[h]	7 d	n/a	n/a	n/a	n/a	(5)
Unspecified	UN	1, 2 mg/mL	NS	n/a	n/a	7 d	28 d	n/a	n/a	n/a	n/a	(3)
Vial, Glass	TR	1 mg/mL	NS, LR, D5W, D5NS, D5LR	n/a	n/a	n/a	24 hr	n/a	n/a	n/a	n/a	(3)
	UN	10 mg/mL[e][g]	NS	n/a	3.0[f]	5 m[c]	24 m[c]	n/a	n/a	n/a	n/a	(4)
	NYC	50 mg/mL	Undiluted	n/a	n/a	8 wk[c]	n/a	n/a	n/a	n/a	n/a	(6)
	CSP	50 mg/mL	Undiluted	n/a	n/a	4 m[c]	n/a	n/a	n/a	n/a	n/a	(7)
	UN	20 mg/mL	Undiluted	n/a	n/a	7 d[c]	n/a	n/a	n/a	n/a	n/a	(8)

Flush Compatibility: Sodium chloride 0.9%, D5W, Lactated Ringer's.[3]

Special Considerations: n/a

Notes

[a] Methylparaben added as a preservative to prevent antimicrobial growth.[1]

[b] Loss in potency < 10% after 45 days at 25°C and < 1% after 90 days at 4°C.[1]

[c] Protected from light.[2,6–8]

[d] Exposed to fluorescent light.[1]

[e] Methyl-4-hydroxybenzoate added as a preservative to prevent antimicrobial growth.[4]

[f] Hydrochloric acid added to adjust pH to 3.0 (corrected solution).[4]

[g] Initial nominal concentration, 10.46 mg anhydrous compound per mL (excess of 4.6%), corresponding to 11.5 mg of succinylcholine chloride dihydrate per mL.[4]

[h] Protected from light and exposed to light.[5]

DOI 10.37573/9781585286720.174

REFERENCES

1. Storms ML, Stewart JT, Warren FW. Stability of succinylcholine chloride injection at ambient temperature and 4 deg C in polypropylene syringes. *Int J Pharm Compd*. 2003; 7(1):68-70.
2. Pramar YV, Moniz D, Hobbs D. Chemical stability and adsorption of succinylcholine chloride injections in disposable plastic syringes. *J Clin Pharm Ther*. 1994; 19(3):195-8.
3. ASHP's Interactive Handbook on Injectable Drugs, 2020. Bethesda, MD: American Society of Health-System Pharmacists; Accessed December 2020.
4. Schmutz CW, Muhlebach SF. Stability of succinylcholine chloride injection. *Am J Hosp Pharm*. 1991; 48(3):501-6.
5. Boulay D, Antier D, Laffon M. Stability and sterility of succinylcholine chloride. *Int J Obstet Anesth*. 2010; 19(3):349-50.
6. De Winter S, Vanbrabant P, Vi NT, et al. Impact of temperature exposure on stability of drugs in a real-world out-of-hospital setting. *Ann Emerg Med*. 2013; 62(4):380-87 e1.
7. De Winter S, Bronselaer K, Vanbrabant P, et al. Stability of Drugs Used in Helicopter Air Medical Emergency Services: An Exploratory Study. *Air Med J*. 2016; 35(4):247-50.
8. Gammon DL, Su S, Jordan J, et al. Alteration in prehospital drug concentration after thermal exposure. *Am J Emerg Med*. 2008; 26(5):566-73.

SUFentanil Citrate

Storage Conditions

	Drug Manufacturer	Concentration	Diluents	Osmolality (mOsm/kg)	pH	Temperature Room	Temperature Refrig	Temperature Frozen	Post-thaw Temp Room	Post-thaw Temp Refrig	Body Temp	Refer.
CONTAINER												
Bag, Polypropylene	JN	0.4 mcg/mL	NS[i]	n/a	5.3	30 d[j](k)	n/a	n/a	n/a	n/a	n/a	(1)(6)
	JN	4 mcg/mL	Undiluted [o]	n/a	4.9	30 d[j](k)	n/a	n/a	n/a	n/a	n/a	(1)(6)
Bag, Polyvinyl Chloride (PVC)	JN	1 mcg/mL	NS[l]	n/a	[m]	n/a	n/a	4 m[a]	n/a	10 wk[a]	n/a	(7)
	JN	12 mcg/mL	NS[n]	n/a	[m]	43 d	43 d	n/a	n/a	n/a	n/a	(1)
	JC	0.5, 0.75, 1 mcg/mL	NS[b]	n/a	[m]	4 d	n/a	n/a	n/a	n/a	n/a	(1)
Syringe, Polypropylene	JN	2 mcg/mL	NS	n/a	[m]	24 hr	n/a	n/a	n/a	n/a	n/a	(1)
	JN	1 mcg/mL	NS	n/a	5.7	72 hr	23 d	n/a	n/a	n/a	n/a	(4)
	JN	1 mcg/mL	NS[c]	n/a	4.8	28 d	28 d	n/a	n/a	n/a	28 d	(4)
Vial, Glass	JN	5 mcg/mL	NS	n/a	5.9-6.5	n/a	21 d	n/a	n/a	n/a	21 d[d]	(1)(2)
	JC	0.5, 0.75, 1 mcg/mL	NS[b]	n/a	[m]	4 d	n/a	n/a	n/a	n/s	n/a	(1)
OTHER INFUSION CONTAINERS												
CADD® Cassette (Smiths Medical)	JN	5 mcg/mL	D5W	n/a	4.5-5.1	n/a	30 d	n/a	n/a	n/a	30 d[d]	(1)(3)
	JN	5 mcg/mL	NS	n/a	5.1-5.4	n/a	21 d	n/a	n/a	n/a	n/a	(2)
	JN	5 mcg/mL	NS[g]	n/a	[m]	n/a	30 d	n/a	n/a	n/a	30 d[d]	(1)(3)
	JN	20 mcg/mL	NS	n/a	[m]	n/a	10 d	n/a	n/a	n/a	n/a	(1)(5)
	JN	20 mcg/mL	NS[f]	n/a	[m]	10 d[e]	10 d	n/a	n/a	n/a	10 d[e]	(1)(5)
	JC	50 mcg/mL	Undiluted	n/a	[m]	14 d	14 d	n/a	n/a	n/a	n/a	(1)
Polyethylene-High Density (Eur. Ph.)	JN	5 mcg/mL	NS	n/a	5.7-6.3	n/a	21 d	n/a	n/a	n/a	21 d[d]	(1)(2)
SynchroMed™ II Implantable Pump (Medtronic)	BB	1,000 mcg/mL	unspec.[p]	n/a	n/a	n/a	n/a	n/a	n/a	n/a	40 d[h]	(1)

Flush Compatibility: Sodium chloride 0.9%.[1]

Special Considerations: Store product protected from light. SUFentanil adsorbs to PVC-lined containers, sets, and filters and polyethylene tubing.[1] Intraspinal infusion requires the use of preservative-free diluents and drug products.

DOI 10.37573/9781585286720.175

Notes

[a] Thawed in a validated cycle microwave prior to refrigerated storage for up to 10 wk.[(7)]

[b] Solution contained: ropivacaine (ASZ) 2 mcg/mL.[(1)]

[c] Solution contained: levobupivacaine (AB) 1 mg/mL.[(4)]

[d] Storage temperature: 32°C.

[e] SUFentanil concentration decreases below acceptable limits in the absence of the bupivacaine additive due to the stabilizing effect and buffering capacity of bupivacaine HCl.[(5)]

[f] Solution contained: bupivacaine HCl 3 mg/mL.

[g] Solution contained: bupivacaine HCl (AST) 2 mg/mL.

[h] 10% loss of ziconotide at 33 d; no SUFentanil loss at 40 d.[(1)]

[i] Solution contained: ropivacaine HCl (ASZ) 1 mg/mL (diluted in NS) or 2 mg/mL.[(6)]

[j] Storage temperature: 30°C.

[k] Protected from light.

[l] Solution contained: levobupivacaine (ABV) 1.25 mg/mL.[(7)]

[m] pH of the undiluted solution is 3.5-6.[(1)]

[n] Solution contained: bupivacaine HCl (AST) 40 mcg/mL.

[o] Solution contained: ropivacaine (ASZ) 2 mg/mL.[(6)]

[p] Drug powder dissolved in ziconotide acetate 25 mcg/mL injection.

REFERENCES

1. ASHP's Interactive Handbook on Injectable Drugs, 2020. Bethesda, MD: American Society of Health-System Pharmacists; Accessed August 2020.
2. Roos PJ, Glerum JH, Meilink JW. Stability of sufentanil citrate in a portable pump reservoir, a glass container and a polyethylene container. *Pharm Weekbl Sci*. 1992; 14(4):196-200.
3. Roos PJ, Glerum JH, Schroeders MJ. Effect of glucose 5% solution and bupivacaine hydrochloride on absorption of sufentanil citrate in a portable pump reservoir during storage and simulated infusion by an epidural catheter. *Pharm World Sci*. 1993; 15(6):269-75.
4. Jappinen A, Turpeinen M, Kokki H, et al. Stability of sufentanil and levobupivacaine solutions and a mixture in a 0.9% sodium chloride infusion stored in polypropylene syringes. *Eur J Pharm Sci*. 2003; 19(1):31-6.
5. Brouwers JRB, Van Doorne H, Meevis RF, et al. Stability of sufentanil citrate and sufentanil citrate/bupivacaine mixture in portable infusion pumps. *EHP*. 1995;1(1):12-4.
6. Oster Svedberg K, McKenzie J, Larrivee-Elkins C. Compatibility of ropivacaine with morphine, sufentanil, fentanyl, or clonidine. *J Clin Pharm Ther*. 2002; 27(1):39-45.
7. Boitquin LP, Hecq JD, Vanbeckbergen DF, et al. Stability of sufentanil citrate with levobupivacaine HCl in NaCl 0.9% infusion after microwave freeze-thaw treatment. *Ann Pharmacother*. 2004; 38(11):1836-9.

Sulfamethoxazole – Trimethoprim

Storage Conditions

						Temperature			Post-thaw Temp			
	Drug Manufacturer[f]	Concentration[e]	Diluents[d]	Osmolality (mOsm/kg)	pH	Room	Refrig	Frozen	Room	Refrig	Body Temp	Refer.
CONTAINER												
Bag, Polyvinyl Chloride (PVC)	ES	1.08, 1.60 mg/mL	NS, D5W	n/a	8.94-9.81	24 hr	n/a	n/a	n/a	n/a	n/a	(6)
Syringe, Polypropylene	ES	16 mg/mL	Undiluted[a]	n/a	[b]	60 hr[g]	n/a	n/a	n/a	n/a	n/a	(1)
Unspecified	RC	0.64, 0.8 mg/mL	NS, D5W, ½NS, D5½NS, LR	n/a	[b]	24 hr	n/a	n/a	n/a	n/a	n/a	(1)
Vial, Glass	RC, BW	0.64 mg/mL	D5W, NS	[c]	8.75-9.51	48 hr	n/a	n/a	n/a	n/a	n/a	(3)
	RC	0.64, 0.8, 1.07, 1.6 mg/mL	NS, D5W, ½NS, D5½NS	n/a	8.49-9.69	24 hr	n/a	n/a	n/a	n/a	n/a	(5)
	RC	0.64, 0.8, 1.07 mg/mL	LR	n/a	8.79-9.56	24 hr	n/a	n/a	n/a	n/a	n/a	(5)
	RC	1.6 mg/mL	LR	n/a	9.64-9.70	12 hr	n/a	n/a	n/a	n/a	n/a	(5)

Flush Compatibility: Sodium chloride 0.9%, heparin.[1]

Special Considerations: Concentrations are stated as the trimethoprim (TMP) component of the 1:5 fixed ratio with sulfamethoxazole (SMZ) (i.e., 16 mg/mL TMP:80 mg/mL SMZ).[2] Dosing is based on the trimethoprim component. Product labeling states that unit-dose glass, polyvinyl chloride, and polyolefin containers may be used for final dilution. Do not refrigerate admixtures.[2]

Notes

[a] Not for direct injection; must be diluted per product labeling prior to infusion.[2]

[b] pH of undiluted solution is 9.5-10.5.[2] The pH of diluted solution ranged from 9.09-9.37.[4]

[c] The osmolalities of co-trimoxazole (BW) 0.8, 1.1, and 1.6 mg/mL (trimethoprim component) in D5W are 541, 669, and 798 mOsm/kg, respectively. The osmolality of 1.6 mg/mL (trimethoprim component) in NS is 833 mOsm/kg.[1]

[d] Manufacturer recommends only D5W for dilution and infusion.[2]

[e] Final Concentrations: 1:10 = 1.60 mg/mL TMP:8 mg/mL SMZ; 1:15 = 1.07 mg/mL* TMP:5.33 mg/mL SMZ; 1:20 = 0.8 mg/mL TMP:4 mg/mL SMZ; 1:25 = 0.64 mg/mL TMP:3.2 mg/mL SMZ. (*Rounded to two decimal places.)[1]

[f] Sulfamethoxazole and trimethoprim injection USP (Teva) contains benzyl alcohol 10 mg/mL as a preservative.[2]

[g] Exposed to fluorescent light during daylight hours.[1]

DOI 10.37573/9781585286720.176

REFERENCES

1. ASHP's Interactive Handbook on Injectable Drugs, 2020. Bethesda, MD: American Society of Health-System Pharmacists; Accessed December 2020.
2. Sulfamethoxazole and Trimethoprim Injection [package insert]. North Wales, PA: Teva Pharmaceuticals USA, Inc.; September 2020.
3. Jarosinski PF, Kennedy PE, Gallelli JF. Stability of concentrated trimethoprim-sulfamethoxazole admixtures. *Am J Hosp Pharm*. 1989; 46(4):732-7.
4. Khaleel I, Zaidi STR, Shastri MD, et al. Investigations into the physical and chemical stability of concentrated co-trimoxazole intravenous infusions. *Eur J Hosp Pharm*. 2018; 25(e2):e102-e08.
5. Deans KW, Lang JR, Smith DE. Stability of trimethoprim-sulfamethoxazole injection in five infusion fluids. *Am J Hosp Pharm*. 1982; 39(10):1681-4.
6. Curtis J, Edwards D. Stability of Trimethoprim in Admixtures of Trimethoprim Sulfamethoxazole Prepared in Polyvinylchloride Bags and Glass Bottles. *Canadian J Hosp Pharm*. 2002; 55.

Tacrolimus

Storage Conditions

	Drug Manufacturer	Concentration	Diluents	Osmolality (mOsm/kg)	pH	Temperature			Post-thaw Temp		Body Temp	Refer.
						Room	Refrig	Frozen	Room	Refrig		
CONTAINER												
Bag, Polyolefin	ASP	0.002-0.008 mg/mL	NS	n/a	n/a	9 d[a]	9 d[a](d)	n/a	n/a	n/a	n/a	(3)(5)
	FUJ	0.02 mg/mL	D5W	n/a	n/a	24 hr[f]	n/a	n/a	n/a	n/a	n/a	(1)
	ASP	0.01 mg/mL	D5W, NS	n/a	n/a	28 hr[e]	20 hr	n/a	n/a	n/a	n/a	(4)(6)
	ASP	0.001, 0.01, 0.1 mg/mL	D5W	n/a	n/a	48 hr[f]	n/a	n/a	n/a	n/a	n/a	(2)(4)(6)
	ASP	0.001 mg/mL	NS	n/a	n/a	24 hr[f]	n/a	n/a	n/a	n/a	n/a	(4)(6)
	ASP	0.01, 0.1 mg/mL	NS	n/a	n/a	48 hr[f]	n/a	n/a	n/a	n/a	n/a	(2)(4)(6)
Syringe, Plastic (Unspecified)	FUJ[c]	0.1 mg/mL	NS	n/a	n/a	24 hr[d]	n/a	n/a	n/a	n/a	n/a	(1)
Vial, Glass	FUJ[b]	0.1 mg/mL	D5W	n/a	n/a	48 hr	n/a	n/a	n/a	n/a	n/a	(1)
	FUJ	0.01 mg/mL	NS	n/a	n/a	48 hr	n/a	n/a	n/a	n/a	n/a	(1)

Flush Compatibility: Sodium chloride 0.9%, heparin.

Special Considerations: Tacrolimus should be kept in a pH between 2 and 6 as the rate of decomposition increases at higher pH values. Tacrolimus should not be co-infused with in solutions with a pH above 9 (e.g. ganciclovir or acyclovir). PVC containers should be avoided due to potential leaching of diethylhexyl phthalate (DEHP) plasticizer and decreased stability of the drug.[1]

Notes

a Container information: Excel® is a copolymer of ethylene and propylene (BRN).[3]

b Tacrolimus (FUJ) 0.1 mg/mL in D5W infused though PVC IV tubing and fat emulsion tubing showed no loss. It showed 2.5% loss in PVC anesthesia extension tubing.[2]

c Packaged as 20 mL in 30 mL syringe.[2]

d Protected from light.

e No loss at 20 hours at 2-8°C followed by 28 hours at 20-25°C.[1]

f Container information: VisIV™ is a polyolefin (ICU).[6]

DOI 10.37573/9781585286720.177

REFERENCES

1. ASHP's Interactive Handbook on Injectable Drugs, 2021. Bethesda, MD: American Society of Health-System Pharmacists; Accessed December 2020.
2. Taormina D, Abdallah HY, Venkataramanan R, et al. Stability and sorption of FK 506 in 5% dextrose injection and 0.9% sodium chloride injection in glass, polyvinyl chloride, and polyolefin containers. *Am J Hosp Pharm*. 1992; 49(1):119-22.
3. B. Braun Medication Information Letter (Ref#: N/A) [personal communication]. Bethlehem, PA: B. Braun Medical, Inc.; 2016:5.
4. Aloumanis V, Ben M, Kupiec TC, et al. Drug Compatibility with a New Generation of VISIV Polyolefin Infusion Solution Containers. *Int J Pharm Compd*. 2009; 13(2):162-5.
5. Myers AL, Zhang Y, Kawedia JD, et al. Stability of tacrolimus injection diluted in 0.9% sodium chloride injection and stored in Excel bags. *Am J Health Syst Pharm*. 2016; 73(24):2083-88.
6. Trissel LA, Xu QA, Baker M. Drug compatibility with new polyolefin infusion solution containers. *Am J Health Syst Pharm*. 2006; 63(23):2379-82.

Tedizolid Phosphate

Storage Conditions

						Temperature			Post-thaw Temp			
	Drug Manufacturer	Concentration	Diluents	Osmolality (mOsm/kg)	pH	Room	Refrig	Frozen	Room	Refrig	Body Temp	Refer.
CONTAINER												
Bag, Polypropylene	MSD	0.8 mg/mL[a]	NS	n/a	n/a	28 d[b]	28 d[b]	28 d[b]	n/a	n/a	n/a	(1)
Vial, Glass	ME	50 mg/mL	SWFI	n/a	n/a	24 hr	24 hr	n/a	n/a	n/a	n/a	(2)

Flush Compatibility: Sodium chloride 0.9%.[2]

Special Considerations: Must reconstitute lyophilized powder with sterile water for injection and subsequently dilute only in sodium chloride 0.9% for intravenous infusion. Do not invert vial to withdraw; withdraw using needle long enough to reach the bottom of the vial. Incompatible with solutions containing divalent ions (i.e., Ca^{2}+, Mg^{2}+), including Lactated Ringer's Injection and Hartmann's Solution.[2]

Notes

[a] Solution contained: rifAMPin 2.4 mg/mL or meropenem 4 mg/mL. Tedizolid remained stable throughout the 28 day study period. RifAMPin and meropenem remained stable for 7 hours RT and 6 days RF.[1]

[b] Protected from light.

REFERENCES

1. Ezquer-Garin C, Ferriols-Lisart R, Martinez-Lopez LM, et al. Stability of tedizolid phosphate-sodium rifampicin and tedizolid phosphate-meropenem admixtures in intravenous infusion bags stored at different temperatures. *Pharmazie*. 2020; 75(5):172-76.
2. Sivextro® (Tedizolid Phosphate) Injection [package insert]. Whitehouse Station, NJ: Merck Sharp & Dohme Corp.; October 2020.

DOI 10.37573/9781585286720.178

Telavancin Hydrochloride

Storage Conditions

						Temperature			Post-thaw Temp			
	Drug Manufacturer	Concentration	Diluents	Osmolality (mOsm/kg)	pH	Room	Refrig	Frozen	Room	Refrig	Body Temp	Refer.
CONTAINER												
Bag, Polyvinyl Chloride (PVC)	ASP	0.6, 8 mg/mL	NS, D5W, LR	n/a	[e]	48 hr	14 d[c]	n/a	n/a	n/a	n/a	(2)
	BV	0.6, 8 mg/mL	D5W, NS	n/a	[e]	n/a	n/a	32 d[c]	n/a	n/a	n/a	(2)(4)
Bag, Polyolefin	BV	0.6, 8 mg/mL	D5W, NS	n/a	[e]	n/a	n/a	32 d[c]	n/a	n/a	n/a	(2)(4)
Bag, Plastic (Unspecified)	ASP	0.6, 8 mg/mL[a]	NS, D5W, LR	n/a	[e]	12 hr[b]	7 d[b]	32 d[c]	n/a	n/a	n/a	(1)
Vial, Glass	ASP	15 mg/mL	D5W, NS, SWFI	n/a	[d]	12 hr[b]	7 d[b][c]	n/a	n/a	n/a	n/a	(2)(3)
OTHER INFUSION CONTAINERS												
Homepump Eclipse® / Homepump® (Halyard)	ASP	0.6, 8 mg/mL	NS, D5W, LR, SWFI	n/a	[e]	n/a	8 d[c]	n/a	n/a	n/a	n/a	(2)(5)
INTERMATE™ (Baxter)[f]	ASP	0.6, 8 mg/mL	NS, D5W, LR, SWFI	n/a	[e]	n/a	8 d[c]	n/a	n/a	n/a	n/a	(2)(5)

Flush Compatibility: Sodium chloride 0.9%.[1]

Special Considerations: Store original vials at refrigerated temperature. Excursions to ambient temperature are acceptable; avoid excessive heat. Reconstitute with NS, SWFI, or D5W.[1]

Notes

[a] When mixed according to the package insert.[1]

[b] Total time in vial plus the time in the infusion bag should not exceed 12 hr at room temperature and 7 d refrigerated.[1,3]

[c] Protected from light.[2]

[d] pH of reconstituted solution in vial is 4-5.[1,3]

[e] pH diluted (per package insert) to 0.6 mg/mL was 4.6-5.7; pH diluted to 8 mg/mL was 4.4-4.9.[2]

[f] INTERMATE™/INFUSOR™ Portable Elastomeric Infusion System devices are no longer available in the United States.

REFERENCES

1. Vibativ® (Telavancin) Injection [package insert]. Nashville, TN: Cumberland Pharmaceuticals Inc.; January 2021.
2. Telavancin Stability Medication Information Letter (Ref#: PRJ/38809) [personal communication]. South San Francisco, CA: Theravance Biopharma; 2015:6.
3. ASHP's Interactive Handbook on Injectable Drugs, 2020. Bethesda, MD: American Society of Health-System Pharmacists; Accessed January 2021.
4. Gu Z, Wong A, Raquinio E, et al. Stability of Reconstituted Telavancin Drug Product in Frozen Intravenous Bags. *Hosp Pharm*. 2015; 50(7):609-14.
5. Sand P, Aladeen T, Kirkegaard P, et al. Chemical Stability of Telavancin in Elastomeric Pumps. *Curr Ther Res Clin Exp*. 2015; 77:99-104.

DOI 10.37573/9781585286720.179

Thiotepa

Storage Conditions

						Temperature			Post-thaw Temp			
	Drug Manufacturer	Concentration	Diluents	Osmolality (mOsm/kg)	pH	Room	Refrig	Frozen	Room	Refrig	Body Temp	Refer.
CONTAINER												
Bag, Polyolefin	IMM	5 mg/mL	D5W	[c]	[b]	72 hr	14 d	n/a	n/a	n/a	n/a	(2)
Bag, Polyvinyl Chloride (PVC)	UN	0.25 mg/mL	NS	[c]	[b]	7 d	n/a	n/a	n/a	n/a	n/a	(1)
	IMM	0.5 mg/mL	NS	[c]	[b]	n/a	48 hr[a]	n/a	n/a	n/a	n/a	(2)
	IMM	1, 3 mg/mL	NS	[c]	[b]	24 hr	48 hr	n/a	n/a	n/a	n/a	(2)
	IMM	5 mg/mL	D5W	[c]	[b]	72 hr	14 d	n/a	n/a	n/a	n/a	(2)
	AMB	0.5-1 mg/mL	NS	[c]	[b]	4 hr	24 hr	n/a	n/a	n/a	n/a	(2)
Syringe, Plastic (Unspecified)	IMM	10 mg/mL[d]	SWFI	[c]	[b]	24 hr	24 hr[a]	n/a	n/a	n/a	n/a	(2)

Flush Compatibility: Sodium chloride 0.9%, heparin.[2]

Special Considerations: Reconstituted solution should be clear. Filtration through a 0.22-micron filter prior to administration eliminates haze and does not affect potency. Do not use solutions that are grossly opaque or contain precipitate after filtration. Dilute prior to administration. Store at 2°C to 8°C, do not freeze.[3] Protect intact vials and reconstituted solutions from light until used.[2]

Notes

[a] Storage temperature: 8°C.[2]

[b] pH of reconstituted solution 10 mg/mL (approx.) in SWFI is 5.5-7.5.[2,3]

[c] Dilutions of 0.5 and 1 mg/mL in NS are 277 and 269 mOsm/kg. Dilutions of 3 and 5 mg/mL in NS are hypotonic.[2]

[d] Dilute prior to administration.[3]

REFERENCES

1. Vyas HM, Baptista RJ, Mitrano FP, et al. Drug stability guidelines for a continuous infusion chemotherapy program. *Hosp Pharm*. 1987; 22(7):685-7.
2. ASHP's Interactive Handbook on Injectable Drugs, 2020. Bethesda, MD: American Society of Health-System Pharmacists; Accessed July 2020.
3. Tepadina® (Thiotepa) Injection [package insert]. Bridgewater, NJ: Amneal Pharmaceuticals, LLC.; April 2020.

DOI 10.37573/9781585286720.180

Tigecycline

Storage Conditions

						Temperature			Post-thaw Temp			
	Drug Manufacturer	Concentration	Diluents	Osmolality (mOsm/kg)	pH	Room	Refrig	Frozen	Room	Refrig	Body Temp	Refer.
CONTAINER												
Bag, Unspecified	ACD, FRK, WY	0.5, 1 mg/mL	D5W, NS	n/a	n/a	18 hr[a]	48 hr	n/a	n/a	n/a	n/a	(1)
OTHER INFUSION CONTAINERS												
Easypump® ST/LT (B. Braun)	UN	0.5, 1 mg/mL	NS	n/a	n/a	24 hr[b]	48 hr[b]	n/a	n/a	n/a	n/a	(4)
SMARTeZ® (Progressive Medical)	UN	0.5, 1 mg/mL	NS	n/a	n/a	24 hr	48 hr	n/a	n/a	n/a	n/a	(3)

Flush Compatibility: Sodium chloride 0.9%, heparin.[2]

Special Considerations: The reconstituted solution should be yellow to orange in color; if not, the solution should be discarded.[1]

Notes

[a] The solution may be stored for up to 24 hr at room temperature, not to exceed 25°C, including up to 6 hr reconstituted in the vial, and the remaining time in the IV bag.[1]

[b] Combined storage conditions of refrigerated and room temperature tested.[4]

REFERENCES

1. Tygacil® (Tigecycline) Injection [package insert]. Philadelphia, PA: Wyeth Pharmaceuticals, LLC.; November 2020.
2. ASHP's Interactive Handbook on Injectable Drugs, 2020. Bethesda, MD: American Society of Health-System Pharmacists; Accessed July 2020.
3. *SMARTeZ® - Stability Data for Drugs Using Elastomeric Infusion Pumps*, 2020. Fenton, MO: Progressive Medical, Inc.; Updated May 2020.
4. *Drug Stability for Easypump® ST/LT*, 2020. Bethlehem, PA: B. Braun USA; Updated June 2020.

DOI 10.37573/9781585286720.181

Tobramycin Sulfate

Storage Conditions

	Drug Manufacturer	Concentration	Diluents	Osmolality (mOsm/kg)	pH	Temperature Room	Temperature Refrig	Temperature Frozen	Post-thaw Temp Room	Post-thaw Temp Refrig	Body Temp	Refer.
CONTAINER												
Bag, Ethylene Vinyl Acetate (EVA)	UN	0.95 mg/mL	NS	[h]	[a]	7 d[b]	30 d[b]	n/a	n/a	n/a	n/a	(4)
Bag, Polyvinyl Chloride (PVC)	LI	0.2, 1 mg/mL	D5W, D5NS, NS, D10W	[h]	[a]	48 hr	n/a	n/a	n/a	n/a	n/a	(1)
	DI	1.2 mg/mL	D5W, NS	[h]	[a]	48 hr	48 hr[b]	n/a	n/a	n/a	n/a	(1)
	DI	2.4 mg/mL	D5W, NS	[h]	[a]	n/a	n/a	28 d	n/a	n/a	n/a	(1)
	LI	3.2 mg/mL	D5W	n/a	[a]	n/a	n/a	30 d	24 hr	n/a	n/a	(1)
Syringe, Plastic (Unspecified)	LI	40 mg/mL	SWFI	n/a	[a]	60 d[f]	60 d[f]	n/a	n/a	n/a	n/a	(1)
Syringe, Polypropylene	APP	12.5 mg/mL	NS, SWFI	n/a	[a]	14 d	14 d	n/a	n/a	n/a	n/a	(7)
	APP	12.5 mg/mL	D5W	n/a	[a]	12 d	14 d	n/a	n/a	n/a	n/a	(7)
	DI	30 mg/mL	NS	[h]	[a]	48 hr	n/a	n/a	n/a	n/a	n/a	(1)
Vial, Glass	LI	2.8, 3.2, 5.2, 6 mg/mL	D10W	[h]	[a]	n/a	30 d[b]	n/a	n/a	n/a	n/a	(1)
OTHER INFUSION CONTAINERS												
CADD® Cassette (Smiths Medical)	MAR	1, 10 mg/mL	NS	[h]	[a]	72 hr	14 d	n/a	n/a	n/a	n/a	(1)
Dosi-Fuser® (Leventon)	LI	0.5-4.8 mg/mL	D5W, NS	[h]	[a]	24 hr[d]	10 d[d]	n/a	n/a	n/a	n/a	(6)
	HOS	1-7.5 mg/mL	NS	[h]	[a]	n/a	22 d	n/a	n/a	n/a	n/a	(6)
Easypump® ST/LT (B. Braun)	UN	0.2, 10 mg/mL	NS	[h]	[a]	24 hr	14 d	n/a	n/a	n/a	n/a	(5)
Homepump Eclipse® / Homepump® (Halyard)	UN	0.2 mg/mL	NS	n/a	[a]	24 hr	7 d	n/a	n/a	n/a	n/a	(3)
	UN	0.8 mg/mL	NS	315	[a]	24 hr	14 d	n/a	n/a	n/a	n/a	(1)(3)
INFUSOR™ (Baxter)[g]	LI	0.8-2.4 mg/mL	NS	[h]	[a]	21 d[c]	19 d[c]	n/a	n/a	n/a	n/a	(2)

DOI 10.37573/9781585286720.182

Storage Conditions

	Drug Manufacturer	Concentration	Diluents	Osmolality (mOsm/kg)	pH	Temperature Room	Temperature Refrig	Temperature Frozen	Post-thaw Temp Room	Post-thaw Temp Refrig	Body Temp	Refer.
OTHER INFUSION CONTAINERS												
INTERMATE™ (Baxter)[g]	LI	0.5 mg/mL	D5W	n/a	[a]	48 hr[e]	7 d	n/a	n/a	n/a	n/a	(2)
	LI	0.5-4.8 mg/mL	NS	[h]	[a]	24 hr	10 d	n/a	n/a	n/a	n/a	(2)
	LI	0.5-4.8 mg/mL	D5W	[h]	[a]	n/a	10 d	n/a	n/a	n/a	n/a	(2)
	LI	0.5-5 mg/mL	NS	[h]	[a]	48 hr[e]	7 d	n/a	n/a	n/a	n/a	(2)
	LI	0.5-5 mg/mL	D5W	[h]	[a]	24 hr[e]	7 d	n/a	n/a	n/a	n/a	(2)
	LI	4.8 mg/mL	D5W	n/a	[a]	n/a	n/a	30 d	24 hr	n/a	n/a	(2)
SMARTeZ® (Progressive Medical)	UN	0.2, 10 mg/mL	NS	n/a	[a]	24 hr[d]	14 d[d]	n/a	n/a	n/a	n/a	(8)

Flush Compatibility: Sodium chloride 0.9%. Incompatible with heparin.[1]

Special Considerations: n/a

Notes

[a] pH of the undiluted solution is 3-6.5.[1]

[b] Protected from light.[1,4]

[c] 19 d refrigerated followed by 21 d at room temperature.[2]

[d] Manufacturer extrapolated data from other sources.[6,8]

[e] Following 7 d refrigerated.[2]

[f] Primary reference authors note that the manufacturer does not recommend storage in plastic syringes due to possible incompatibility with plunger heads.[1]

[g] INTERMATE™/INFUSOR™ Portable Elastomeric Infusion System devices are no longer available in the United States.

[h] The osmolality of tobramycin sulfate 1 mg/mL in D5W is 254 mOsm/kg, and 288 mOsm/kg in NS. The osmolality of tobramycin sulfate 2.5 mg/mL in D5W is 261 mOsm/kg, and 283 mOsm/kg in NS. The osmolality of tobramycin sulfate 10 mg/mL is 133 mOsm/kg by freezing point depression, and 213 mOsm/kg by vapor pressure.[1]

REFERENCES

1. ASHP's Interactive Handbook on Injectable Drugs, 2020. Bethesda, MD: American Society of Health-System Pharmacists; Accessed September 2020.
2. Stabforum - Stability Database: Tobramycin, Ontario, Canada: Baxter Healthcare; Accessed January 2021.
3. *Stability Data for Drugs Using Homepump Disposable Ambulatory Infusion Systems (MK-00314 rev 3)*, 2015. Alpharetta, GA: Halyard Health; Updated June 2015.
4. Xu QAP, Trissel LABR, Saenz CA, et al. Stability of Gentamicin Sulfate and Tobramycin Sulfate in AutoDose Infusion System Bags. *Int J Pharm Compd*. 2002; 6(2):152-4.
5. *Drug Stability for Easypump® ST/LT*, 2020. Bethlehem, PA: B. Braun USA; Updated June 2020.
6. *Drug Stability Table - Dosi-Fuser® Elastomeric Pump (S-CL-00-001v16)*, 2021. Barcelona, Spain: Leventon SAU; Updated May 2021.
7. Fugit KD, Anderson BD. Antibiotic Stability in Freedom 60 Syringe Report by HealthTek™ and the University of Kentucky, Lexington. Chester, NY: RMS Medical Products; 2015.
8. *SMARTeZ® - Stability Data for Drugs Using Elastomeric Infusion Pumps*, 2020. Fenton, MO: Progressive Medical, Inc.; Updated May 2020.

Tocilizumab

Storage Conditions

						Temperature			Post-thaw Temp			
	Drug Manufacturer	Concentration	Diluents	Osmolality (mOsm/kg)	pH	Room	Refrig	Frozen	Room	Refrig	Body Temp	Refer.
CONTAINER												
Bag, Polyethylene	GEN	[b]	NS	n/a	[c]	24 hr[a]	24 hr[a]	n/a	n/a	n/a	n/a	(1)
	GEN	[b]	½NS	n/a	[c]	4 hr[a]	24 hr[a]	n/a	n/a	n/a	n/a	(1)
Bag, Polyolefin	RC[d]	4, 6 mg/mL	NS	n/a	[c]	n/a	24 hr[a]	n/a	n/a	n/a	n/a	(2)
	RC[e]	4, 6 mg/mL	NS	n/a	[c]	n/a	24 hr[a]	n/a	n/a	n/a	n/a	(2)
Bag, Polypropylene	GEN	[b]	NS	n/a	[c]	24 hr[a]	24 hr[a]	n/a	n/a	n/a	n/a	(1)
	GEN	[b]	½NS	n/a	[c]	4 hr[a]	24 hr[a]	n/a	n/a	n/a	n/a	(1)
Bag, Polyvinyl Chloride (PVC)	GEN	[b]	NS	n/a	[c]	24 hr[a]	24 hr[a]	n/a	n/a	n/a	n/a	(1)
	GEN	[b]	½NS	n/a	[c]	4 hr[a]	24 hr[a]	n/a	n/a	n/a	n/a	(1)
Vial, Glass	GEN	[b]	NS	n/a	[c]	24 hr[a]	24 hr[a]	n/a	n/a	n/a	n/a	(1)
	GEN	[b]	½NS	n/a	[c]	4 hr[a]	24 hr[a]	n/a	n/a	n/a	n/a	(1)

Flush Compatibility: Sodium chloride 0.9%.[1]

Special Considerations: For preparation of final administration solution, withdraw a volume of NS equal to the volume of the dose of tocilizumab, then slowly add the medication to the infusion bag or vial; mix gently and avoid foaming.[1]

Notes

[a] Protected from light.[1,2]

[b] Dose diluted in 50 mL or 100 mL NS.[1]

[c] pH of undiluted 20 mg/mL solution is approximately 6.5.[1]

[d] RoActemra® for infusion (RC).[2]

[e] RoActemra® Prefilled Syringe 162 mg (RC).[2]

REFERENCE

1. Actemra® (Tocilizumab) Injection [package insert]. South San Francisco, CA: Genentech, Inc.; May 2020.
2. Navas N, Hermosilla J, Torrente-Lopez A, et al. Use of subcutaneous tocilizumab to prepare intravenous solutions for COVID-19 emergency shortage: Comparative analytical study of physicochemical quality attributes. *J Pharm Anal*. 2020; 10(6):532-45.

DOI 10.37573/9781585286720.183

Topotecan Hydrochloride

Storage Conditions

						Temperature			Post-thaw Temp			
	Drug Manufacturer	Concentration	Diluents	Osmolality (mOsm/kg)	pH	Room	Refrig	Frozen	Room	Refrig	Body Temp	Refer.
CONTAINER												
Bag, Polyolefin	SKB	50 mcg/mL	D5W, NS	n/a	3.31-3.58[d]	24 hr	7 d[a]	n/a	n/a	n/a	n/a	(2)(4)
Bag, Polyvinyl Chloride (PVC)	SKB	10, 25, 50 mcg/mL	D5W, NS	n/a	[d]	28 d[a]	28 d[a]	n/a	n/a	n/a	n/a	(3)(4)
	SKB	10 mcg/mL	NS	n/a	[d]	17 d[f]	n/a	n/a	n/a	n/a	n/a	(3)(4)
	SKB	25, 50 mcg/mL	D5W, NS	n/a	3.31-3.58[d]	24 hr	7 d[a]	n/a	n/a	n/a	n/a	(2)(4)
Vial, Glass	SKB	50 mcg/mL	NS, D5W	n/a	3.31-3.58[d]	24 hr	7 d[a]	n/a	n/a	n/a	n/a	(2)(4)
	SKB	1,000 mcg/mL	SWFI	n/a	3.1[d]	28 d	28 d	n/a	n/a	n/a	28 d[c]	(1)(4)
	SKB	1,000 mcg/mL	SWFI	n/a	[d]	28 d[a]	28 d[a]	n/a	n/a	n/a	n/a	(3)(4)
OTHER INFUSION CONTAINERS												
INFUSOR™ (Baxter)[e]	SKB	10, 25, 50 mcg/mL	D5W, NS	n/a	[d]	28 d[a]	28 d[a]	n/a	n/a	n/a	5 d[a][b]	(3)(4)

Flush Compatibility: D5W, Sodium chloride 0.9%.[5]

Special Considerations: Store unopened vials in original carton to protect from light.[5]

Notes

[a] Protected from light.

[b] Stored at room temperature followed by 5 days at 37°C.

[c] Storage temperature: 30°C.

[d] pH of reconstituted product is 2.5-3.5.[4]

[e] INFUSOR™ Portable Elastomeric Infusion System devices are no longer available in the United States.

[f] 10% loss in 17 days due to photodegradation in mixed daylight and fluorescent light.

REFERENCES

1. Patel K, Craig SB, McBride MG, et al. Microbial inhibitory properties and stability of topotecan hydrochloride injection. *Am J Health Syst Pharm*. 1998; 55(15):1584-7.
2. Craig SB, Bhatt UH, Patel K. Stability and compatibility of topotecan hydrochloride for injection with common infusion solutions and containers. *J Pharm Biomed Anal*. 1997; 16(2):199-205.
3. Krämer I, Thiesen J. Stability of topotecan infusion solutions in polyvinylchloride bags and elastomeric portable infusion devices. *J Oncol Pharm Pract*. 1999; 5(2):75-82.
4. ASHP's Interactive Handbook on Injectable Drugs, 2020. Bethesda, MD: American Society of Health-System Pharmacists; Accessed December 2020.
5. Hycamtin® (Topotecan Hydrochloride) Injection [package insert]. East Hanover, NJ: Novartis Pharmaceuticals Corporation; June 2020.

DOI 10.37573/9781585286720.184

Tranexamic Acid

Storage Conditions

						Temperature			Post-thaw Temp			
	Drug Manufacturer	Concentration	Diluents	Osmolality (mOsm/kg)	pH[f]	Room	Refrig	Frozen	Room	Refrig	Body Temp	Refer.
CONTAINER												
Bag, Polyethylene	PF	10, 20 mg/mL	NS	n/a	n/a	7 d	7 d[c]	n/a	n/a	n/a	n/a	(2)
Bag, Polyolefin[a]	MYL	15.4 mg/mL	NS	n/a	[b]	90 d[c]	90 d[c]	n/a	n/a	n/a	n/a	(1)
Bag, Polypropylene	PF	10, 20 mg/mL	NS	n/a	n/a	7 d	7 d[c]	n/a	n/a	n/a	n/a	(2)
	PF	10, 20 mg/mL	D5W	n/a	n/a	24 hr	24 hr[c]	n/a	n/a	n/a	n/a	(2)
Bag, Polyvinyl Chloride (PVC)	PF	10, 20 mg/mL	D5W	n/a	n/a	24 hr	24 hr[c]	n/a	n/a	n/a	n/a	(2)
	PF	10, 20 mg/mL	NS	n/a	n/a	7 d	7 d[c]	n/a	n/a	n/a	n/a	(2)
	PF	10, 20 mg/mL	LR	n/a	n/a	7 d	7 d[c]	n/a	n/a	n/a	n/a	(2)
Vial, Glass[d]	MYL	20 mg/mL	NS	n/a	[e]	180 d[c]	n/a	n/a	n/a	n/a	n/a	(1)
	PF	10, 20 mg/mL	D5W	n/a	n/a	24 hr	24 hr[c]	n/a	n/a	n/a	n/a	(2)
	PF	10, 20 mg/mL	NS	n/a	n/a	24 hr	7 d[c]	n/a	n/a	n/a	n/a	(2)

Flush Compatibility: Sodium chloride 0.9%, heparin.[2]

Special Considerations: Intact vials and ampules are preservative free, and should be stored at controlled room temperature, protected from light and freezing.[2]

Notes

[a] Container information: PAB® (BRN) is a copolymer of ethylene and propylene.

[b] pH of 6.2-7.4 at controlled room temperature, and pH of 6.7-7.6 at refrigerated temperature.[1]

[c] Protected from light.

[d] Clear Type 1 borosilicate glass 50 mL vials with intact elastomeric, Flourotec-coated stoppers, held in place by aluminum seals.[1]

[e] pH of 6.9-7.4 at controlled room temperature.[1]

[f] pH of undiluted product is 6.5-8.0.[2]

REFERENCES

1. McCluskey SV, Sztajnkrycer MD, Jenkins DA, et al. Stability of tranexamic acid in 0.9% sodium chloride, stored in type 1 glass vials and ethylene/propylene copolymer plastic containers. *Int J Pharm Compd*. 2014; 18(5):432-7.
2. ASHP's Interactive Handbook on Injectable Drugs, 2020. Bethesda, MD: American Society of Health-System Pharmacists; Accessed September 2020.

DOI 10.37573/9781585286720.185

Trastuzumab

Storage Conditions

	Drug Manufacturer	Concentration	Diluents	Osmolality (mOsm/kg)	pH	Temperature Room	Temperature Refrig	Temperature Frozen	Post-thaw Temp Room	Post-thaw Temp Refrig	Body Temp	Refer.
CONTAINER												
Bag, Polyethylene	GEN	Various[a]	NS	n/a	[d]	n/a	24 hr	n/a	n/a	n/a	n/a	(1)
Bag, Polyolefin	GEN	1.5 mg/mL[i]	NS	n/a	[d]	24 hr[e]	n/a	n/a	n/a	n/a	n/a	(2)
	GEN	1.5 mg/mL[f][i]	NS	n/a	[d]	24 hr[e]	n/a	n/a	n/a	n/a	n/a	(2)
	GEN	3 mg/mL[i]	NS	n/a	[d]	24 hr[e]	24 hr	n/a	n/a	n/a	n/a	(2)
	GEN	2.3 mg/mL[g][i]	NS	n/a	[d]	24 hr[e]	24 hr	n/a	n/a	n/a	n/a	(2)
	GEN	0.8, 2.4 mg/mL	NS	n/a	[d]	6 m[c]	6 m[c]	n/a	n/a	n/a	n/a	(4)
Bag, Polyvinyl Chloride (PVC)	GEN	3 mg/mL[i]	NS	n/a	[d]	24 hr[e]	24 hr	n/a	n/a	n/a	n/a	(2)
	GEN	2.3 mg/mL[g][i]	NS	n/a	[d]	24 hr[e]	24 hr	n/a	n/a	n/a	n/a	(2)
	GEN	Various[a]	NS	n/a	[d]	n/a	24 hr	n/a	n/a	n/a	n/a	(1)
Bag, Unspecified	GEN	0.4, 1, 4 mg/mL	NS	n/a	5.8-6.2	n/a	28 d	n/a	n/a	n/a	n/a	(3)
Vial, Glass	GEN	21 mg/mL	BWFI[b]	n/a	6	n/a	28 d[b]	n/a	n/a	n/a	n/a	(1)(2)
OTHER INFUSION CONTAINERS												
INTERMATE™ (Baxter)[h]	RC	0.3-4 mg/mL	NS	n/a	n/a	24 hr	n/a	n/a	n/a	n/a	n/a	(5)

Flush Compatibility: Sodium chloride 0.9%.[1]

Special Considerations: Do not freeze reconstituted or diluted solutions. Do not mix with dextrose 5% solution; dilute required dosage of reconstituted solution in 250 mL of NS. Do not shake vial during reconstitution. Gently invert IV bag to mix solution. Do not confuse Trastuzumab (Herceptin®) with ADO-Trastuzumab Emtansine (Kadcyla®); these have different physicochemical properties and clinical indications.[1]

Notes

[a] Dose diluted in 250 mL sodium chloride 0.9%.[1]

[b] BWFI. If reconstituted with preservative-free SWFI, use immediately and discard unused portion.[1]

[c] Protected from light.[4]

[d] pH of product reconstituted with SWFI or BWFI to 21 mg/mL is approximately 6.0.[1]

DOI 10.37573/9781585286720.186

[e] Storage temperature: 30°C.[2]

[f] Solution contained: pertuzumab 1.5 mg/mL (approx.).[2]

[g] Solution contained: pertuzumab 2.7 mg/mL (approx.).[2]

[h] INTERMATE™/INFUSOR™ Portable Elastomeric Infusion System devices are no longer available in the United States.

[i] Approximate concentration based on diluent volume and volume of admixed medication(s).

REFERENCES

1. Herceptin® (Trastuzumab) Injection [package insert]. South San Francisco, CA: Genentech, Inc.; February 2021.
2. Glover ZW, Gennaro L, Yadav S, et al. Compatibility and stability of pertuzumab and trastuzumab admixtures in i.v. infusion bags for coadministration. *J Pharm Sci*. 2013; 102(3):794-812.
3. Pabari RM, Ryan B, Ahmad W, et al. Physical and structural stability of the monoclonal antibody, trastuzumab (Herceptin(R)), intravenous solutions. *Curr Pharm Biotechnol*. 2013; 14(2):220-5.
4. Paul M, Vieillard V, Da Silva Lemos R, et al. Long-term physico-chemical stability of diluted trastuzumab. *Int J Pharm*. 2013; 448(1):101-4.
5. Stabforum - Stability Database: Trastuzumab, Ontario, Canada: Baxter Healthcare; Accessed February 2021.

Treprostinil Sodium

Storage Conditions

	Drug Manufacturer	Concentration	Diluents	Osmolality (mOsm/kg)	pH	Temperature Room	Temperature Refrig	Temperature Frozen	Post-thaw Temp Room	Post-thaw Temp Refrig	Body Temp	Refer.
CONTAINER												
Bag, Polyvinyl Chloride (PVC)	UT	≥ 0.004 mg/mL	SWFI, NS	n/a	[c]	4 hr	24 hr	n/a	n/a	n/a	48 hr[a]	(2)
	UT	1, 2.5, 5, 10 mg/mL	Undiluted	n/a	[c]	n/a	n/a	n/a	n/a	n/a	4 m	(2)
	UT	≥ 0.004 mg/mL	[d]	n/a	n/a	14 d	n/a	n/a	n/a	n/a	48 hr[a]	(2)
Syringe, Polypropylene	UT	≥ 0.004 mg/mL	SWFI, NS	n/a	[c]	4 hr	24 hr	n/a	n/a	n/a	48 hr[a]	(2)
	UT	≥ 0.004 mg/mL	[d]	n/a	n/a	14 d	n/a	n/a	n/a	n/a	48 hr[a]	(2)
	UT	1, 2.5, 5, 10 mg/mL	Undiluted	n/a	[c]	n/a	n/a	n/a	n/a	n/a	4 m	(2)
Vial, Glass	UT	≥ 0.004 mg/mL	SWFI, NS	n/a	[c]	4 hr	24 hr	n/a	n/a	n/a	48 hr[a]	(2)
	UT	≥ 0.004 mg/mL	[d]	n/a	n/a	14 d	n/a	n/a	n/a	n/a	48 hr[a]	(2)
	UT	1, 2.5, 5, 10 mg/mL	Undiluted	n/a	[c]	n/a	n/a	n/a	n/a	n/a	4 m	(2)
OTHER INFUSION CONTAINERS												
CADD® Cassette (Smiths Medical)	UT	0.004, 0.13 mg/mL	NS, SWFI	n/a	6.5-7	n/a	n/a	n/a	n/a	n/a	48 hr[a]	(1)(3)
	UT	0.004, 0.13 mg/mL	[d]	n/a	10.4-10.6	n/a	n/a	n/a	n/a	n/a	52 hr[a]	(4)
	UT	0.02, 0.13 mg/mL	D5W	n/a	6.7-7.1	n/a	n/a	n/a	n/a	n/a	48 hr[a]	(1)(3)
MiniMed™ Syringe (Medtronic)	UT	1, 2.5, 5, 10 mg/mL	Undiluted	n/a	[c]	60 d	60 d[b]	60 d[b]	n/a	n/a	60 d[b]	(1)

Flush Compatibility: Sodium chloride 0.9%.[2]

Special Considerations: Vial should be used for no more than 30 days after initial entry into the vial.[2]

Notes

[a] Storage temperature: 40°C.

[b] Protected from light.

[c] pH of undiluted solution is 6-7.2.[2]

[d] High-pH glycine diluent (Sterile Diluent for Remodulin®, Sterile Diluent for Flolan®, or Sterile Diluent for Epoprostenol Sodium).[2]

DOI 10.37573/9781585286720.187

REFERENCES

1. ASHP's Interactive Handbook on Injectable Drugs, 2020. Bethesda, MD: American Society of Health-System Pharmacists; Accessed August 2020.
2. Remodulin® (Treprostinil) Injection [package insert]. Research Triangle Park, NC: United Therapeutics Corporation; July 2019.
3. Phares KR, Weiser WE, Miller SP, et al. Stability and preservative effectiveness of treprostinil sodium after dilution in common intravenous diluents. *Am J Health Syst Pharm*. 2003; 60(9):916-22.
4. Zaccardelli D, Phares K, Jeffs R, et al. Stability and antimicrobial effectiveness of treprostinil sodium in Sterile Diluent for Flolan. *Int J Clin Pract*. 2010; 64(7):885-91.

Valproate Sodium

Storage Conditions

CONTAINER	Drug Manufacturer	Concentration	Diluents	Osmolality (mOsm/kg)	pH	Temperature: Room	Temperature: Refrig	Temperature: Frozen	Post-thaw Temp: Room	Post-thaw Temp: Refrig	Body Temp	Refer.
Bag, Polyethylene	SW	1.6 mg/mL	D5W, NS, LR	n/a	[a]	6 d	n/a	n/a	n/a	n/a	n/a	(2)
Bag, Polyvinyl Chloride (PVC)	SW	1.6 mg/mL	D5W, NS, LR	n/a	[a]	6 d	n/a	n/a	n/a	n/a	n/a	(2)
	FRK	unspec.	D5W, NS, LR	n/a	[a]	24 hr	n/a	n/a	n/a	n/a	n/a	(1)
Syringe, Polypropylene	SAA	20 mg/mL	NS	n/a	[a]	n/a	30 d[b]	n/a	n/a	n/a	n/a	(3)
	MYL	12 mg/mL	NS	n/a	[a]	48 hr	n/a	n/a	n/a	n/a	n/a	(2)
Vial, Glass	FRK	unspec.	D5W, NS, LR	n/a	[a]	24 hr	n/a	n/a	n/a	n/a	n/a	(1)
	SW	1.6 mg/mL	D5W, NS, LR	n/a	[a]	6 d	n/a	n/a	n/a	n/a	n/a	(2)

Flush Compatibility: Sodium chloride 0.9%.[1]

Special Considerations: n/a

Notes

[a] pH of undiluted solution is 7.6.[2]

[b] Protected from light.[2]

REFERENCES

1. Valproate Sodium Injection [package insert]. Lake Zurich, IL: Fresenius Kabi USA, LLC.; May 2019.
2. ASHP's Interactive Handbook on Injectable Drugs, 2020. Bethesda, MD: American Society of Health-System Pharmacists; Accessed December 2020.
3. Lardinois B, Baltzis A, Braibant M, et al. Long-term Physicochemical Stability of Concentrated Solutions of Sodium Valproate in Polypropylene Syringes for Administration in the Intensive Care Unit. *Int J Pharm Compd*. 2019; 23(4):320-23.

DOI 10.37573/9781585286720.188

Vancomycin Hydrochloride

Storage Conditions

Container	Drug Manufacturer	Concentration	Diluents	Osmolality (mOsm/kg)	pH	Temperature: Room	Temperature: Refrig	Temperature: Frozen	Post-thaw Temp: Room	Post-thaw Temp: Refrig	Body Temp	Refer.
CONTAINER												
Bag, Polyolefin	QLM	2 mg/mL	D5W, NS	n/a	[e]	48 hr	48 hr	n/a	n/a	n/a	n/a	(1)
	GSK	10 mg/mL	D5W	n/a	[e]	n/a	23 d	n/a	n/a	n/a	n/a	(1)
	MYL	10 mg/mL	D5W	n/a	[e]	n/a	43 d	n/a	n/a	n/a	n/a	(1)
Bag, Polyvinyl Chloride (PVC)	LI	5 mg/mL	D5W, NS	249, 291	[e]	17 d	n/a	n/a	n/a	n/a	n/a	(1)
	LI	5, 10 mg/mL	D5W	249	[e]	n/a	58 d	n/a	n/a	n/a	n/a	(1)
	LI	5 mg/mL	D5W, NS	249, 291	[e]	24 hr	n/a	n/a	n/a	n/a	n/a	(1)
	QLM	8 mg/mL	D5W, NS	n/a	[e]	24 hr	n/a	n/a	n/a	n/a	n/a	(1)
	QLM	5 mg/mL	D5W, NS	249, 291	[e]	48 hr	7 d[h]	n/a	n/a	n/a	n/a	(1)
	QLM	2 mg/mL	D5W, NS	n/a	[e]	48 hr	48 hr	n/a	n/a	n/a	n/a	(1)
	BRK	1 mg/mL	LR[o]	n/a	n/a	n/a	9 d	n/a	n/a	n/a	n/a	(4)
Syringe, Plastic (Unspecified)	LI	10 mg/mL	D5W, NS, SWFI	n/a	[e]	29 d[a]	12 wk	n/a	n/a	n/a	n/a	(1)
Syringe, Polypropylene	UN	5 mg/mL	D5W, NS	249, 291	[e]	14 d	6 m[b]	n/a	n/a	n/a	n/a	(1)
	MYL	41.66 mg/mL	D5W, NS	n/a	[e]	48 hr	n/a	n/a	n/a	n/a	n/a	(12)
	SZ	25-60 mg/mL[m]	NS	[i]	[k]	24 hr	n/a	n/a	n/a	n/a	n/a	(8)
	SZ	80 mg/mL[m]	NS	[i]	[k]	22 hr[l]	n/a	n/a	n/a	n/a	n/a	(8)
	SZ	62.5, 83.3 mg/mL	D5W	[n]	3.3	48 hr	n/a	n/a	n/a	n/a	n/a	(5)
	SZ	62.5 mg/mL	NS	[n]	3.6	48 hr	n/a	n/a	n/a	n/a	n/a	(5)
	SZ	83.3 mg/mL	NS	[n]	3.6	24 hr	n/a	n/a	n/a	n/a	n/a	(5)
Unspecified	FRK, HOS	4 mg/mL	[p]	n/a	[e]	n/a	4 d	n/a	n/a	n/a	n/a	(1)
	MYL	5 mg/mL	D5LR, D5NS, LR	n/a	[e]	n/a	4 d	n/a	n/a	n/a	n/a	(1)
	FRK, HOS	4 mg/mL	D5W, NS	n/a	[e]	n/a	14 d	n/a	n/a	n/a	n/a	(1)
	MYL	5 mg/mL	D5W, NS	249, 291	[e]	n/a	14 d	n/a	n/a	n/a	n/a	(1)
	LI	5 mg/mL	D5W, NS	249, 291	[e]	7 d	7 d	n/a	n/a	n/a	n/a	(1)
	LI	4, 5 mg/mL	D5W	249	[e]	17 d	n/a	n/a	n/a	n/a	n/a	(1)
	LI	4, 5 mg/mL	NS	291	[e]	24 d	30 d	n/a	n/a	n/a	n/a	(1)

DOI 10.37573/9781585286720.189

Storage Conditions

	Drug Manufacturer	Concentration	Diluents	Osmolality (mOsm/kg)	pH	Temperature			Post-thaw Temp		Body Temp	Refer.
						Room	Refrig	Frozen	Room	Refrig		
CONTAINER												
Vial, Glass	LI	5 mg/mL	D5W, NS	249, 291	[e]	17 d	9 wk	9 wk	n/a	n/a	n/a	(1)(11)
	QLM	2 mg/mL	D5W, NS	n/a	[e]	48 hr	48 hr	n/a	n/a	n/a	n/a	(1)
OTHER INFUSION CONTAINERS												
Accufusor® (Vygon)	HOS	1, 5 mg/mL	D5W, NS	n/a	[e]	7 d	31 d	n/a	n/a	n/a	n/a	(1)
CADD® Cassette (Smiths Medical)	AB	20, 40 mg/mL	D5W	n/a	[e]	4 d	30 d	n/a	n/a	n/a	n/a	(1)
	ES	10 mg/mL	NS, SWFI	n/a	[e]	24 hr	24 hr	n/a	n/a	n/a	n/a	(1)(13)
Dosi-Fuser® (Leventon)	LI	10-20 mg/mL	D5W, NS	n/a	[e]	24 hr[d]	10 d[d]	30 d[d]	24 hr[d]	n/a	n/a	(10)
	HIK	20 mg/mL	D5W, NS	n/a	[e]	72 hr	28 d	31 d	n/a	n/a	n/a	(10)
Easypump® ST/LT (B. Braun)	UN	15 mg/mL	D5W, NS	n/a	[e]	48 hr[d]	14 d[d]	n/a	n/a	n/a	n/a	(7)
	UN	15 mg/mL	NS	n/a	[e]	48 hr[d]	30 d[d]	n/a	n/a	n/a	n/a	(7)
	UN	4 mg/mL	D5W, NS	n/a	[e]	4 d[d]	21 d[d]	n/a	n/a	n/a	n/a	(7)
Homepump Eclipse® / Homepump® (Halyard)	UN	5 mg/mL	D5W	n/a	[e]	17 d[d]	9 wk[d]	n/a	n/a	n/a	n/a	(3)
	UN	5 mg/mL	NS	n/a	[e]	24 hr[d]	14 d[d]	n/a	n/a	n/a	n/a	(3)
	UN	5, 10, 15 mg/mL	NS	n/a	[e]	24 hr[d]	28 d[d]	n/a	n/a	n/a	n/a	(3)
INFUSOR™ (Baxter)[g]	LI	10-20 mg/mL	D5W	n/a	[e]	72 hr[f]	17 d	n/a	n/a	n/a	n/a	(2)
	ACT	5-10 mg/mL	NS	n/a	[e]	n/a	48 hr	n/a	n/a	n/a	24 hr[j]	(2)
	HOS	5-20 mg/mL	NS	n/a	[e]	6 hr	14 d	n/a	n/a	n/a	42 hr[j]	(2)
INTERMATE™ (Baxter)[g]	LI	10-20 mg/mL	D5W, NS	n/a	[e]	24 hr	10 d	30 d	24 hr	n/a	n/a	(2)
	LI	10-20 mg/mL	D5W	n/a	[e]	n/a	n/a	31 d	24 hr	n/a	n/a	(2)
	LI	15 mg/mL	SWFI	n/a	[e]	n/a	10 d	n/a	n/a	n/a	n/a	(2)
	ACT	5-10 mg/mL	NS	n/a	[e]	24 hr	48 hr	n/a	n/a	n/a	n/a	(2)
	HOS	5-20 mg/mL	NS	n/a	[e]	24 hr	14 d	n/a	n/a	n/a	n/a	(2)
SMARTeZ® (Progressive Medical)	UN	5 mg/mL	NS	n/a	[e]	24 hr[d]	14 d[d]	n/a	n/a	n/a	n/a	(9)
	UN	15 mg/mL	NS	n/a	[e]	48 hr[d]	30 d[d]	n/a	n/a	n/a	n/a	(9)
COMMERCIAL PREPARATIONS (RTU)												
GALAXY™ Plastic Container (Baxter)	BA	5 mg/mL	D5W, NS	iso	3-5	n/a	n/a	[c]	72 hr[c]	30 d[c]	n/a	(1)(6)

Flush Compatibility: Sodium chloride 0.9%. Incompatible with heparin.[(1)]

Special Considerations: Administer higher concentrations via a central line to avoid irritation.

Notes

[a] Chemical degradation was dependent on the diluent. This is the shortest time in which the drug degraded 10%.[(1)]

[b] Stored refrigerated followed by 48 hours at room temperature.[(1)]

[c] Frozen expiration date per manufacturer's label. Do not extrapolate commercial premix stability data to extemporaneously compounded solutions. Thaw at room temperature or under refrigeration. Do not force thaw. Do not refreeze.[(1,6)]

[d] Manufacturer extrapolated data from other sources.

[e] pH of a 5% solution in SWFI is 2.5-4.5.[(1)]

[f] Following 17 d refrigerated storage.[(2)]

[g] INTERMATE™/INFUSOR™ Portable Elastomeric Infusion System devices are no longer available in the United States.

[h] Protected from light.[(1)]

[i] Reconstituted the vancomycin with either SWFI or NS. Osmolality at baseline was as follows (measured in mOsmol/kg): 25 mg/mL: SWFI 176, NS 319; 40 mg/mL: SWFI 95, NS 323; 60 mg/mL: SWFI 74, NS 351; 80 mg/mL: SWFI 72, NS 349.[(8)]

[j] Storage temperature: 33°C.[(2)]

[k] pH of 5.1 for SWFI and 5.6 for NS.[(8)]

[l] A visible precipitate was observed at 22 hours in the vancomycin reconstituted with NS. The sample reconstituted with SWFI was stable for 24 hours.[(8)]

[m] Must be infused with a 0.2 micron filter as the number of particles exceeding 10 and 25 microns exceeded the summary of product characteristics.[(8)]

[n] Osmolality was 363-383 mOsm/kg at 62.5 mg/mL and 379-409 mOsm/kg at 83.3 mg/mL.[(5)]

[o] Solution contained: cefepime 2 mg/mL.[(4)]

[p] Diluents: D5LR, D5NS, Isolyte E, NMD5W, LR.[(1)]

REFERENCES

1. ASHP's Interactive Handbook on Injectable Drugs, 2020. Bethesda, MD: American Society of Health-System Pharmacists; Accessed September 2020.
2. Stabforum - Stability Database: Vancomycin, Ontario, Canada: Baxter Healthcare; Accessed February 2021.
3. *Stability Data for Drugs Using Homepump Disposable Ambulatory Infusion Systems (MK-00314 rev 3)*, 2015. Alpharetta, GA: Halyard Health; Updated June 2015.
4. Shakeraneh P, Robinson R, Kufel WD, et al. Chemical and Physical Stability of an Admixture Containing Cefepime and Vancomycin in Lactated Ringer Solution. *Hosp Pharm*. 2020; 0(0):0018578719901278.
5. d'Huart E, Vigneron J, Charmillon A, et al. Physicochemical Stability of Vancomycin at High Concentrations in Polypropylene Syringes. *Can J Hosp Pharm*. 2019; 72(5):360-68.
6. Vancomycin Injection in GALAXY™ Plastic Container (PL 2501) [package insert]. Deerfield, IL: Baxter Healthcare Corporation; January 2021.
7. *Drug Stability for Easypump® ST/LT*, 2020. Bethlehem, PA: B. Braun USA; Updated June 2020.
8. Masse M, Genay S, Martin Mena A, et al. Evaluation of the stability of vancomycin solutions at concentrations used in clinical services. *Eur J Hosp Pharm*. 2020; 27(e1):e87-e92.
9. *SMARTeZ® - Stability Data for Drugs Using Elastomeric Infusion Pumps*, 2020. Fenton, MO: Progressive Medical, Inc.; Updated May 2020.
10. *Drug Stability Table - Dosi-Fuser® Elastomeric Pump (S-CL-00-001v16)*, 2021. Barcelona, Spain: Leventon SAU; Updated May 2021.
11. Das Gupta V, Stewart KR, Nohria S. Stability of vancomycin hydrochloride in 5% dextrose and 0.9% sodium chloride injections. *Am J Hosp Pharm*. 1986; 43(7):1729-31.
12. Godet M, Simar J, Closset M, et al. Stability of Concentrated Solution of Vancomycin Hydrochloride in Syringes for Intensive Care Units. *Pharm Technol Hosp Pharm*. 2018; 3(1):23-30.
13. *Pharmaceutical report on chemical and physical stability of drugs commonly used with CADD® infusion pumps (IN193109GB-122019)*, 2019. Minneapolis, MN: Smiths Medical ASD, Inc.; Updated December 2019.

VinBLAStine Sulfate

Storage Conditions

	Drug Manufacturer	Concentration	Diluents	Osmolality (mOsm/kg)	pH	Temperature: Room	Temperature: Refrig	Frozen	Post-thaw Temp: Room	Post-thaw Temp: Refrig	Body Temp	Refer.
CONTAINER												
Bag, Polyvinyl Chloride (PVC)	LI	0.1 mg/mL	NS, D5W	n/a	[b]	n/a	7 d[a]	n/a	n/a	n/a	n/a	(6)
	LI	0.15 mg/mL	NS	n/a	[b]	8 d	n/a	n/a	n/a	n/a	n/a	(1)
Syringe, Polypropylene	DB	1 mg/mL	SWFI	n/a	[b]	30 d[a]	30 d	n/a	n/a	n/a	n/a	(2)
	LI	1 mg/mL	NS	n/a	[b]	30 d[a]	n/a	n/a	n/a	n/a	n/a	(3)(6)
	DB	1 mg/mL	unspec.	n/a	[b]	23 d[a]	31 d[a]	n/a	n/a	n/a	n/a	(6)
Test Tube, Polypropylene	LI	0.02 mg/mL	D5W, LR, NS	n/a	[b]	21 d[a]	21 d[a]	n/a	n/a	n/a	n/a	(4)(6)
Unspecified	LI	0.02 mg/mL	D5W, LR, NS	n/a	[b]	n/a	n/a	28 d	n/a	n/a	n/a	(4)(6)
Vial, Glass	UN	0.05 mg/mL	NS	n/a	[b]	21 d[a]	21 d[a]	n/a	n/a	n/a	n/a	(6)
	LI	1 mg/mL	SWFI	n/a	[b]	n/a	21 d[a]	n/a	n/a	n/a	n/a	(4)
OTHER INFUSION CONTAINERS												
Dosi-Fuser® (Leventon)	UN	0.015 mg/mL	NS	n/a	[b]	n/a	11 wk[e]	n/a	n/a	n/a	48 hr[e]	(7)
	UN	1 mg/mL	NS	n/a	[b]	21 d	21 d	n/a	n/a	n/a	n/a	(7)
INFUSOR™ (Baxter)[d]	LI	0.015 mg/mL	NS	n/a	[b]	n/a	11 wk[c]	n/a	n/a	n/a	48 hr[c]	(5)

Flush Compatibility: Sodium chloride 0.9%, heparin.[6]

Special Considerations: Affix warning sticker to individual dosage container stating: FOR INTRAVENOUS USE ONLY – FATAL IF GIVEN BY OTHER ROUTES.[6]

Notes

[a] Protected from light.

[b] pH of undiluted solution is 3.5-5.[6]

[c] Storage at 5°C for 11 weeks, followed by 48 hr at 33°C.[5]

[d] INTERMATE™/INFUSOR™ Portable Elastomeric Infusion System devices are no longer available in the United States.

[e] Manufacturer extrapolated data from other sources.[7]

DOI 10.37573/9781585286720.190

REFERENCES

1. Vyas HM, Baptista RJ, Mitrano FP, et al. Drug stability guidelines for a continuous infusion chemotherapy program. *Hosp Pharm*. 1987; 22(7):685-7.
2. Weir PJ, Ireland DS. Chemical stability of cytarabine and vinblastine injections. *Br J Pharm Prac*. 1990; 12:53-4,60.
3. Girona V, Prat J, Pujol M, et al. Stability of vinblastine sulphate in 0.9% sodium chloride in polypropylene syringes. *Boll Chim Farm*. 1996; 135(7):413-4.
4. Beijnen JH, Vendrig DE, Underberg WJ. Stability of vinca alkaloid anticancer drugs in three commonly used infusion fluids. *J Parenter Sci Technol*. 1989; 43(2):84-7.
5. Stabforum - Stability Database: Vinblastine, Ontario, Canada: Baxter Healthcare; Accessed December 2020.
6. ASHP's Interactive Handbook on Injectable Drugs, 2020. Bethesda, MD: American Society of Health-System Pharmacists; Accessed December 2020.
7. *Drug Stability Table - Dosi-Fuser® Elastomeric Pump (S-CL-00-001v16)*, 2021. Barcelona, Spain: Leventon SAU; Updated May 2021.

VinCRIStine Sulfate

Storage Conditions

	Drug Manufacturer	Concentration	Diluents	Osmolality (mOsm/kg)	pH	Temperature: Room	Temperature: Refrig	Temperature: Frozen	Post-thaw Temp: Room	Post-thaw Temp: Refrig	Body Temp	Refer.
CONTAINER												
Bag, Polyolefin	LI	0.001 mg/mL	NS[u]	n/a	[i]	72 hr	n/a	n/a	n/a	n/a	n/a	(16)
	LI	0.0014 mg/mL	NS[v]	n/a	[i]	72 hr	n/a	n/a	n/a	n/a	n/a	(16)
	LI	0.0016 mg/mL	NS[w]	n/a	[i]	72 hr[c]	n/a	n/a	n/a	n/a	n/a	(16)
	LI	0.005 mg/mL	NS[g]	n/a	[i]	n/a	124 hr[c]	n/a	n/a	n/a	124 hr[c][f]	(6)(8)
	LI	0.01 mg/mL	NS[j]	n/a	[i]	n/a	124 hr[c]	n/a	n/a	n/a	124 hr[c][f]	(6)(8)
	LI	0.016 mg/mL	NS[d]	n/a	[i]	n/a	124 hr[c]	n/a	n/a	n/a	124 hr[f]	(6)(8)
	UN	0.02 mg/mL	D5W	n/a	[i]	24 hr	n/a	n/a	n/a	n/a	n/a	(6)
Bag, Polyvinyl Chloride (PVC)	LI	0.01, 0.02, 0.04, 0.06, 0.08, 0.12 mg/mL	NS	n/a	[i]	48 hr[e]	7 d[e]	n/a	n/a	n/a	n/a	(6)(7)
	LI	0.02 mg/mL	D5W, NS	n/a	[i]	n/a	7 d[c]	n/a	n/a	n/a	n/a	(5)(6)
	UN	0.02 mg/mL	D5W	n/a	[i]	24 hr	n/a	n/a	n/a	n/a	n/a	(6)
	LI	0.028 mg/mL	NS	n/a	[i]	5 d[t]	24 hr	n/a	n/a	n/a	n/a	(15)
	LI	0.036 mg/mL	NS[a]	n/a	3.5-3.6	n/a	7 d[b][c]	n/a	n/a	n/a	4 d[b]	(1)(6)
Syringe, Polypropylene	LI	0.025, 0.05, 0.1, 0.15 mg/mL	NS	n/a	[i]	48 hr[e]	7 d[e]	n/a	n/a	n/a	n/a	(6)(7)
Test Tubes, Polypropylene	LI	0.02 mg/mL	D5W, LR, NS	n/a	[i]	21 d[c]	21 d[c]	n/a	n/a	n/a	n/a	(2)(6)
Unspecified	LI	0.033 mg/mL	D2.5½NS, NS[k]	n/a	[i]	14 d[c]	n/a	14 d[c]	n/a	n/a	14 d[c][l]	(6)(14)
	LI	0.02 mg/mL	D5W, LR, NS	n/a	[i]	n/a	n/a	24 d	n/a	n/a	n/a	(2)(6)
Vial, Glass	UN	0.02 mg/mL	D5W	n/a	[i]	24 hr	n/a	n/a	n/a	n/a	n/a	(6)
	LI	1 mg/mL	SWFI	n/a	[i]	n/a	21 d[c]	n/a	n/a	n/a	n/a	(2)
OTHER INFUSION CONTAINERS												
Dosi-Fuser® (Leventon)	LI	0.04-0.2 mg/mL	NS	n/a	[i]	10 d[n]	n/a	n/a	n/a	n/a	n/a	(9)
	LI	0.2 mg/mL	NS	n/a	[i]	10 d[n]	29 d[n]	n/a	n/a	n/a	n/a	(9)
	TE	1 mg/mL	NS	n/a	[i]	21 d	25 d	n/a	n/a	n/a	n/a	(9)

DOI 10.37573/9781585286720.191

Storage Conditions

	Drug Manufacturer	Concentration	Diluents	Osmolality (mOsm/kg)	pH	Temperature Room	Temperature Refrig	Temperature Frozen	Post-thaw Temp Room	Post-thaw Temp Refrig	Body Temp	Refer.
OTHER INFUSION CONTAINERS												
Easypump® ST/LT (B. Braun)	UN	1 mg/mL	NS	n/a	n/a	21 d	n/a	n/a	n/a	n/a	n/a	(11)
Graseby™ 9000 Cassette (Graseby Medical)	FAU	0.0002 mg/mL	SWFI[h]	n/a	4.7-4.95	n/a	14 d[c]	n/a	n/a	n/a	7 d[c]	(4)(6)
INFUSOR™ (Baxter)[m]	HOS	0.005 mg/mL	NS[o]	n/a	4.25-4.28	n/a	14 d	n/a	n/a	n/a	7 d[r]	(12)
	HOS	0.01 mg/mL	NS[p]	n/a	4.16-4.20	n/a	14 d	n/a	n/a	n/a	7 d	(12)
	LI	0.014 mg/mL	NS[s]	n/a	[i]	24 hr	5 d	n/a	n/a	n/a	n/a	(15)
	HOS	0.016 mg/mL	NS[q]	n/a	4.12-4.21	n/a	14 d	n/a	n/a	n/a	7 d[r]	(12)
	LI	0.036 mg/mL	NS[a]	n/a	3.5-3.6	n/a	7 d[b](c)	n/a	n/a	n/a	4 d[b]	(1)(6)
	LI	0.04-0.2 mg/mL	NS	n/a	[i]	10 d	n/a	n/a	n/a	n/a	n/a	(3)
	LI	0.2 mg/mL	NS	n/a	[i]	n/a	29 d	n/a	n/a	n/a	n/a	(3)
SMARTeZ® (Progressive Medical)	UN	1 mg/mL	NS	n/a	n/a	21 d[n]	n/a	n/a	n/a	n/a	n/a	(13)

Flush Compatibility: Sodium chloride 0.9%, heparin.[6]

Special Considerations: Affix special warning sticker to individual dosage container stating: FOR INTRAVENOUS USE ONLY — FATAL IF GIVEN BY OTHER ROUTES.[6,7,10]

Notes

[a] Solution contained: DOXOrubicin (NY) 1.67 mg/mL.[1,6]

[b] Storage temperature: 4°C for 7 days, followed by 4 days at 35°C.[1]

[c] Protected from light.

[d] Solution contained: DOXOrubicin (PHU) 400 mcg/mL and etoposide phosphate (BMS) 2,000 mcg/mL.[6,8]

[e] Storage temperature: 4°C for 7 days, followed by 48 hours at room temperature (23°C).[6,7]

[f] Storage temperature: 35-40°C.[6,8]

[g] Solution contained: DOXOrubicin (PHU) 120 mcg/mL and etoposide phosphate (BMS) 600 mcg/mL.[6,8]

[h] Solution contained: DOXOrubicin (PHU) 2 mg/mL.[4,6]

[i] pH of undiluted solution is 4-5.[10]

[j] Solution contained: DOXOrubicin (PHU) 240 mcg/mL and etoposide phosphate (BMS) 1,200 mcg/mL.[6,8]

[k] Solution contained: DOXOrubicin (FA) 1.4 mg/mL.[6,14]

[l] Storage temperature: 30°C and 37°C.[6]

[m] INTERMATE™/INFUSOR™ Portable Elastomeric Infusion System devices are no longer available in the United States.

[n] Manufacturer extrapolated data from other sources.

[o] Solution contained: DOXOrubicin (ARR) 120 mcg/mL and etoposide phosphate (BMS) 600 mcg/mL.[(12)]

[p] Solution contained: DOXOrubicin (ARR) 240 mcg/mL and etoposide phosphate (BMS) 1,200 mcg/mL.[(12)]

[q] Solution contained: DOXOrubicin (ARR) 400 mcg/mL and etoposide phosphate (BMS) 2,000 mcg/mL.[(12)]

[r] Storage temperature: 35°C after 14 d at 4°C.[(12)]

[s] Solution contained: ondansetron 0.48 mg/mL and DOXOrubicin 0.4 mg/mL at 5 days at 4°C followed by 24 hours at 24°C.[(15)]

[t] Storage temperature: 4°C for 24 hours, followed by 5 days at 30°C.[(15)]

[u] Solution contained: DOXOrubicin (PHU) 25 mcg/mL and etoposide (BMS) 125 mcg/mL.[(16)]

[v] Solution contained: DOXOrubicin (PHU) 35 mcg/mL and etoposide (BMS) 175 mcg/mL.[(16)]

[w] Solution contained: DOXOrubicin (PHU) 40 mcg/mL and etoposide (BMS) 200 mcg/mL at 31-33°C.[(16)]

REFERENCES

1. Nyhammar EK, Johansson SG, Seiving BE. Stability of doxorubicin hydrochloride and vincristine sulfate in two portable infusion-pump reservoirs. *Am J Health Syst Pharm*. 1996; 53(10):1171-3.
2. Beijnen JH, Vendrig DE, Underberg WJ. Stability of vinca alkaloid anticancer drugs in three commonly used infusion fluids. *J Parenter Sci Technol*. 1989; 43(2):84-7.
3. Stabforum - Stability Database: Vincristine, Ontario, Canada: Baxter Healthcare; Accessed February 2021.
4. Priston M, Sewell G. Stability of three cytotoxic drug infusions in the Graseby 9000 ambulatory infusion pump. *J Oncol Pharm Pract*. 1998; 4(3):143-49.
5. Dine T, Luyckx M, Cazin JC, et al. Stability and compatibility studies of vinblastine, vincristine, vindesine and vinorelbine with PVC infusion bags. *Int J Pharm*. 1991; 77(2):279-85.
6. ASHP's Interactive Handbook on Injectable Drugs, 2020. Bethesda, MD: American Society of Health-System Pharmacists; Accessed August 2020.
7. Trissel LA, Zhang Y, Cohen MR. The Stability of Diluted Vincristine Sulfate Used as a Deterrent to Inadvertent Intrathecal Injection. *Hosp Pharm*. 2001; 36(7):740-45.
8. Yuan P, Grimes GJ, Shankman SE, et al. Compatibility and stability of vincristine sulfate, doxorubicin hydrochloride, and etoposide phosphate in 0.9% sodium chloride injection. *Am J Health Syst Pharm*. 2001; 58(7):594-8.
9. *Drug Stability Table - Dosi-Fuser® Elastomeric Pump (S-CL-00-001v16)*, 2021. Barcelona, Spain: Leventon SAU; Updated May 2021.
10. VinCRIStine Sulfate Injection, USP [package insert]. Lake Forest, IL: Hospira, Inc.; March 2021.
11. *Drug Stability for Easypump® ST/LT*, 2020. Bethlehem, PA: B. Braun USA; Updated June 2020.
12. Svirskis D, Behera S, Naidoo N, et al. Stability of vincristine sulfate, doxorubicin hydrochloride and etoposide phosphate admixtures in polyisoprene elastomeric pump supporting transition of the EPOCH regimen to outpatient care. *J Oncol Pharm Pract*. 2019; 25(4):831-40.
13. *SMARTeZ® - Stability Data for Drugs Using Elastomeric Infusion Pumps*, 2020. Fenton, MO: Progressive Medical, Inc.; Updated May 2020.
14. Beijnen JH, Neef C, Meuwissen OJ, et al. Stability of intravenous admixtures of doxorubicin and vincristine. *Am J Hosp Pharm*. 1986; 43(12):3022-7.
15. Stewart JT, Warren FW, King DT, et al. Stability of ondansetron hydrochloride, doxorubicin hydrochloride, and dacarbazine or vincristine sulfate in elastomeric portable infusion devices and polyvinyl chloride bags. *Am J Health Syst Pharm*. 1997; 54(8):915-20.
16. Wolfe JL, Thoma LA, Du C, et al. Compatibility and stability of vincristine sulfate, doxorubicin hydrochloride, and etoposide in 0.9% sodium chloride injection. *Am J Health Syst Pharm*. 1999; 56(10):985-9.

Vinorelbine Tartrate

Storage Conditions

	Drug Manufacturer	Concentration	Diluents	Osmolality (mOsm/kg)	pH	Temperature Room	Temperature Refrig	Temperature Frozen	Post-thaw Temp Room	Post-thaw Temp Refrig	Body Temp	Refer.
CONTAINER												
Bag, Polyvinyl Chloride (PVC)	PRF	0.5-2 mg/mL	D5W, NS, D5½NS, ½NS, R, LR	n/a	[c]	24 hr	24 hr	n/a	n/a	n/a	n/a	(4)
	PRF	0.5 mg/mL	D5W	n/a	[c]	n/a	7 d[a]	n/a	n/a	n/a	n/a	(2)
	PRF	0.5 mg/mL	NS	n/a	[c]	n/a	3 d[a]	n/a	n/a	n/a	n/a	(2)
	GW	0.5, 2 mg/mL	D5W, NS	n/a	[c]	5 d	n/a	n/a	n/a	n/a	n/a	(1)
Syringe, Polypropylene	PRF	1.5-3 mg/mL	D5W, NS	n/a	[c]	24 hr	24 hr	n/a	n/a	n/a	n/a	(4)
OTHER INFUSION CONTAINERS												
INTERMATE™ (Baxter)[b]	PRF	0.1-2 mg/mL	D5W, NS	n/a	[c]	24 hr	21 d[d]	n/a	n/a	n/a	n/a	(3)

Flush Compatibility: Sodium chloride 0.9%.[1]

Special Considerations: Store vials protected from light, refrigerate, do not freeze.[4] If dispensed in a syringe containing an individual dosage, label the syringe with this statement: WARNING — FOR IV USE ONLY! FATAL if given intrathecally.[1]

Notes

[a] Protected from light.[2]

[b] INTERMATE™/INFUSOR™ Portable Elastomeric Infusion System devices are no longer available in the United States.

[c] pH of undiluted solution is 3.5.[1]

[d] 21 days refrigerated, followed by 24 hours at room temperature.[3]

REFERENCES

1. ASHP's Interactive Handbook on Injectable Drugs, 2020. Bethesda, MD: American Society of Health-System Pharmacists; Accessed August 2020.
2. Dine T, Luyckx M, Cazin JC, et al. Stability and compatibility studies of vinblastine, vincristine, vindesine and vinorelbine with PVC infusion bags. *Int J Pharm*. 1991; 77(2):279-85.
3. Stabforum - Stability Database: Vinorelbine, Ontario, Canada: Baxter Healthcare; Accessed February 2021.
4. Navelbine® (Vinorelbine Tartrate) Injection [package insert]. Pierre Fabre Pharmaceuticals, Inc.; March 2014.

DOI 10.37573/9781585286720.192

Voriconazole

Storage Conditions

	Drug Manufacturer	Concentration	Diluents	Osmolality (mOsm/kg)	pH	Temperature			Post-thaw Temp		Body Temp	Refer.
						Room	Refrig	Frozen	Room	Refrig		
CONTAINER												
Bag, Polyolefin	PF	2 mg/mL	NS	n/a	5.7	8 d[c]	8 d[c]	n/a	n/a	n/a	n/a	(4)
	PF	2 mg/mL	NS	n/a	n/a	n/a	32 d	n/a	n/a	n/a	n/a	(1)
	PF	2 mg/mL	D5W	n/a	4.8	5 d[c]	6 d[c]	n/a	n/a	n/a	n/a	(4)
Bag, Polyvinyl Chloride (PVC)	PF	0.5 mg/mL	NS	n/a	5.6-5.9	<48 hr[b][c][d]	11 d[a][c]	n/a	n/a	n/a	n/a	(2)
	PF	0.5 mg/mL	D5W	n/a	4.2-4.4	<48 hr[b][c][d]	9 d[a][c]	n/a	n/a	n/a	n/a	(2)
	PF	4 mg/mL	D5W	n/a	n/a	n/a	15 d	n/a	n/a	n/a	n/a	(1)
Unspecified	PF	0.5-5 mg/mL	NS, LR, D5LR, D5½NS, D5W, ½NS, D5NS	n/a	n/a	[b]	24 hr[b]	n/a	n/a	n/a	n/a	(3)
OTHER INFUSION CONTAINERS												
INTERMATE™ (Baxter)[e]	PF	2 mg/mL	D5W, NS	n/a	6.1, 5.6	4 hr	4 d	n/a	n/a	n/a	4 hr	(1)(5)

Flush Compatibility: Sodium chloride 0.9%, heparin.[1,6]

Special Considerations: Manufacturer recommends removing and discarding volume of infusion diluent equal to the volume of 10 mg/mL concentrate to be added in order to achieve recommended final concentration range. Do not use vial if vacuum does not draw in diluent. [3]

Notes

[a] There was evidence of drug sorption by PVC bags at the end of the stability study.

[b] Manufacturer recommends using immediately due to preservative free formulation, however the reconstituted solution is stable for 24 hr if refrigerated.[3]

[c] Protected from light.

[d] Based on analysis at time 0 and 2 d interval post preparation. The voriconazole content dropped down to 88.3 and 86.6% in NS or D5W respectively at 2 days.[4]

[e] INTERMATE™/INFUSOR™ Portable Elastomeric Infusion System devices are no longer available in the United States.

DOI 10.37573/9781585286720.193

REFERENCES

1. ASHP's Interactive Handbook on Injectable Drugs, 2020. Bethesda, MD: American Society of Health-System Pharmacists; Accessed August 2020.
2. Adams AI, Morimoto LN, Meneghini LZ, et al. Treatment of invasive fungal infections: stability of voriconazole infusion solutions in PVC bags. *Braz J Infect Dis*. 2008; 12(5):400-4.
3. Vfend® (Voriconazole) Injection [package insert]. New York, NY: Roerig Div Pfizer, Inc.; September 2020.
4. Sahraoui L, Chiadmi F, Schlatter J, et al. Stability of voriconazole injection in 0.9% sodium chloride and 5% dextrose injections. *Am J Health Syst Pharm*. 2006; 63(15):1423-6.
5. Harmanjeet H, Zaidi STR, Ming LC, et al. Physicochemical stability of voriconazole in elastomeric devices. *Eur J Hosp Pharm*. 2018; 25(e2):e88-e92.
6. Cayo L. Compatibility of Commonly Used IV Drugs. *Pharm Pract News*. 2018; SE2018:31-8.

Ziconotide Acetate

Storage Conditions

	Drug Manufacturer	Concentration	Diluents	Osmolality (mOsm/kg)	pH	Temperature			Post-thaw Temp		Body Temp	Refer.
						Room	Refrig	Frozen	Room	Refrig		
CONTAINER												
Bag, Polyolefin	EI	0.2 mcg/mL	NS[a]	n/a	[c]	14 d	n/a	n/a	n/a	n/a	n/a	(1)
Syringe, Plastic (Unspecified)	EI	0.1, 0.25, 0.5, 0.75 mcg/mL	NS[o]	1030	3.46	n/a	30 d	n/a	n/a	n/a	n/a	(6)
	EI	0.1, 0.25, 0.5, 0.75 mcg/mL	NS	308	6.11	n/a	30 d	n/a	n/a	n/a	n/a	(6)
	ELN	25 mcg/mL	[d]	n/a	[c]	n/a	28 d	n/a	n/a	n/a	n/a	(9)
Vial, Plastic (Unspecified)	ELN	25 mcg/mL	[h]	n/a	5.8	n/a	30 d[b]	n/a	n/a	n/a	30 d[b]	(4)
	ELN	25 mcg/mL	[j]	n/a	6.0	n/a	30 d[b]	n/a	n/a	n/a	n/a	(4)
	ELN	25 mcg/mL	[d]	n/a	[c]	n/a	28 d	n/a	n/a	n/a	28 d	(7)
Vial, Polymethylpentene	ELN	25 mcg/mL	[e]	n/a	[c]	n/a	25 d	n/a	n/a	n/a	n/a	(8)
	ELN	25 mcg/mL	[f]	n/a	[c]	n/a	17 d	n/a	n/a	n/a	n/a	(8)
	ELN	25 mcg/mL	[g]	n/a	[c]	n/a	22 d	n/a	n/a	n/a	22 d	(5)
OTHER INFUSION CONTAINERS												
SynchroMed® II Implantable Pump (Medtronic)	ELN	25 mcg/mL	[g]	n/a	[c]	n/a	n/a	n/a	n/a	n/a	22 d	(5)
	ELN	25 mcg/mL	[d]	n/a	[c]	n/a	n/a	n/a	n/a	n/a	28 d	(7)
	ELN	25 mcg/mL	[i]	n/a	[c]	n/a	n/a	n/a	n/a	n/a	26 d	(9)
	ELN	25 mcg/mL	[e]	n/a	[c]	n/a	n/a	n/a	n/a	n/a	19 d	(8)
	ELN	25 mcg/mL	[k]	n/a	[c]	n/a	n/a	n/a	n/a	n/a	34 d	(9)
	ELN	25 mcg/mL	[l]	n/a	[c]	n/a	n/a	n/a	n/a	n/a	19 d	(9)
	ELN	25 mcg/mL	[f]	n/a	[c]	n/a	n/a	n/a	n/a	n/a	8 d	(8)
	ELN	25 mcg/mL	[m]	n/a	[c]	n/a	n/a	n/a	n/a	n/a	33 d	(9)
	ELN	25 mcg/mL	[h]	n/a	5.8	n/a	n/a	n/a	n/a	n/a	12 d[b]	(4)
	ELN	25 mcg/mL	[j]	n/a	6.0	n/a	n/a	n/a	n/a	n/a	20 d[b]	(4)
	ELN	25 mcg/mL	Undiluted	n/a	[c]	n/a	n/a	n/a	n/a	n/a	15 wk[b]	(3)
	ELN	25 mcg/mL	NS	n/a	[c]	n/a	n/a	n/a	n/a	n/a	53 d[b]	(3)
	ELN	25 mcg/mL	[n]	n/a	[c]	n/a	n/a	n/a	n/a	n/a	6 d	(7)
	ELN	100 mcg/mL	Undiluted	n/a	[c]	n/a	n/a	n/a	n/a	n/a	158 d[b]	(3)

DOI 10.37573/9781585286720.194

Flush Compatibility: n/a

Special Considerations: Refrigerate diluted and undiluted product. Protect from light and freezing. For intrathecal use only.[2]

Notes

[a] Solution contained: morphine sulfate 2 mg/mL (LAV) and ropivacaine 6 mg/mL (FRE).

[b] Data is from previously exposed (i.e. rinsed and/or infused) pumps tested in vitro.

[c] pH of undiluted solution is 4-5.[2]

[d] Solution contained: cloNIDine HCl (dissolved powder) 2 mg/mL (BB).

[e] Solution contained: HYDROmorphone HCl (dissolved powder) 35 mg/mL (BB).

[f] Solution contained: morphine sulfate (dissolved powder) 35 mg/mL (BB).

[g] Solution contained: bupivacaine HCl (dissolved powder) 5 mg/mL (BB).

[h] Solution contained: commercial Lioresal Intrathecal® (baclofen) 1.5 mg/mL (SAO).

[i] Solution contained: fentaNYL citrate (dissolved powder) 1 mg/mL (BB).

[j] Solution contained: baclofen (dissolved powder) 2 mg/mL (BB).

[k] Solution contained: morphine sulfate (dissolved powder) 10 mg/mL (BB).

[l] Solution contained: morphine sulfate (powder) 20 mg/mL (BB).

[m] Solution contained: SUFentanil citrate (powder) 1 mg/mL (BB).

[n] Solution contained: cloNIDine HCl (dissolved powder) 2 mg/mL (BB) and morphine sulfate (dissolved powder) 35 mg/mL (BB).

[o] Solution contained: ropivacaine 7.5 mg/mL (ASZ), morphine sulfate 7.5 mg/mL (LAV) and cloNIDine 15 mcg/mL (BI).

REFERENCES

1. Robert J, Sorrieul J, Rossignol E, et al. Chemical Stability of Morphine, Ropivacaine, and Ziconotide in Combination for Intrathecal Analgesia. *Int J Pharm Compd*. 2017; 21(4):347-51.
2. Prialt® (Ziconotide) Injection [package insert]. Lake Forest, IL: TerSera Therapeutics; August 2019.
3. Shields DE, Liu W, Gunning K, et al. Statistical evaluation of the chemical stability of ziconotide solutions during simulated intrathecal administration. *J Pain Symptom Manage*. 2008; 36(1):e4-6.
4. Shields D, Montenegro R, Aclan J. Chemical stability of admixtures combining ziconotide with baclofen during simulated intrathecal administration. *Neuromodulation*. 2007; 10 Suppl 1:12-7.
5. Shields D, Montenegro R, Aclan J. Chemical stability of an admixture combining ziconotide and bupivacaine during simulated intrathecal administration. *Neuromodulation*. 2007; 10 Suppl 1:1-5.
6. Dupoiron D, Richard H, Chabert-Desnot V, et al. In vitro stability of low-concentration ziconotide alone or in admixtures in intrathecal pumps. *Neuromodulation*. 2014; 17(5):472-82; discussion 82.
7. Shields D, Montenegro R. Chemical stability of ziconotide-clonidine hydrochloride admixtures with and without morphine sulfate during simulated intrathecal administration. *Neuromodulation*. 2007; 10 Suppl 1:6-11.
8. Shields D, Montenegro R, Ragusa M. Chemical Stability of Admixtures Combining Ziconotide with Morphine or Hydromorphone During Simulated Intrathecal Administration. *Neuromodulation*. 2005; 8(4):257-63.
9. ASHP's Interactive Handbook on Injectable Drugs, 2020. Bethesda, MD: American Society of Health-System Pharmacists; Accessed July 2020.

Zidovudine

Storage Conditions

	Drug Manufacturer	Concentration	Diluents	Osmolality (mOsm/kg)	pH	Temperature: Room	Temperature: Refrig	Temperature: Frozen	Post-thaw Temp: Room	Post-thaw Temp: Refrig	Body Temp	Refer.
CONTAINER												
Bag, Polyvinyl Chloride (PVC)	BW	4 mg/mL	D5W, NS	n/a	[a]	8 d	8 d	n/a	n/a	n/a	n/a	(1)
OTHER INFUSION CONTAINERS												
Dosi-Fuser® (Leventon)	WEL	4 mg/mL	D5W	n/a	[a]	8 d[b]	8 d[b]	n/a	n/a	n/a	n/a	(2)

Flush Compatibility: Sodium chloride 0.9%, heparin.[1]

Special Considerations: Dilute in D5W to a concentration no greater than 4 mg/mL.[1]

Notes

[a] pH of undiluted solution is 5.5.[1]

[b] Manufacturer extrapolated data from other sources.

REFERENCES

1. ASHP's Interactive Handbook on Injectable Drugs, 2020. Bethesda, MD: American Society of Health-System Pharmacists; Accessed December 2020.
2. *Drug Stability Table - Dosi-Fuser® Elastomeric Pump (S-CL-00-001v16)*, 2021. Barcelona, Spain: Leventon SAU; Updated May 2021.

DOI 10.37573/9781585286720.195

Zoledronic Acid

Storage Conditions

	Drug Manufacturer	Concentration	Diluents	Osmolality (mOsm/kg)	pH	Temperature Room	Temperature Refrig	Temperature Frozen	Post-thaw Temp Room	Post-thaw Temp Refrig	Body Temp	Refer.
CONTAINER												
Bag, Polyethylene	NVA	0.03-0.04 mg/mL	NS, D5W	n/a	[d]	[a]	24 hr	n/a	n/a	n/a	n/a	(1)(2)
Bag, Polypropylene	NVA	0.03-0.04 mg/mL	NS, D5W	n/a	[d]	[a]	24 hr	n/a	n/a	n/a	n/a	(1)(2)
Bag, Polyvinyl Chloride (PVC)	NVA	0.03-0.04 mg/mL	NS, D5W	n/a	[d]	[a]	24 hr	n/a	n/a	n/a	n/a	(1)(2)
OTHER INFUSION CONTAINERS												
INFUSOR™ (Baxter)[f]	NVA	0.04 mg/mL	D5W	n/a	n/a	24 hr	n/a	n/a	n/a	n/a	24 hr[e]	(4)
COMMERCIAL PREPARATIONS (RTU)												
Vial, Glass	NVA	0.05 mg/mL	RTU[b]	n/a	6-7	[c]	24 hr[c][g]	n/a	n/a	n/a	n/a	(3)
	NVA	0.04 mg/mL	RTU[b]	n/a	[d]	[c]	24 hr[c][g]	n/a	n/a	n/a	n/a	(1)

Flush Compatibility: Sodium chloride 0.9%.[1,3]

Special Considerations: Infuse in a separate line from all other medication. Do not mix with calcium or other divalent cation-containing solutions (e.g., LR.).[1,2,4] Administer solutions at room temperature.[1,3] Manufacturer recommends not preparing in syringes to avoid inadvertent injection.[1]

Notes

[a] Manufacturer recommends immediate use after dilution if not refrigerated; time between reconstitution, dilution, refrigerated storage, and end of administration must not exceed 24 hr.[1,2]

[b] All formulations of zoledronic acid contain various amounts of mannitol.

[c] Expiration date per manufacturer's label. After opening, may be refrigerated for 24 hr prior to administration.[1,3]

[d] pH of 0.7% solution in SWFI is 2.[1,3] pH of 0.05 mg/mL RTU is 6 to7.[3] pH of 0.04 mg/mL RTU is 5.5 to 6.5.[5] The reconstituted zoledronic acid concentrate for injection has a pH from 5.7 to 6.7.[5]

[e] 24 hr at 33°C following 24 hr at 25°C.[4]

[f] INTERMATE™/INFUSOR™ Portable Elastomeric Infusion System devices are no longer available in the United States.

[g] Do not extrapolate commercial premix stability data to extemporaneously prepared solutions.

DOI 10.37573/9781585286720.196

REFERENCES

1. Zometa® (Zoledronic Acid) Injection [package insert]. East Hanover, NJ: Novartis Pharmaceuticals Corporation; June 2020.
2. Zometa® Reconstitution, Stability, Storage and Administration Medication Information Letter (Ref#: 1-202375596) [personal communication]. East Hanover, NJ: Novartis Pharmaceuticals Corporation; 2008:4.
3. Reclast® (Zoledronic Acid) Injection [package insert]. East Hanover, NJ: Novartis Pharmaceuticals Corporation; April 2020.
4. Stabforum - Stability Database: Zoledronic Acid, Ontario, Canada: Baxter Healthcare; Accessed January 2021.
5. ASHP's Interactive Handbook on Injectable Drugs, 2020. Bethesda, MD: American Society of Health-System Pharmacists; Accessed August 2020.

PART III

APPENDICES

APPENDIX A: MANUFACTURER AND COMPENDIUM ABBREVIATIONS[7]

A

AAB	Apoteket AB
AAP	AAPER Alcohol & Chemical Co
AB	Abbott
ABI	Abic Ltd.
ABV	AbbVie
ABX	Abraxis
ACC	American Critical Care
ACD	Accord Healthcare
ACN	Actelion
ACT	Actavis
AD	Adria
ADM	ADMA Biologics, Inc.
AGT	Aguettant
AH	Allen & Hanburys
AHP	Ascot Hospital Pharmaceuticals
AKN	Akorn
ALP	Alpharma
ALT	Altana-Nycomed
ALV	Alveda Pharma
ALZ	Alza
AM	ASTA Medica
AMB	Amneal Biosciences
AMD	Amdipharm
AMG	Amgen
AMP	Amphastar
AMR	American Regent
AMS	Amerisource
AND	Andromaco
ANT	Antigen
AP	Asta-Pharma
APC	Apothecon
APO	Apotex
APP	American Pharmaceutical Partners
APT	Aspen Triton
AQ	American Quinine
AR	Armour
ARD	Ardeapharm
AS	Arnar-Stone
ASC	Ascot
ASH	Ash-Stevens
ASM	AstraMedica
ASN	Aspen Pharmacare Holdings
ASP	Astellas Pharma
AST	Astra
ASZ	AstraZeneca
AT	Alpha Therapeutic
AUB	Aurobindo
AUR	Auromedics
AVD	Avadel Legacy Pharmaceuticals
AVE	Aventis
AVG	Alvogen
AW	Asta Werke
AY	Ayerst

B

BA	Baxter
BAN	Banyu Pharmaceuticals
BAX	Baxalta, Inc.
BAY	Bayer
BB	B & B Pharmaceuticals
BC	Bencard
BCT	BioCryst Pharmaceuticals
BD	Becton, Dickinson and Company
BE	Beecham
BED	Bedford
BEH	Behring
BEL	R. Bellon
BFM	Bieffe Medital
BGD	Biogen-Idec
BI	Boehringer Ingelheim
BIO	Bioniche Pharma
BK	Berk
BKN	Baker Norton
BM	Boehringer Mannheim
BMS	Bristol-Myers Squibb
BN	Breon
BP	British Pharmacopeia
BPC	British Pharmaceutical Codex
BPH	Biotest Pharmaceuticals

DOI 10.37573/9781585286720.PT3001

BPL	Bio Products Laboratories
BR	Bristol
BRD	Bracco Diagnostics
BRK	Breckenridge Pharmaceutical, Inc.
BRN	B. Braun
BRT	Britianna
BT	Boots
BTK	Biotika
BV	Ben Venue
BW	Burroughs Wellcome
BX	Berlex

C

CA	Calmic
CAD	Cadence Pharmaceuticals
CAN	Cangene bioPharma, Inc.
CAR	Cardinal Health
CBH	CSL Behring
CE	Carlo Erba
CEL	Celltrion
CEN	Centocor
CER	Cerenex
CET	Cetus
CG	Ciba Geigy
CGC	Ciba Geigy Canada, LTD
CH	Lab. Choay Societe Anonyme
CHI	Chiron
CHS	Chiesi
CI	Ciba
CIS	CIS US
CL	Clintec
CLA	Claris Lifesciences
CMB	Cumberland
CN	Cannaught
CNF	Centrafarm
CO	Cole
COM	CommScope
COR	COR Therapeutics
COV	Covis
CP	Continental Pharma
CPF	Coop. Pharmaceutique Francaise
CPP	CP Pharmaceuticals
CR	Critikon
CRC	Caraco
CSL	CSL Ltd.
CSP	CSP Benelux
CTI	Cell Therapeutics Inc.
CU	Cutter
CUB	Cubist
CUP	Cura Pharmaceuticals
CUR	Curomed
CY	Cyanamid

D

DAK	Dakota
DB	David Bull Laboratories
DCC	Dupont Critical Care
DI	Dista
DIA	Diamant
DIO	Diosynth
DM	Dome
DME	Dupont Merck Pharma
DMX	Dumex
DRA	Dr. Rentschler Arzneimittel
DRT	Durata Therapeutics
DRX	Draxis
DSM	DSM Pharmaceuticals
DU	DuPont
DUR	Dura
DVL	David Vult Laboratories
DW	Delta West

E

EA	Eaton
EBE	Ebewe
ECL	Éclat
EI	Eisai
EL	Enzon, Inc.
ELN	Elan
EN	Endo
ENZ	Enzon
ERF	Erfa
ERM	Erempharma
ERS	E. R. Squibb & Sons, LLC.
ES	Elkins-Sinn
ESL	ESI Lederie
ESP	ESP Pharma
EST	Esteve
EV	Evans
EX	Essex
EXL	Exela

F

FA	Farmitalia
FAN	Fandre Laboratories
FAU	Faulding
FC	Frosst & Cie
FED	Federa
FER	Ferring
FGN	Fagron
FI	Fisons
FL	Funk Labs
FLU	Fluka Co.
FOR	Forest Laboratories
FP	Faro Pharma
FRE	Fresenius
FRK	Fresenius Kabi
FUJ	Fujisawa

G

GAL	Galenova, Inc.
GEI	Geistich Pharma
GEM	Geneva-Marsam
GEN	Genentech
GG	Geigy
GIL	Gilead
GIU	Giulini
GL	Glaxo
GNS	Gensia-Sicor
GO	Goedecke
GRI	Grifols
GRP	Gruppo
GRU	Grunenthal S.A. Sint-Stevens-Woluwe
GSK	GlaxoSmithKline
GVA	Geneva
GW	Glaxo Wellcome
GZ	Genzyme

H

HAE	Haemonetics
HAG	Hanseler AG
HB	Hoechst-Biotika
HC	Hillcross
HE	Hengrui Medicine Co.
HER	Heritage
HIK	Hikma
HMR	Hoechst Marion Roussel
HO	Hoechst-Roussel
HOS	Hospira
HP	Hisun Pharmaceuticals
HQS	HQ Specialty Pharma
HR	Horner
HY	Hyland

I

ICI	ICI Pharmaceuticals
ICN	ICN Pharmaceuticals
ICU	ICU Medical, Inc.
IDX	Interstate Drug Exchange, Inc.
IMM	Immunex
IMS	IMS Ltd.
IN	Intra
INT	Intermune
IV	Ives
IVX	Ivex
IX	Invenex

J

JAZ	Jazz
JC	Janssen-Cilag
JHP	JHP Pharmaceuticals
JIH	Jiangsu Henfrui Medicine
JJ	Johnson & Johnson
JN	Janssen
JP	Jones Pharma

K

KA	Kabi
KED	Kedrion
KEY	Key Pharmaceuticals
KN	Knoll Pharmaceutical Company
KP	Kabi Pharmacia
KV	Kabi-Vitrum
KY	Kyowa

L

LA	Lagap
LAV	Lavoisier Pharmaceutical
LB	Leadiant Biosciences
LE	Lederle
LEI	Leiras, Finland
LEM	Lemmon
LEO	Leo Laboratories
LFB	Laboratorie Français du Fractionnement et des Biotechnologies

LI	Lilly
LME	Laboratoire Meram
LUN	Lundbeck
LY	Lyphomed
LZ	Labaz Laboratories

M

MA	Mallinckrodt
MAC	Maco Pharma
MAR	Marsam
MAY	Mayne Pharma
MB	May & Baker
MCD	Merck Chibret Dohme
MCO	Monico spa
MDI	Medimmune
MDX	Medex
ME	Merck
MED	Medac Pharma, Inc.
MEL	Melinta Therapeutics
MG	McGaw
MGI	MGI Pharma
MI	Miles
MIL	Millimed
MJ	Mead Johnson
MM	Merrimack
MMD	Marion Merrell Dow
MMT	Meridian Medical Technologies
MN	McNeil
MOL	Molteni Farmaceutici
MON	Monarch
MRD	Merrell-Dow
MRN	Merrell-National
MSD	Merck Sharp & Dohme
MTN	Marathon
MUN	Mundi Pharma
MY	Maney
MYL	Mylan
MYR	Mayrhofer Pharmazeutika

N

NA	National
NAB	Nabi
NAP	NAPP Pharmaceuticals
NCI	National Cancer Institute
NE	Norwich-Eaton
NF	National Formulary
NIN	Ningbo Team
NL	Normon Laboratories
NO	Nordic
NOP	Novopharm
NOV	Novo Pharm
NP	Nycomed-Pharma
NVA	Novartis
NVC	Novocol Chemical Mfg. Co., Inc.
NVN	Novo Nordisk
NVP	Nova Plus
NVX	Novex Pharma
NYC	Nycomed

O

OB	Ortho Biotech
OCT	Octapharma
OHM	Ohmeda
OM	Omega
OMJ	OMJ Pharmaceuticals
OMN	Ortho-McNeil
ON	Orion
OR	Organon
ORC	Orchid
ORP	Orphan Medical
ORT	Ortho
OTS	Otsuka

P

PAD	Paddock
PAL	Paladin
PAN	Panpharma Laboratory
PAR	Par
PB	Pohl-Boskamp
PCC	Piramal Critical Care, Inc.
PD	Parke-Davis
PE	Pentagone
PF	Pfizer
PFM	Pfrimmer
PH	Pharmacia
PHC	Pharmachemie
PHS	Pharmascience
PHT	Pharma-Tek
PHU	Pharmacia & Upjohn
PHX	Phoenix
PNN	Pantheon
PNT	Parenta

PO	Poulenc
PP	Pharmaceutical Partners
PPC	Pharmaceutical Partners of Canada
PPR	Premier Pro Rx
PR	Pasadena Research
PRF	Pierre Fabre
PRK	Parkfields
PRM	Premier
PRP	Premier Pro
PS	ProStrakan Pharmaceuticals
PUR	Purdue Pharma, LP
PX	Pharmax

Q

QI	Qilu
QLM	Qualimed Labs
QU	Quad

R

RB	Robins
RBP	Ribosepharm
RC	Roche
REC	Recordati
REN	Renaudin
RI	Riker
RKB	Reckitt & Benckhiser
RKC	Reckitt & Colman
RMS	Repro-Med Systems
RNB	Ranbaxy Laboratories
ROR	Rorer
ROX	Roxane Labs
RP	Rhône-Poulenc
RPR	Rhône-Poulenc-Rorer
RR	Roerig
RS	Roussel
RU	Rugby

S

SA	Sankyo
SAA	Sanofi Aventis
SAB	Sabex
SAG	Sageant
SAN	Sanofi
SAO	Saol Therapeutics
SB	Sintetica Bioren
SC	Schering
SCI	Scios
SCN	Schein
SCS	SCS Pharmaceuticals
SE	Searle
SEQ	Sequus
SER	Servier
SGS	SangStat
SGT	Sagent
SH	Spectrum Healthcare
SHI	Shionogi
SHN	Shyndec Pharmaceutical Co.
SHP	Shanghai Harvest Pharma
SI	Sigma
SIA	Siam Pharmaceutical
SIC	Sicor
SIG	Sigma Tau
SJN	Samjin Pharmaceutical Co., Ltd.
SKB	SmithKline Beecham
SKF	Smith Kline & French
SM	Smith
SMX	SteriMax
SN	Smith + Nephew
SO	SoloPak
SP	Spectrum Pharmaceuticals
SQ	Squibb
SS	Sanofi-Synthelabo
ST	Sterilab
STE	Stella
STP	Sterop
STR	Sterling
STS	Steris
STU	Stuart
SUN	Sun
SV	Savage
SW	Sanofi Winthrop
SX	Sabex
SY	Syntex
SYN	Synergen
SYO	Synthelabo
SZ	Sandoz

T

TAK	Takeda
TAL	Talon Theraputics
TAP	TAP Holdings
TAR	Targanta Therapeutics

TAS	Talecris
TAY	Taylor
TE	Teva
TEC	Teclapharm
TES	Tesaro
TL	Tillotts
TLP	Therabel Lucien Pharma
TMC	The Medicines Company
TO	Torigian
TPI	Tetraphase Pharmaceuticals, Inc.
TR	Travenol
TYS	Tayside Pharmaceuticals

U

UCB	UCB
UN	Unknown
UP	Upjohn
USB	US Bioscience
USP	United States Pharmacopeia
USV	USV Pharmaceuticals
UT	United Therapeutics

V

VFP	Vifor Pharma
VHA	VHA Plus
VI	Vitarine
VIC	Vicuron Pharmaceuticals
VT	Vitrum

W

WAS	Wasserman
WAT	Watson
WAY	Wyeth-Ayerst
WB	Winthrop-Breon
WC	Warner-Chilcott
WED	Weddel
WEL	Wellcome
WG	WG Critical Care
WI	Winthrop
WL	Warner Lambert
WOC	Wockhardt
WW	West-Ward
WY	Wyeth

X

XGN	X-Gen
XU	Xudong Pharmaceutical Co.

Y

YAM	Yamanouchi

Z

ZEN	Zeneca
ZLB	ZLB Biopharma
ZNS	Zeneus Pharma
ZY	ZyGenerics

APPENDIX B: GLOSSARY OF TERMS

Absorption: Form of sorption where there is diffusion and retention of a drug molecule within the matrix of the container or administration set material.[6]

Accuracy: A measure of the volume or weight of an ingredient to determine that the correct quantities of nutrients, electrolytes, or other components are delivered.[3]

Adsorption: Form of sorption where there is a weak and reversible interaction between a drug in solution and the container surface that causes the drug to bind to the surface of the container or administration set.

Aggregation: Process by which dispersed droplets come together but do not fuse. May be redispersed with gentle agitation.

Agitation: Mixing to evenly disperse a drug or solution.

Antibiotic lock technique (ALT): Instillation of a high concentration of antibiotic, usually at least 1000-times higher than the pathogen minimum inhibitory concentration, as a means to penetrate or disrupt biofilms and eradicate or prevent the growth of bacteria in a central venous catheter.

Beyond-use date: The date, or the hour and date, beyond which the preparation must not be used and must be discarded. The beyond-use date or BUD is determined from the date/time that preparation of the CSP is initiated. The BUD is not intended to limit the time during which the CSP is administered (e.g., infused).[1]

Central venous access device (CVAD): A central venous access device (CVAD) is a catheter whose tip terminates in the lower segment of the superior vena cava. CVADs may be utilized for administration of any type of infusion therapy. The large diameter and high flow of blood permits administration of medications with high osmolality, concentration and/or viscosity, parenteral nutrition, chemotherapy, blood products, and medications with vesicant properties.

Closure: Seal on a sterile container that prevents leakage, tampering, or entry of contaminants. A closure is part of a container.[3]

Coalescence: The fusion of droplets leading to a decreased number of droplets and an increase in droplet size.

Commercial product: A drug product manufactured in large quantities intended for commercial sale.

Compounded sterile preparation (CSP): A preparation intended to be sterile that is created by combining, admixing, diluting, pooling, reconstituting, repackaging, or otherwise altering a drug product or bulk drug substance.[1]

DOI 10.37573/9781585286720.PT3002

Compounding record: A detailed record that provides specific compounding instructions, describes how the CSP was prepared, and documents the entire process. Compounding records are specific to each compounding event.

Concentration: Amount of active ingredient in a volume of solution (e.g., mg/mL).

Container: That which holds the preparation and is or may be in direct contact with the preparation. The closure is part of the container.[3]

Cracking: Coalescence of an emulsion continues to a point of complete separation and an oily layer is seen at the top.

Creaming: Formation of a layer of aggregates at the emulsion surface.

Degradation: Chemical and physical changes of a drug during storage resulting in modified pharmacological outcomes, altering the therapeutic or toxic profile.

Diluent: Ingredient in a compounded sterile preparation that lacks pharmacologic activity but is necessary for the dissolution of drug(s) to be administered parenterally.

Dissolution: The process of dissolving one substance into another. A dissolution test measures the amount of drug that goes into solution over time.

Elastomeric container: Containers made of materials obtained by vulcanization (cross-linking) polymerization, polyaddition, or polycondensation of macromolecular organic substances (elastomers). Formulations contain natural or synthetic elastomers and inorganic and organic additives to aid or control vulcanization, impart physical and chemical properties or color, or stabilize the container formulation.[2]

Emulsion: A dosage form consisting of a two-phase system composed of at least two immiscible liquids, one of which is dispersed as droplets with the other liquid, generally stabilized with one or more emulsifying agents.[5] Oil-in-water mixture requiring an emulsifying agent to disperse the oil phase into the aqueous phase.

Evaporation: Loss of water through the container material.

Expiration date: Date that identifies the time during which a conventionally manufactured drug product, active ingredient, or added substance can be expected to meet the requirements of a compendial monograph, if one exists, or maintain expected quality provided it is kept under the specified storage conditions. Expiration dates are assigned by manufacturers and are not the same as beyond-use dates (BUDs).[1]

Extended stability: The maximum time period in which 90% or greater of a labeled active ingredient is measurable in the solution and container specified, under the stated storage conditions. An exception applies to coagulation factors, which are considered stable when at least 80% of the factor activity is retained.

Extrapolation: The prediction or estimation of a variable beyond the given data set by observing its relation with other variables in the existing data set.

Flocculation: Process by which dispersed droplets come together, but do not fuse, and may be redispersed with gentle agitation.

Hydrolysis: The chemical process of drug degradation by water. For aqueous solutions, pH, presence of acids or bases, drug concentration, and temperature are all factors that could affect the rate of hydrolysis.

Inert: Chemically inactive, and does not contain additives or other compounds that may potentially migrate into the finished preparation.

Infusate: A fluid given parenterally for a therapeutic purpose.

Leaching: Components of the plastic formulation (such as from a container) migrate into the infusate, contaminating the drug solution.

Lipophilic: The ability of a compound to dissolve in lipid-containing solutions.

Lock: The final step in intravenous therapy administration when the vascular access device (VAD) will remain in place for future therapy to prevent occlusion or infection of a catheter between uses.

Master formulation record: A detailed record that provides specific compounding instructions and describes how the CSP was prepared. Master formulation records should contain sufficient detail to be used on their own without additional verbal explanation.

Microbial contamination: Introduction of infectious material into a sterile solution.

Midline catheter: Midline catheters measure 38 inches with the tip terminating in veins located between the elbow and shoulder. Midline catheter duration of therapy is typically 1 to 4 weeks. This type of catheter is an alternative to PICCs for certain indications, and intravenous solutions appropriate for administration into the peripheral vasculature.

Osmolality: The measure of particles of solute per kilogram of solvent (mOsm/kg), and contributes to the osmotic pressure of a solution.

Osmolarity: The measure of particles of solute per liter of solution (mOsm/L), and contributes to the osmotic pressure of a solution.

Overfill: Addition of a sufficient amount of excess solution to allow for water vapor transmission losses out of the container over the shelf life of the product, and to account for the variation in the amount of solution dispensed by compounding or administration devices. USP <1151>, *Pharmaceutical Dosage Forms*, recommends an excess volume of 2% of the labeled container size for mobile liquids.[5]

Oxidation: The chemical process of drug degradation by oxygen. Factors that affect the rate of oxidation include the presence of oxygen, light, heavy metal ions, temperature, pH, and the presence of other drugs or chemicals that act as oxidizing agents.

Parenteral nutrition: Intravenous administration of nutrition, which may include protein, carbohydrates, fats, minerals, electrolytes, and vitamins.

Peripheral catheter: Peripheral catheters are usually 1 to 1.5 inches in length with the tip terminating in a peripheral vein. This type of catheter should not be used for continuous infusions of vesicants, parenteral nutrition, or infusates > 900 mOsm/L. The anticipated duration of therapy is generally less than 6 days.

Peripherally inserted central catheter (PICC): A peripherally inserted central catheter (PICC) is a type of non-tunneled CVAD that is inserted in the antecubital space into the basilic, brachial, or cephalic veins and advanced within the blood vessel to achieve central placement.

Permeation: Loss of container contents by allowing vapor, water, or drug molecules to migrate through the wall of the container.

Peroxidation: Peroxidation of lipids occurs as a free radical-mediated chain of reactions that results in an oxidative degradation of lipid emulsions.

Plasticizer: Component added to a plastic material to make it softer and more flexible.

Precipitation: Reaction upon mixing of drugs or solutions resulting in insoluble particulates that may be observed as crystals, haziness, or turbidity.

Preservative: A substance added to inhibit microbial growth.[1]

Product: A commercially manufactured sterile drug or nutrient that has been evaluated for safety and efficacy by the US Food and Drug Administration (FDA). Products are accompanied by full prescribing information, which is commonly known as the FDA-approved manufacturer's labeling or product package insert.

Ready-to-use (RTU): Commercially manufactured product that does not require additional compounding prior to administration.

Reconstitution: The process of adding a diluent to a conventionally manufactured product to prepare a sterile solution or suspension.[1]

Shearing: Occurs from differences of fluid velocity in moving liquids between the solution and the surface, such as a solution going through syringes and administration sets. It may promote interfacial reactions for solid-liquid (adsorption, leaching), gas-liquid (air-bubble entrapment), and oil-water (silicon lubricants).

Sorption: Drug loss from a solution intended to be administered by adsorption to the surface or absorption into the matrix of the container material, administration set, or filter.[3]

Stability: The extent to which a product or preparation retains physical and chemical properties and characteristics within specified limits throughout its expiration or BUD.[1]

Standard operating procedure (SOP): Written procedures describing operations, testing, sampling, interpretation of results, and corrective actions that relate to the operations that are taking place.[4]

Sterility: The absence of viable microorganisms.[1]

Temperature excursion: Occurs when a temperature reading is outside the recommended range for the medication as defined in the manufacturer's package insert.

Turbidity: Cloudiness or haziness of a solution caused by large numbers of individual particles.

Vascular access device (VAD): Vascular access devices are flexible catheters inserted into a vein to deliver infusion therapy.

Vial-bag connector: Specialized point-of-care activated devices and bags that allow for the connection of a vial of medication to a small volume infusion container.

Visual inspection: Immediately after compounding, and as a condition of release, each CSP unit, where possible, should be inspected against a lighted white or black background or both for evidence of visible particulates or other foreign matter. Prerelease inspection also includes container-closure integrity and any other apparent visual defect. When CSPs are not distributed promptly after preparation, a pre-distribution inspection is conducted to ensure that a CSP with defects, such as precipitation, cloudiness, and leakage, which may develop between the time of release and the time of distribution, is not released.

REFERENCES

1. USP <797> Pharmaceutical Compounding - Sterile Preparations. In: *2020: USP Compounding Compendium*. Rockville, MD: The United States Pharmacopeial Convention; 2020:40-74.
2. USP <381> Elastomeric Closures for Injections. In: *2020: USP Compounding Compendium*. Rockville, MD: The United States Pharmacopeial Convention; 2020:208-14.
3. Glossary. In: Buchanan EC, Schneider PJ, Forrey RA eds. *Compounding Sterile Preparations*. 4th ed. Bethesda, MD: American Society of Health-System Pharmacists; 2017:551-66.
4. USP <800> Hazardous Drugs - Handling in Healthcare Settings. In: *2020: USP Compounding Compendium*. Rockville, MD: The United States Pharmacopeial Convention; 2020:74-92.
5. USP <1151> Pharmaceutical Dosage Forms. In: *2020: USP Compounding Compendium*. Rockville, MD: The United States Pharmacopeial Convention; 2020:408-30.
6. Bing CD. Storage and beyond-use dating. In: Buchanan EC, Schneider PJ, Forrey RA eds. *Compounding Sterile Preparations*. 4th ed. Bethesda, MD: American Society of Health-System Pharmacists; 2017:213-26.
7. ASHP's Interactive Handbook on Injectable Drugs, 2020. Bethesda, MD: American Society of Health-System Pharmacists; Accessed February 2021.

Index

Page numbers followed by f *denotes a figure, the letter* n *denotes an endnote, and the letter* t *denotes a table.*

A

B

DOI 10.37573/9781585286720.BM

C

D

E

F

G

H

I

K

L

M

N

O

P

Q

R

S

T

U

V

W

Z